Neurology for the Boards
Second Edition

Neurology for the Boards
Second Edition

James D. Geyer, M.D.
Neurology Consultants of Tuscaloosa
Tuscaloosa, Alabama

Janice M. Keating, M.D.
Department of Neurology
Cooper Clinic
Fort Smith, Arkansas

Daniel C. Potts, M.D.
Neurology Consultants of Tuscaloosa
Tuscaloosa, Alabama

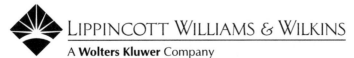

LIPPINCOTT WILLIAMS & WILKINS
A **Wolters Kluwer** Company

Philadelphia · Baltimore · New York · London
Buenos Aires · Hong Kong · Sydney · Tokyo

Acquisitions Editor: Anne M. Sydor
Developmental Editor: Anjou K. Dargar
Production Editor: Emily Lerman
Manufacturing Manager: Tim Reynolds
Cover Designer: Patricia Gast
Compositor: Lippincott Williams & Wilkins Desktop Division
Printer: Maple Press

© 2002 by LIPPINCOTT WILLIAMS & WILKINS
530 Walnut Street
Philadelphia, PA 19106 USA
LWW.com

Printed in the USA

Library of Congress Cataloging-in-Publication Data
Geyer, James D.
Neurology for the boards / James D. Geyer, Janice M. Keating, Daniel C. Potts.—2nd ed.
  p. ; cm.
Includes index.
ISBN 0-7817-3719-2 (alk. paper)
1. Neurology—Outlines, syllabi, etc. 2. Physicians—Licenses—United States—Examinations—Study guides. 1. Keating, Janice M. II. Potts, Daniel C. III. Title.
[DNLM: 1. Nervous System Diseases—Outlines. 2. Nervous System—Outlines. WL 18.2 G397n 2002]
RC357.G485 2002
616.8—dc21
                                                                    2002017856

Care has been taken to confirm the accuracy of the information presented and to describe generally accepted practices. However, the authors and publisher are not responsible for errors or omissions or for any consequences from application of the information in this book and make no warranty, expressed or implied, with respect to the currency, completeness, or accuracy of the contents of the publication. Application of this information in a particular situation remains the professional responsibility of the practitioner.

The authors and publisher have exerted every effort to ensure that drug selection and dosage set forth in this text are in accordance with current recommendations and practice at the time of publication. However, in view of ongoing research, changes in government regulations, and the constant flow of information relating to drug therapy and drug reactions, the reader is urged to check the package insert for each drug for any change in indications and dosage and for added warnings and precautions. This is particularly important when the recommended agent is a new or infrequently employed drug.

Some drugs and medical devices presented in this publication have Food and Drug Administration (FDA) clearance for limited use in restricted research settings. It is the responsibility of the health care provider to ascertain the FDA status of each drug or device planned for use in their clinical practice.

10 9 8 7 6 5 4 3 2

Dedicated to our beautiful children: Sydney and Emery, Claire and Benjamin, and Julia and Maria

This text is also commemorated to the memory of our mentor–John N. Whitaker, M.D.

Contents

Foreword

The practitioners of neurological medicine must have at their command a large body of knowledge ranging from elements of basic neuroscience to in-depth accounts of the clinical features of a wide variety of disorders affecting one or more areas in the central and peripheral nervous systems. While some of this information is used in a nonverbal fashion as the practitioner applies it in patient care, there is also the need to be able to recall the information quickly for review at all levels of training, examination, and teaching.

Drs. James Geyer, Janice Keating, and Daniel Potts were outstanding members of the Neurology Training Program at the University of Alabama at Birmingham during the years 1994 to 1997. In addition to their own responsibilities in clinical care and in meeting educational standards, they were each active in their roles as Senior and Chief Resident in assisting others in learning about neurology. In the summer of 1996, at the transition of their second and third years of residency, they presented a draft of this book, which now appears in published form. I was struck by the fact that the authors covered the clinical applications of this material in greater depth than has been achieved in books and learning programs currently available.

As both writers and consumers of the information they prepared for lectures to medical students, housestaff, and fellows, the authors recognized the need to have a concise record of information that was sufficiently thorough, was rapidly accessible, and could be used efficiently by the individual who wants to review and test his/her base of knowledge. The information listed is what most would underline or highlight in other textbooks. *Neurology for the Boards* has been arranged based on the experience of the authors as they acquired, and then sought to retrieve and solidify in their own minds, the information contained in this book. Thus, the audience projected is most likely those who already have read or used, at least once, the information contained in the book, and now seek rapidly to review it. Those preparing for examinations, such as the annual in-service examination, the board examination, or—as soon will be required—an examination for recertification, may find this a useful book. I readily admit that I find it to be a quick review myself for rounds and conferences dealing with disorders that I do not see frequently.

For whatever influence I may have had on the authors in their learning neurology and writing this book, I am honored to write this foreword. As Drs. Geyer, Keating, and Potts point out in their acknowledgments, this book represents the product of a number of individuals. However, the compilation and presentation are original and reflect the diligent efforts of the authors.

John N. Whitaker, M.D.
Department of Neurology
University of Alabama, Birmingham
December, 1997

Preface

Neurology covers a broad spectrum of disease processes, including neurodegenerative disorders, neuro-oncology, neuromuscular disease, neuro-immunology, epilepsy, cerebrovascular disease, metabolic disorders, sleep disorders, and pain. These diseases are often complicated by, or directly associated with, general medical or psychiatric conditions. Furthermore, the evaluation of neurologic disorders ranges from the neurologic examination to technically complex procedures such as video electroencephalography, repetitive nerve stimulation tests, and cerebral angiography.

The initial goal of this book was to produce a concise yet comprehensive tool for our own use (both for board review and for patient care). The essential background information, including neuro-anatomy and basic science, is covered in the first sections. This is followed by a review of the diseases and syndromes, as well as their evaluation and treatment.

This book was designed specifically as an aid in preparation for the American Board of Psychiatry and Neurology certification examination, and as a reference tool for patient evaluation and management. It is not meant to replace the more detailed classic texts of neurology. It does, however, provide a concise review of the clinically important aspects of neurology, as well as much of the esoteric minutiae beloved by the board examiners.

All diagrams and illustrations are modified from original drawings by Dr. Janice Keating. The drawings are not drawn to scale or to anatomic accuracy. They are simplified diagrams designed to facilitate the learning of complex neurologic pathways and functional anatomy.

The book has been "field tested" by residents and medical students at the University of Alabama at Birmingham. The residents who have used the book found it very useful both for residency in-service training examinations and for board review. Residents and students alike felt that it provided a good overview of patient evaluation and management. Their patience and feedback is greatly appreciated.

The practicing neurologist should also find this book useful for board recertification and as an office reference tool. The recertification examinations require current knowledge of neurologic disease and management, even of the subspecialist.

Neurology for the Boards provides the core material condensed into a single source. We sincerely hope that it helps the reader prepare not only for board examinations, but also for the more important task of providing excellent medical care.

Acknowledgments

This book is the product of the efforts of many people. The entire faculty of the Department of Neurology at the University of Alabama at Birmingham contributed either directly or indirectly to the creation of this text. Faculty members from the University of Michigan also contributed to the material for this text. Much of the book was derived from the lectures, informal discussions, and bedside teaching of UAB faculty. We extend special thanks to the Chairman of the UAB Department of Neurology, John N. Whitaker, M.D. Dr. Whitaker's guidance and support throughout our residency laid the groundwork for this project.

We also thank Dr. Tom Emig who wrote the section on the thalamus and Dr. Katherine Daru who wrote the section on muscle physiology. We are also indebted to those residents who preceded us in our training at UAB for their contributions to this project.

Special thanks to our spouses, Stephenie, Bill, and Ellen. Their unconditional love and support throughout residency helped make all of this a reality. We also thank Anne Sydor, Ph.D., and everyone at Lippincott Williams & Wilkins for the encouragement and guidance we received.

Neurology for the Boards
Second Edition

1

Embryology and Development

I. Divisions
   A. Prosencephalon
      1. Telencephalon—cortex, amygdala, caudate, putamen
      2. Diencephalon—thalamus, hypothalamus, globus pallidus
   B. Mesencephalon—midbrain
   C. Rhombencephalon
      1. Metencephalon—pons, cerebellum
      2. Myelencephalon—medulla
II. Basal and Alar Plates
   A. Basal Plate (ventral)
      1. Anterior horn cells
      2. Motor nuclei of cranial nerves
   B. Alar Plate (dorsal)
      1. Dorsal sensory horn
      2. Sensory nuclei in brain stem
      3. Cerebellum (from rhombic lips)
      4. Inferior olive
      5. Quadrigeminal plate (superior and inferior colliculi)
      6. Red nucleus
   C. Sulcus Limitans
      1. Boundary between basal and alar plates
III. Neural Tube Formation
   A. Fusion begins on day 22 in region of the lower medulla.
   B. Fusion begins at the fourth somite.
   C. Anterior neuropore closes on day 25.
   D. Posterior neuropore closes on day 27.
   E. Neural crest cells give rise to
      1. Dorsal root ganglion
      2. Melanocytes
      3. Sensory ganglia of cranial nerves
      4. Adrenal medulla
      5. Autonomic ganglia
      6. Cells of the pia/arachnoid
      7. Schwann cells
      8. Preganglionic sympathetic neurons

IV. Caudal Neural Tube Formation (Secondary Neurulation)
   A. Forms on days 28 to 32
   B. Forms sacral/coccygeal segments, filum terminale, ventriculus terminalis
V. Disorders of Primary Neurulation
   A. Anencephaly
      1. Failure of anterior neuropore closure (<24 days)
      2. Effects forebrain and variable portions of brain stem
         a. Holoacrania—to foramen magnum
         b. Meroacrania—slightly higher than foramen magnum
      3. 75% are stillborn.
      4. Most common in whites, Irish, females, children born to either very old or very young mothers
      5. Risk in subsequent pregnancies is 5% to 7%.
   B. Myeloschisis
      1. Failure of posterior neuropore closure
      2. Associated with iniencephaly—malformation of skull base
      3. Most are stillborn.
   C. Encephalocele
      1. Restricted defect in anterior neural tube closure
      2. 75% occipital
      3. 50% with hydrocephalus
   D. Myelomeningocele
      1. Restricted defect in posterior neural tube closure
      2. 80% lumbar
      3. 90% have hydrocephalus if lumbar region is involved.
      4. 60% have hydrocephalus if another region is involved.
      5. Symptoms include motor, sensory, and sphincter dysfunction.
   E. Arnold-Chiari Malformation
      1. Type I
         a. Isolated displacement of the cerebellar tonsils into the cervical canal
         b. Kinked cervical cord
      2. Type II
         a. Displacement of the cerebellum into cervical canal
         b. Displacement of the medulla and fourth ventricle into the cervical canal
         c. Long, thin medulla and pons, tectum deformity
         d. Skull base and upper cervical spine defects
         e. Hydrocephalus due to fourth ventricle obstruction or aqueductal stenosis
         f. 100% with myelomeningocele
         g. 96% with cortex malformations (heterotopias, polymicrogyria)
         h. 76% with brain stem malformations (hypoplasia of cranial nerves, pons)
         i. 72% with cerebellar dysplasia
         j. 30% with thoracolumbar kyphoscoliosis

        k. 30% with diastematomyelia (bifid cord)

        l. Syringomyelia

    3. Type III

        a. All the above plus encephalocele (occipital)

  F. Meckel's Syndrome

    1. Associated with maternal hyperthermia or fever on days 20 to 26

    2. Includes encephalocele, microcephaly, microphthalmia, cleft lip, polydactyly, polycystic kidneys, ambiguous genitalia.

  G. Neural Tube Defects

    1. Causes

        a. Chromosomal abnormalities (trisomy 13, 18)

        b. Teratogens (thalidomide, valproate, phenytoin)

        c. Single mutant gene (Meckel's syndrome)

        d. Multifactorial

    2. Diagnosis

        a. Increased alpha-fetoprotein

        b. Increased acetylcholinesterase

        c. Ultrasound

    3. Prevention—folate

    4. Recurrence rate—2% to 3%

VI. Disorders of Secondary Neurulation—Occult Dysraphic States

  A. General Information

    1. Intact dermal layer over lesion

    2. 80% have an overlying dermal lesion (dimple, hairy tuft, lipoma, hemangioma).

    3. Frequent tethered spinal cord

    4. 100% have abnormal conus and filum.

    5. 90% have vertebral defects.

    6. 4% have siblings with a disorder of primary neurulation.

  B. Caudal Regression Syndrome

    1. 20% are infants of diabetic mothers.

    2. Characterized by dysraphic sacrum and coccyx with atrophic muscle and bone

    3. Symptoms include delayed sphincter control and walking, back and leg pain, scoliosis, pes cavus, leg asymmetry.

  C. Myelocystocele—cystic central canal

  D. Diastematomyelia—bifid cord

  E. Meningocele—rare. No associated hydrocephalus.

  F. Lipomeningocele

  G. Subcutaneous Lipoma/Teratoma

  H. Dermal Sinus

VII. Disorders of Prosencephalic Development

  A. Aprosencephaly—absence of the telencephalon and diencephalon

  B. Atelencephaly—absence of the telencephalon, but normal diencephalon

        1. Intact skull and skin
        2. Associated with cyclopia, absent eyes, abnormal limbs, and genitalia
    C. Holoprosencephaly
        1. Defect in prosencephalic cleavage
        2. 100% anosmia—absent olfactory bulbs and tracts
        3. Single-lobed cerebrum and single ventricle
        4. Hypoplastic or single optic nerve
        5. Absent corpus callosum
        6. Common neuronal migration defects
        7. Facial defects
           a. Ethmocephaly—hypertelorism with proboscis between eyes
           b. Cebocephaly—single nostril
           c. Cyclopia—single eye with or without proboscis
           d. Cleft lip
        8. Clinical features
           a. Seizures
           b. Apnea
           c. Decreased hypothalamic function
           d. Developmental delay
           e. Anosmia
           f. Single maxillary incisor
        9. Chromosomal abnormality
           a. Trisomy 13
           b. Ring 13
       10. Recurrence rate—6%
        11. 2% are infants of diabetic mothers
    D. Agenesis of the Corpus Callosum—frequently associated with
        1. Holoprosencephaly
        2. Absent septum pellucidum
        3. Neuronal migration disorders, schizencephaly
        4. Chiari II malformation
        5. Septooptic dysplasia/septooptohypothalamic dysplasia
        6. Aicardi syndrome
           a. X-linked dominant (only females affected, males die)
           b. Agenesis of the corpus callosum
           c. Neuronal migration defects
           d. Chorioretinal lacunae
           e. **Note:** The X-linked dominant disorders include the following (mnemonic: AIR):
        1. Aicardi syndrome
        2. Incontinentia pigmenti
        3. Rett's syndrome
VIII. Congenital Hydrocephalus
    A. Aqueductal Stenosis—33%

    B. Arnold-Chiari Malformation—28%

    C. Communicating Hydrocephalus—22%

    D. Dandy-Walker Malformation—7%

    E. Other (tumor, vein of Galen, X-linked aqueductal stenosis)

IX. Dandy-Walker Malformation

    A. Secondary to failed or delayed development of the foramen of Magendie

    B. Cystic dilation of the fourth ventricle

    C. Cerebellar Agenesis-maldevelopment of the cerebellar vermis

    D. Hydrocephalus

    E. Associated with

        1. Agenesis of the corpus callosum

        2. Neuronal migration disorders (70%)

        3. Large inion

        4. Large posterior fossa

        5. Cardiac abnormalities

        6. Urinary tract abnormalities

X. Neuronal Proliferation and Migration Disorders

    A. General Information

        1. All neurons and glia are derived from the ventricular and subventricular zones.

        2. Radial glia

            a. Provide positional guidance for migration of neurons from the ventricular surface to the developing cortex.

            b. May serve as precursors to astrocytes and oligodendrocytes.

            c. Persist as Bergmann glia in the mature cerebellum.

        3. Phase I—2 to 4 months neuronal proliferation and generation of radial glia

            a. Phase II—5 to 12 months glial multiplication

    B. Disorders of Proliferation

        1. Microcephaly—decreased size of proliferative units

        2. Radial microbrain—decreased number of proliferative units

        3. Macrencephaly—well formed but large

        4. Unilateral macrencephaly (hemimegencephaly)

XI. Neuronal Migration

    A. General Information

        1. Radial glial cells send foot processes from the ventricular surface to the pial surface, forming a limiting membrane at the pial surface.

        2. Proliferative units of the ventricular zone migrate via the radial glia scaffolding to become the neuronal cell columns.

        3. The later migrating cells take a more superficial position ("inside-out pattern").

        4. Radial glia later differentiate into astrocytes (except in the cerebellum, where the Bergmann glia are located).

        5. Migrational disorders are often associated with agenesis of the corpus callosum, absence of the septum pellucidum, cavum septum pellucidum, copocephaly (large trigones and occipital and temporal horns).

    B. Types

1. Radial—primary mechanism for formation of the cortex and deep nuclei, cerebellar Purkinje cells, and cerebellar nuclei
2. Tangential—originating in the germinal zones of the rhombic lip and migrating to form the external and internal granular layers

C. Disorders
1. Schizencephaly—clefts, space between ventricles and the subarachnoid space. No gliosis. Associated with heterotopias in wall of cleft.
2. Porencephaly—variable communication between the ventricles and the subarachnoid space. Gliosis. Secondary to ischemia later in gestation.
3. Lissencephaly—few or no gyri (smooth brain)
4. Pachygyria—few, broad, thick gyri
5. Polymicrogyria—to many small gyri (wrinkled chestnut)
6. Heterotopias—rests of neurons in the white matter secondary to arrested radial migration. Associated with seizures.
    a. Periventricular
    b. Laminar (in deep white matter)
    c. Bandlike (between cortex and ventricular surface)

D. Miller-Dieker Syndrome
1. Associated with lissencephaly
2. Chromosome 17 deletion in 90% of cases
3. Clinical presentation—microcephaly, seizures, hypotonia, poor feeding, craniofacial defects, cardiac defects, and genital abnormalities

E. Walker-Warburg Syndrome
1. Associated with Fukuyama congenital muscular dystrophy, cerebellar malformation, retinal malformation, macrocephaly

F. Zellweger's Syndrome (Cerebro-Hepato-Renal Syndrome)
1. Autosomal recessive
2. Peroxisomal disorder (increased long-chain fatty acids)
3. Polymicrogyria, heterotopias, seizures, hepatomegaly, renal cysts

XII. Organizational Disorders of the Cortex
A. Mental Retardation—decreased dendritic spines and branching
B. Down's Syndrome
1. Trisomy 21
2. Abnormal dendrites and axons
3. Amyloid, tangles, plaques
C. Fragile X Syndrome
1. Triple repeat disease
2. Most common form of inherited mental retardation
3. Abnormal dendrites
D. Angelman's Syndrome
1. Deletion of chromosome 15q11–13 (mother)
2. Mental retardation, ataxia, seizures, microencephaly, "happy puppet"
E. Prader-Willi Syndrome

      1. Deletion of chromosome 15q11–13 (father)

      2. Hypotonia, hypogonadism, eating disorder

   F. Secondary Disorders

      1. Phenylketonuria (PKU), Zellweger syndrome, rubella, trisomy 13, 15, 18

XIII. Disorders of Myelination

   A. Peripheral Nervous System

      1. The peripheral nervous system myelinates before the central nervous system.

      2. Motor fibers myelinate before sensory fibers.

   B. Central Nervous System

      1. Sensory areas myelinate before motor areas.

      2. Association areas myelinate last.

      3. Most rapid myelination occurs from birth to 2 years of age.

   C. Disorders of Myelination

      1. Aminoacidurias/organic acidopathies

         a. Ketotic hyperglycinemia

         b. Nonketotic hyperglycinemia

         c. PKU

         d. Maple syrup urine disease (MSUD)

         e. Homocysteinuria

      2. Hypothyroidism

      3. Malnutrition

      4. Periventricular leukomalacia

         a. Primarily premature infants

         b. Decreased IQ

         c. Spastic diplegia

      5. Prematurity

XIV. Primitive Reflexes

Reflex	Description	Appears (Gestational Age)	Disappears (Age)
Suck	Suck when finger or pacifier is placed in mouth	32–34 wk	4 mo
Grasp (hand)	Grasps object with hand stimulation	32–34 wk	6 mo
Grasp (foot)	Grasps object with foot stimulation	32-34 wk	10 mo
Moro	Opening of palms, extension and abduction of arms followed by adduction at shoulders, cry when head is allowed to fall backward	34 wk	3 mo
Tonic neck	Turn head, ipsilateral arm and leg extension and contralateral arm and leg flexion	34 wk	6 mo
Landau	With ventral suspension, head, trunk, and hips should extend, legs should flex at knees	3 mo after birth	24 mo
Placing	When dorsal foot is brushed by bed/table, the knee should flex and foot lift as if to step	35 wk	6 wk
Parachute	In prone position baby is suddenly thrust to the floor, arms extend and adduct, fingers spread as if to break the fall	9 mo after birth	Persists
Babinski	Great toe dorsiflexes when lateral aspect of foot is stroked	Birth	10 mo

XV. Normal Developmental Milestones

Smiles responsively	1 month
Visual tracking to 180°	2–3 mo
Rolls over, holds head upright	3 mo
Reaches for objects	3–4 mo
Sits unsupported	6 mo
Thumb finger grasp	8 mo
Crawls	9 mo
Walks with support	10 mo
Pincer grasp	12 mo
Walks alone	12–14 mo
Says 3 words (besides "Mama" and "Dada")	13 mo
Climbs steps	17 mo
Pedals tricycle	3 yr

2

Anatomy

THE CEREBELLUM AND CONNECTIONS

I. External Architecture
  A. Three Lobes—rostral to caudal
    1. Anterior Lobe–functionally known as *paleocerebellum* or *spinocerebellum*
    2. Posterior Lobe—functionally known as *neocerebellum* or *pontocerebellum* or *cerebrocerebellum*
    3. Flocculonodular Lobe—functionally known as *archicerebellum* or *vestibulocerebellum*
  B. Ten lobules—names need not be learned, but **tonsils** are clinically important (i.e., tonsilar herniation).
  C. Two Fissures
    1. Primary—separates anterior and posterior lobes.
    2. Posterolateral—separates posterior and flocculonodular lobes.
  D. Peduncles—connect cerebellum with brain stem.
    1. Superior Cerebellar Peduncle (brachium conjunctivum)—connects cerebellum to midbrain.
    2. Middle Cerebellar Peduncle (brachium pontis)—connects the cerebellum to the pons.
    3. Inferior Cerebellar Peduncle (corpus restiform or restiform body)—connects the cerebellum with the medulla and is the largest peduncle.
  E. The *vermis* ("worm") lies between the two cerebellar hemispheres and is almost circular, its continuity interrupted in ventral sagittal plane only by the fourth ventricle.
  F. The lateral recesses of the fourth ventricle communicate with the subarachnoid space via the foramina of Luschka.
II. Internal Architecture
  A. Nuclei—each hemisphere contains four. The first three are in the roof of the fourth ventricle. These include
    1. Fastigial Nucleus—phylogenetically the oldest. Associated with the archicerebellum (vestibulocerebellum). Receives afferents from flocculonodular lobe and vermis; sends efferents direct via inferior cerebellar peduncle to vestibular nuclei (some fibers cross to contralateral cerebellum, loop around contralateral SCP, and reach vestibular nuclei and reticular formation via the uncinate bundle of Russell). This nucleus controls antigravity and other muscle synergies in standing and walking (proximal muscles).
    2. Globose and Emboliform Nuclei (together known as the *interposed nucleus*)—lie slightly lateral to fastigial nucleus; receive afferents from paravermian region of

paleocerebellum or spinocerebellum; send efferents via superior cerebellar peduncle (SCP) to contralateral red nucleus; concerned mainly with modulation of stretch reflexes (distal muscles).

3. Dentate Nucleus—largest nucleus. Located deep within white matter of cerebellar hemispheres; receives afferents from Purkinje cells of entire neocerebellum and part of paleocerebellum; also afferents from premotor and supplementary motor cortices via pontocerebellar system; efferents course through SCP, cross to opposite side at pontomesencephalic border, and terminate in contralateral red nucleus and ventrolateral thalamus. Helps to initiate and control volitional movements (planning of movements).

4. Vestibular Nuclei—think of these as "displaced" cerebellar nuclei because of association with vestibulocerebellum. Function is to maintain gaze fixation and upright posture.

B. Microscopic Properties—(Fig. 1)

  1. Three cellular layers in the cortex (from outside to inside):

    a. Molecular Layer—containing primarily basket cells, stellate cells, Purkinje cell dendrites, parallel fibers of the granule cells, and dendrites of the Golgi cells

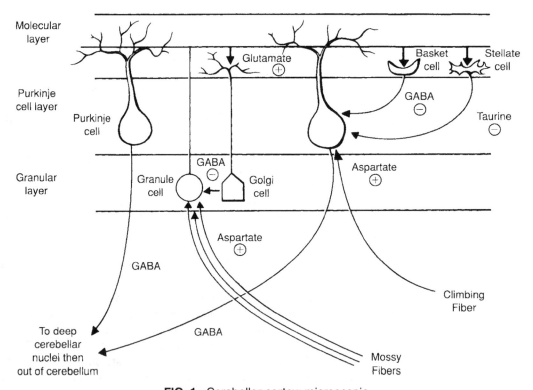

FIG. 1. Cerebellar cortex: microscopic.

   b. Purkinje Cell Layer—containing *only* Purkinje cells
   c. Granular Cell Layer—containing granule cells, Golgi cells, and glomeruli (bulbous expansions of mossy fibers where synaptic contact with granule and Golgi cells is made). This layer contains more neurons than the whole cerebral cortex!
2. Five cell types in the cortex:
   a. Stellate and Basket Cells—local inhibitory interneurons that are excited by granule cells and inhibit Purkinje cells. Basket cells use **GABA**, and stellate cells are thought to use **taurine** as their neurotransmitters.
   b. Purkinje Cells—large neurons that are the *only* cells in the cerebellum capable of transmitting efferent impulses from the cortex; also the only cells projecting out of the cerebellar cortex. These cells use GABA as their neurotransmitter.
   c. Granule Cells—axons project upward to molecular layer as *parallel fibers* (run only parallel to longitudinal axis of each folia). The neurotransmitter is **glutamate**.
   d. Golgi Cells—are located in the granular layer and send dendrites to the molecule layer. They are excited by granular cells and inhibit granule cells. They also are thought to use GABA as their neurotransmitter. They suppress the excitation of granule cells to mossy fiber input and curtail the duration of excitation reaching Purkinje cells.
3. Four afferent fiber types in the cortex:
   a. Three bring information from **outside** the cerebellum:
      (1) Mossy fibers (make up 99% of incoming fibers)—transmit impulses exclusively from spinal cord and the vestibular and pontine nuclei by using granule cells as mediators; enter via all three peduncles. Thought to use **aspartate** as a neurotransmitter.
      (2) Climbing fibers—transmit impulses from inferior olives directly to dendrites of Purkinje cells of the opposite hemisphere. Thought to use aspartate as a neurotransmitter. Stronger excitatory input than mossy fibers and can enhance or inhibit mossy fiber input, thus functioning in motor learning.
      (3) Aminergic afferents—arise in Raphe nuclei and locus ceruleus. Raphe inputs are seratonergic and terminate in granular and molecular layers. Locus ceruleus inputs are noradrenergic and terminate in all three layers. Both inputs have widespread modulatory actions.
   b. One fiber type—parallel fibers (axons of granule cells) originates within the cerebellum.
   Note: Each Purkinje cell receives indirect input from >200,000 mossy fibers and only one climbing fiber. Both fiber types are excitatory.
   Note: When a group of parallel fibers excites a row of Purkinje cells and neighboring basket cells, these basket cells inhibit distant Purkinje cells outside the band of excitation.
C. Contents of the Peduncles
   1. Inferior Cerebellar Peduncle

    a. Contains the following afferents:
       (1) Fibers from vestibular nerve and nucleus, terminating at the flocculonodular lobe (relayed to fastigial nucleus)
       (2) The olivocerebellar tract, originating in contralateral inferior olive and terminating as climbing fibers directly on Purkinje cell dendrites
       (3) Posterior or dorsal spinocerebellar tract, which originates in Clarke's column. Impulses transmitted here originate mainly in muscle spindles and are carried to the paravermian zone of the anterior and posterior lobes of the cerebellum (fastest- conducting fibers in nervous system).
       (4) Fibers originating from accessory cuneate nucleus joining those of posterior spinocerebellar tract. Transmit impulses received by accessory cuneate nucleus from nuclei in middle and rostral portions of cervical cord above Clarke's column (ascend in lateral cuneate fasciculus).
       (5) Fibers from brain stem reticular formation
    b. Contains only one efferent, the fastigiobulbar or cerebellobulbar tract, representing the efferent limb of the vestibulocerebellar feedback circuit through which cerebellum influences spinal cord motor activity via vestibulospinal tract and medial longitudinal fasciculus.

Note: Inferior cerebellar peduncle contains *all* afferents, except the anterior spinocerebellar tract and the pontocerebellar fibers.

  2. Middle cerebellar peduncle contains *only* afferents from the pontine nuclei (second neurons of fibers of the corticopontine tracts).
  3. Superior cerebellar peduncle contains the following:
    a. Only one afferent—the anterior or ventral spinocerebellar tract—which carries impulses from peripheral receptors (primarily Golgi tendon organs) to the paleocerebellum (primarily vermis).
    b. Numerous efferents (most of which eventually reach the cortex). Fibers originating in dentate and interposed nuclei that project through superior to contralateral red nucleus, ventrolateral and centromedian nuclei of thalamus, and brain stem reticular formation.

Note: Two important feedback loops exist, utilizing the SCP for outflow:
    (1) Triangle of Guillain-Mollaret (Fig. 2)—projections from red nucleus descend via the central tegmental tract to the ipsilateral inferior olive, from there to the contralateral cerebellar cortex (climbing fibers through inferior cerebellar peduncle), then to the dentate nucleus, then via the SCP to the contralateral red nucleus. With this circuit the cerebellum indirectly modulates spinal cord motor activity by its connections with the red nucleus and reticular formation, from which the descending rubrospinal and reticulospinal tracts originate. **The effect of cerebellar actions here is ipsilateral because of a double decussation** (dentate to contralateral red nucleus; then rubrospinal fibers cross again in Forel's decussation shortly after leaving red nucleus). Lesions anywhere along this circuit produce *palatal mycoclonus*, one of the few involuntary movements that doesn't go away during sleep (usually due to lesions of the central tegmental tract, which disinhibit the inferior olivary nucleus).

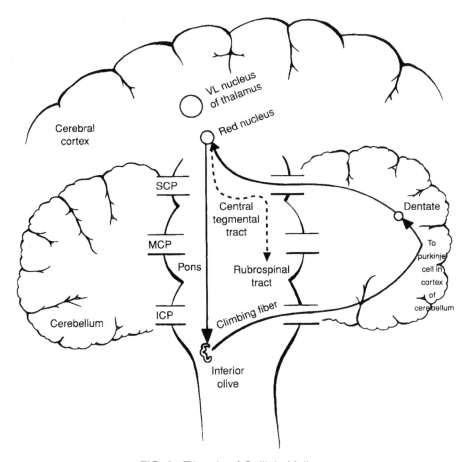

FIG. 2. Triangle of Guillain Mollaret.

(2) Cerebellar feedback circuit via pontine nuclei—cerebral cortex to ipsilateral pontine nuclei (corticopontine fibers) to contralateral cerebellar cortex (mossy fibers via middle CP) to dentate nucleus to contralateral ventrolateral subnucleus (VL) of thalamus to cortex.

III. Blood Supply

A. Superior Cerebellar Arteries—supply the bulk of cerebellum and peduncles; follow pontomesencephalic border, giving off branches to the tectum of the lower midbrain and superior cerebellar peduncles; these vessels run with peduncular fibers to deep nuclei (primarily dentate); supplies ventral vermis and paravermis; continue on to supply rostral vermis and rostroventral portions of both hemispheres; give off small branches to almost every sulcus; cross tentorial margin on way to dorsal and lateral parts of rostral hemispheres.

Note: This feature makes these branches vulnerable to compression. Results in infarction of rostral cortex.

   B. Anterior Inferior Cerebellar Artery (AICA)—branch of basilar; supplies flocculus and
      adjacent convolutions.
      Note: Internal auditory arteries supplying inner ear are usually branches of these.
   C. Posterior Inferior Cerebellar Artery (PICA)—branches of vertebral; some branches go
      to dorsolateral medulla (Wallenberg syndrome), caudal nuclei and inferior vermis, cau-
      dal cerebellum including tonsils
IV. Functional Considerations and Tracts (Fig. 3)
   A. General Information
      1. Cerebellum acts as coordination center for maintenance of equilibrium and muscle
         tone via complex regulatory and feedback mechanisms. Also enables somatic mo-
         tor system to accomplish discrete, skilled movements. It regulates movement and
         posture indirectly by adjusting the output of the major descending motor systems
         of the brain. It is a *comparator*, which compares intention with performance of
         movement and adjusts appropriately.

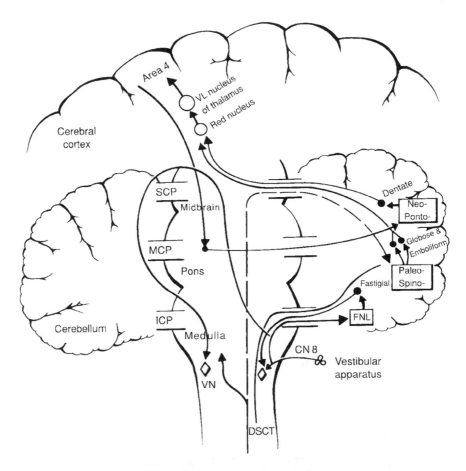

FIG. 3. Pathways of the cerebellum.

B. Vestibulocerebellum (Archicerebellum)
 1. Input—vestibulocerebellar tract (VCT). Impulses from ipsilateral labyrinth travel via cranial nerve (CN) VIII to vestibular nuclei (some go directly as mossy fibers to cerebellar cortex); VCT fibers (mossy fibers) go from vestibular nucleus (VN) to flocculonodular lobe (FNL) via inferior cerebellar peduncle (ICP) to synapse on granule cells, which synapse on Purkinje cells in cortex of FNL. Also receives visual information from the lateral geniculate body, superior colliculus, and striate cortex, relayed via pontine nuclei.
 2. Output—Purkinje cells in FNL send impulses to fastigial nucleus (this nucleus also receives inputs from vermis); from here fibers run via ICP to ipsilateral lateral VN (fastigiobulbar or cerebellobulbar tract). Some fibers cross to the other side of cerebellum, loop around contralateral SCP, and synapse on contralateral VN and reticular formation via the uncinate bundle of Russell. Fibers from VN and reticular formation form vestibulospinal and reticulospinal tracts, respectively, projecting to anterior horn cells.
 3. Function—the maintenance of equilibrium, regardless of movement or body position, by synergistically modulating spinal motor impulses. Also helps govern eye movements during stance and gait.
 4. Lesions of the vestibulocerebellum cause the following:
   a. Distorted equilibrium (on standing—*astasia*; on walking—*abasia*) with truncal ataxia and wide-based gait
   b. Nystagmus
   c. Tendency to fall *toward* side of lesion
C. Spinocerebellum (Paleocerebellum)
 1. Input
   a. Dorsal (posterior) spinocerebellar tract (DSCT)—impulses arising from Golgi tendon organs and muscle spindles travel via type Ia (FAST) fibers in posterior root and form collaterals that synapse on second neurons in Clarke's column (nucleus thoracicus) at medial base of dorsal horn from C8 to L2. Fibers from these neurons form DSCT and ascend ipsilaterally through inferior cerebellar peduncle to synapse on granule cells in the paravermian region (mossy fibers); these synapse on Purkinje cells.
   b. Ventral (anterior) spinocerebellar tract (VSCT)—again, collaterals of Ia afferents synapse on neurons in medial portion of dorsal horns. These second neurons, found throughout the cord, send projections bilaterally, forming the VSCT, which passes through tegmentum of medulla, pons, and midbrain and reaches granule cells of spinocerebellum via the SCPs bilaterally; granule cells go to Purkinje cells. Signals in the VSCT are felt to reflect activity of segmental interneurons that integrate both descending and peripheral inputs. The VSCT neurons are principally driven by central commands that regulate the locomotor cycle. VSCT input allows the cerebellum to monitor spinal circuit operation.
 Note: This is the only afferent tract in the SCP.
   c. Cuneocerebellar Tract—fibers from cervical dorsal roots (conveying position sense and deep sensibility of arms) ascend via cuneate fasciculus to accessory

cuneate nucleus; from here fibers travel with DSCT fibers to reach spinocerebellum via ICP.

Note: These spinal impulses project to cerebellar cortex in a somatotopic pattern.

    d. Inputs from auditory, visual, vestibular systems, as well as primary motor and somatosensory cortices have also been described.

2. Output—Purkinje cells of vermis project to fastigial nucleus (FN), and those of para-vermian region project to globose and emboliform nuclei. Efferents from FN project bilaterally to brain stem reticular formation and lateral vestibular nucleus. Additionally, crossed ascending projections reach the contralateral ventrolateral nucleus of the thalamus and are relayed to the primary motor cortex (axial and proximal muscles). Efferents from the interposed nuclei cross in the decussation of the SCP to terminate on neurons of the magnocellular portion of the contralateral red nucleus. Some of these fibers ascend to the VL thalamic nucleus to synapse on neurons projecting to the limb areas of primary motor cortex. Fibers from the red nucleus cross back to form the descending rubrospinal tract, which modulates the activity of brain stem and spinal motor neurons.

Note: Test questions say only globose, emboliform, and dentate nuclei send projections through the SCP.

Note: There is a double decussation here. Ipsilateral deep cerebellar nuclei go to contralateral red nucleus and thalamus/motor cortex; from there they cross rubrospinal and corticospinal tracts to ipsilateral brain stem and spinal cord motor neurons.

3. Function—influences muscle tone, controlling collaboration between agonist and antagonist muscle groups; modulates activity of antigravity musculature, providing enough tone to maintain equilibrium while standing or walking. Controls the execution of movement.

Note: Spinocerebellum and vestibulocerebellum act together to control muscle tone and to ensure smooth, synergistic coordination of agonists/antagonists subserving gait and stance.

4. Lesions of the spinocerebellum cause the following (ipsilateral):

    a. Truncal and limb ataxia

    b. Proprioceptive errors of limbs

    c. Gait disorders

    d. Scanning speech (vermis)

D. Corticopontocerebellum (Neocerebellum)

1. Input

    a. Corticopontocerebellar Tract—afferents from extensive areas of cerebral cortex, particularly areas 4 and 6, but also premotor and sensory cortices, form the corticopontine tract, passing through internal capsule and crus cerebri to synapse on ipsilateral pontine nuclei.

Note: Frontopontine fibers pass through anterior limb; all other fibers pass through posterior limb of internal capsule. Input crosses midline via pontine bridging fibers and enters contralateral cerebellar hemisphere via the MCP (pontocerebellar tract) to synapse on granule cells, to Purkinje cells.

    b. Olivocerebellar Tract—fibers from inferior olive (climbing fibers) cross midline and enter the contralateral cerebellar hemisphere (posterior lobe) via the ICP to synapse *directly* on Purkinje cell dendrites.

Note: Remember that inferior olives receive input from ipsilateral red nucleus via central tegmental tract (triangle of Guillain-Mollaret).

    2. Output

        a. Dentatorubrothalamic Tract—Purkinje cells of entire neocerebellum and part of paleocerebellum project to dentate nucleus; from here fibers project via SCP to contralateral red nucleus (parvocellular component) and ventrolateral thalamic nucleus (via the SCP decussation); from VL of thalamus, fibers pass through anterior limb of IC to synapse in areas 4 and 6 of motor cortex.

    3. Function—neocerebellum receives information on each planned voluntary movement in advance and corrects by inhibiting some pyramidal and extrapyramidal motor impulses. It helps make complex voluntary movement smooth and precise.

    4. Lesions of the corticoponto cerebellum cause the following:

        a. Ataxia—particularly distal limbs, with deviation of gait and stance toward the lesion

        b. Dysmetria

        c. Asynergia—decomposition of movement

        d. Dysdiadochokinesia

        e. Intention tremor—usually associated with dentate nucleus or SCP lesions

        f. Rebound

        g. Hypotonia (decreased deep tendon reflexes [DTRs])

        h. Delays in movement initiation

        i. Inability to discriminate weight—objects feel lighter in the hand ipsilateral to lesion.

V. Summary Table—Cerebellum and Connections

	Archicerebellum	Paleocerebellum	Neocerebellum
Synonym	Vestibulocerebellum	Spinocerebellum	Cerebrocerebellum/pontocerebellum
Lobe	Flocculonodular	Anterior	Posterior
Nucleus	Fastigial/vestibular	Globose/emboliform	Dentate
In-Peduncle	Inferior	Inferior/superior	Middle
Out-Peduncle	Inferior	Superior	Superior
Function	Equilibrium	Muscle tone	Compares planned to actual move
	Posture	Movement execution	Smooth precise movements
	Eye movement	Stretch reflexes	

THALAMUS

Function/Functional Subdivisions

Major relay and processing area for all sensory modalities (except olfaction) and motor input reaching cortex. Also important to autonomic function and arousal.

    I. Specific Relay Nuclei—modality specific (sensory and motor), topologically arranged, has discrete cortical projections (reciprocal). Examples: VPM, VPL, IC, VL, VA.

II. Nonspecific Nuclei—multimodal activation, widespread cortical projection, do not receive input from ascending tracts, involved with arousal. Examples: CM, parafascicular nucleus (Pf).

III. Association Nuclei—varied afferents/efferents to broad regions of association cortex. Examples: dorsal tier of lateral mass, anterior, dorsomedial.

IV. Subcortical Nuclei—project mostly to other thalamic nuclei. Example: reticular nucleus.

Anatomy: Dorsal portion of diencephalon (other parts are hypothalamus, subthalamus, epithalamus) is divided by internal medullary laminae into medial and lateral masses, anterior nucleus, and intralaminar nuclei.

I. Medial Mass—only one major nucleus—dorsomedial
   A. Small-cell (parvocellular) component has reciprocal projection to prefrontal cortex, is involved with abstract thinking and long-term, goal-directed behavior.
   B. Large-cell (magnocellular) part interrelates with hypothalamus, amygdala, frontal lobe, and is involved with olfactory activity.

II. Lateral Mass
   A. Dorsal Tier—related to the association cortex, involved with integration of sensory information.
      1. Lateral Dorsal (LD): caudal extension of anterior thalamic nuclei, interconnects with cingulate gyrus.
      2. Lateral Posterior (LP): interconnects with precuneus and receives input from superior colliculus.
      3. Pulvinar: connects reciprocally with large association areas of parietal, temporal, occipital cortex. Also receives input from superior colliculus, reticular system, cerebellum.
   B. Ventral Tier—posterior nuclei are concerned with all sensory modalities except olfaction; more anterior nuclei also have motor input and output.
      1. Ventral anterior (VA): large-cell component receives input from substantia nigra. Small-cell portion receives input from globus pallidus. Output primarily to premotor cortex (area 6) for integration of movement.
      2. Ventral lateral (VL): similar to VA with large- and small-cell components and similar input, but also has major cerebellar input and projects reciprocally with primary motor cortex (area 4).
      3. Ventral posterior (VP): main somatosensory and taste region, arranged somatotopically.
         a. Ventral posterior medial (VPM): receives input from head through secondary trigeminal tracts and taste input from nucleus of solitary tract (located most medially). Projects to postcentral gyrus (areas 5, 2, and 1).
         b. Ventral posterior lateral (VPL): medial lemniscus system, spinothalamic tract from body input here. Lower dermatomes are located more laterally. Projects to cortex areas 3, 2, 1.
      4. Metathalamic nuclei
         a. Medial geniculate body (MGB): lies adjacent to superior colliculus, receives bilateral input from inferior colliculi and projects to auditory cortex of superior temporal gyrus (Heschl, area 41).

     b. Lateral geniculate body (LGB): six cell layers (three for each eye with 2, 3, 5 uncrossed); therefore no cell in LGB receives bipolar input. Projects to visual cortex (area 17) through retrolenticular limb of internal capsule and optic radiations (geniculocalcarine projections).

III. Anterior Thalamic Nucleus: actually a complex of three nuclei, input from mammilothalamic tract, with reciprocal output to cingulate gyrus, hypothalamus. Very important limbic system relay.

IV. Intralaminar Nuclei: small collection of nerve cells, functionally the rostral extent of the ascending reticular system.
    A. Centromedian Nucleus (CM): input from globus pallidus and output to caudate and putamen.
    B. Parafascicular Nucleus (Pf): input is from anterolateral system and cortical area 6, with output to caudate, putamen, and other thalamic nuclei.

V. Thalamic Reticular Nucleus: thin layer of cells between the posterior limb of internal capsule and external medullary laminae of thalamus. Does not project to cortex but does receive cortical input. Projects to other thalamic nuclei, brain stem reticular system, and itself. Nearly all thalamic efferents to cortex pass through here; therefore may be important regulator of thalamic function.

Blood Supply

I. Posteromedial Arteries (Thalamoperforating): branches of posterior cerebral and posterior communicating arteries. Supply anterior and medial portions of thalamus.

II. Posterolateral Arteries (Thalamogeniculate): branches of PCA that supply posterior thalamus (pulvinar) and lateral nuclei, including geniculate bodies.

III. Posterior Choroidal Artery—branch of the PCA that supplies choroid plexus of third ventricle and posterior thalamus.

IV. Anterior Choroidal Artery: branch of the ICA that supplies subthalamus and ventral thalamus.

Clinical Correlates

I. Thalamic Aphasia: due to lesion of left thalamus, reflecting left hemisphere, producing deficits in language production, syntax, reception, or expression.

II. Nondominant Thalamic Lesions: may produce contralateral neglect and difficulties with spatial relationships.

III. Ventral Posterior Lesions: produces contralateral sensory loss to all modalities. Also may have thalamic pain syndrome in affected areas as "anesthesia dolorosa" in D'Jerene-Roussy syndrome.

IV. Lateral Geniculate Lesion: causes contralateral homonymous hemianopia. May accompany thalamic sensory or capsular stroke.

V. Bilateral Thalamic Lesions: most often vascular from anomalous blood supply; can impair consciousness and higher function.

HYPOTHALAMUS

I. Anatomy
   A. The hypothalamus has direct connections with the posterior lobe of the pituitary (the neurohypophysis).
   B. Supraoptic Nucleus—secretes *vasopressin* (antidiuretic hormone [ADH]).
   C. Paraventricular Nucleus—secretes *oxytocin*.
   D. Axons from the supraoptic and paraventricular nuclei project to the posterior lobe of the pituitary, and from here, the hormones (ADH and oxytocin, respectively) have direct access to the bloodstream.
II. Clinical Presentations
   A. Diabetes Insipidus—can result from damage to osmoreceptors in the sulpraoptic nucleus.
   B. The hypothalamus regulates body temperature and food intake.
      1. Stimulation of the lateral nuclei → hunger, gluttony
      2. Stimulation of the ventromedial nuclei → satiety, decreased appetite

LIMBIC SYSTEM

I. General Information
   A. A collection of interconnected but not contiguous structures in the telencephalon.
   B. Together with the hypothalamus and reticular formation, functions to maintain homeostasis, emotional and motivational states, arousal, memory, and learning.
   C. The limbic pathways interrelate the telencephalon and diencephalon with medial midbrain structures.
II. Components of the Limbic System
   A. Hippocampal Formation
      1. Dentate gyrus
         a. Has a three-layered cortex—molecular layer, granule cell layer, polymorphic cell layer
      2. Hippocampus (Ammon's horn)
         a. Also has a three-layered cortex: molecular layer, granule cell layer, polymorphic cell layer.
         b. Forms the floor of the temporal horn of the lateral ventricle.
         c. Covered by white matter called the *alveus*, which contains efferents from the hippocampus and subiculum, then forms the *fimbria* of the fornix.
      3. Fornix
         a. The main efferent system for the hippocampus.
         b. Contains precommisural and postcommisural fibers (split by the anterior commisure).
            (1) Precommisural fibers → septal area and anterior hypothalamus
            (2) Postcommisural fibers → mammillary bodies
      4. Subiculum
         a. A zone of transition between the hippocampus and the parahippocampal gyrus

5. Parahippocampal gyrus
    a. Part of the limbic system but has a six-layered cortex like the neocortex.
    b. Contains the entorhinal cortex.
B. Amygdala
C. Mammillary Bodies
D. Anterior Nucleus of Thalamus
E. Cingulate Gyrus
F. Entorhinal Cortex
III. Connections of the Limbic System
    A. Circuit of Papez (Fig. 4)
       1. Hippocampus → alveus → fimbrae → fornix → mammillary bodies → anterior nucleus of thalamus → cingulate gyrus → amygdala → back to hippocampus

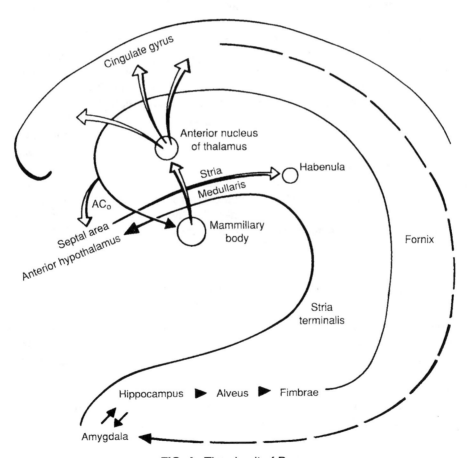

FIG. 4. The circuit of Papez.

      B. Stria Terminalis
        1. From the amygdala → follows curvature of the tail of the caudate nucleus → to septal nuclei and anterior hypothalamus
      C. Stria Medullaris
        1. From septal nuclei and anterior hypothalamus → to habenular nucleus
      D. Mammillo-tegmental Tract
        1. Mammillary bodies → raphe nuclei of midbrain reticular formation
      E. Medial Forebrain Bundle
        1. Septal area and amygdala → raphe nuclei of midbrain reticular formation
  IV. Clinical Correlates
      A. Klüver-Bucy Syndrome—results from bilateral damage to the temporal lobes (herpes encephalitis, Pick's disease, etc.). Classic symptoms: hyperoral, increased appetite, hypersexual, docile.
      B. Korsakoff Psychosis—may result from any disease of the temporal lobes. Common etiologies include thiamine deficiency (associated with Wernicke encephalopathy), third ventricular tumors, infarction (or resection) of inferomedial temporal lobes, and sequelae of herpes simplex virus encephalitis. Classic symptoms: amnesia (retentive memory impaired out of proportion to other cognitive functions), confabulation.
      C. Wernicke Encephalopathy—due to thiamine deficiency, often seen in alcoholics. Pathologic changes occur in the mammillary bodies, dorsomedial nucleus of the thalamus, periaqueductal gray, and oculomotor nuclei. Classic symptoms: mental status change (delirium), ophthalmoparesis, ataxia, nystagmus (mnemonic: MOAN).
      D. Sham Rage—strong emotional outburst produced by stimulation of the amygdala
      E. Hippocampal Sclerosis (mesial temporal sclerosis)—common cause for complex partial seizures (temporal lobe epilepsy)
      F. Limbic Encephalitis—can be due to herpes encephalitis or paraneoplastic disease
      G. Transient Global Amnesia—loss of memory for minutes or hours without recollection of events during this period. Occurs in middle-aged or elderly individuals. Rarely recurs. Pathogenesis unknown; suggested etiologies include ischemia/TIA, migraine, and complex partial seizure.

THE BASAL GANGLIA

  I. Function
      A. To control and regulate the activities of the motor and premotor cortical areas via various reverberating circuits so that voluntary movements can be performed smoothly.
      B. Motor activity is intricately controlled by the interactions of three major regions of the brain: cortex, cerebellum, and basal ganglia (BG).
      C. These three regions influence the lower motor neurons either:
        1. Directly via the *pyramidal system*—the corticobulbar and corticospinal tracts
        2. Indirectly via the *extrapyramidal system*—the basal ganglia
  II. Anatomy
      A. The basal ganglia consist of five subcortical nuclei:
        1. Caudate—develops from the matrix around the lateral ventricle; derived from the telencephalon—part of the neostriatum.

     2. Putamen—developed and derived same as caudate.

     3. Globus pallidus—develops from the matrix around the lateral ventricle; derived from the *diencephalon*—part of the paleostriatum; divided into internal and external segments by the internal medullary lamina

     4. Substantia nigra—also derived from the diencephalon

     5. Subthalamic nucleus of Luys—also derived from the diencephalon

     Note: The claustrum and amygdala were once considered a part of the basal ganglia, but they are now considered part of the limbic system.

III. Terminology

    A. **Striatum** or **Neostriatum** or **Striate Body** = Caudate + Putamen

    B. **Corpus Striatum** = Caudate + Putamen + Globus Pallidus

    C. **Pallidum** or **Paleostriatum** = Globus Pallidus (internal and external segments)

    D. **Lentiform nuclei** = Globus Pallidus + Putamen

    E. **Nucleus Accumbens** or **Fundus of the Striate Body** = where the head of the caudate and the putamen become one structure

IV. Functional Anatomy

    A. The Caudate and Putamen

      1. The caudate and putamen develop from the same telencephalic structures and are composed of identical cell types. They are partially separated by the internal capsule but connected by numerous gray bridges that cross through the internal capsule.

      2. They can be thought of as one entity from a functional standpoint.

      3. **Caudate and putamen serve as the major input nuclei for the basal ganglia** (i.e., they receive most of the input from the cerebral cortex).

      4. The caudate—large, C-shaped mass of gray matter that is closely related to the lateral ventricle and lies lateral to the thalamus.

        a. Composed of three parts:

          (1) Head—forms lateral wall of anterior horn of lateral ventricle.

          (2) Body—long and narrow; forms part of wall of lateral ventricle.

          (3) Tail—curves ventrally and follows the inferior horn of lateral ventricle into the temporal lobe, ends near the amygdala.

      5. The putamen—means "shell" in Latin. (It covers the globus pallidus like a shell.)

        a. Bordered medially by the globus pallidus, laterally by the external capsule.

        b. Putamen + Globus Pallidus = Lentiform nuclei . . . but there is no functional overlap, this is an anatomical term only (because they lie like a lens-shaped wedge between the internal and external capsules). These two structures are very different in phylogenesis, structure, and function.

    B. The Globus Pallidus

      1. Resembles the substantia nigra pars reticulata histologically.

      2. The internal segment of the globus pallidus and the pars reticulata are strikingly similar in structure and function, and can be considered a single structure divided by the internal capsule from a functional standpoint (much like the Caudate and Putamen).

      3. **Pars reticulata and the globus pallidus serve as the major output nuclei of the basal ganglia.**

C. The Substantia Nigra
   1. Means "black substance" in Latin.
   2. Lies in the midbrain and is composed of two zones:
      a. Ventral (pale) zone—*pars reticulata*; resembles internal segment of globus pallidus; is GABA-ergic.
      b. Dorsal (dark) zone—*pars compacta*; comprised of dopaminergic neurons; has reciprocal connections with the striatum.
D. The Subthalamic Nucleus (SN)
   1. Involved in the indirect pathway
V. Basal Ganglia Connections (Fig. 5)
  A. The Direct Pathway
   1. Input to the BG arises from the *entire cortex* and goes to the caudate/putamen.
   2. Cortical projections to the striatum are topographically organized. Specific areas of the cortex project to different parts of the striatum and have specific functions.
      a. Limbic lobes, orbitofrontal areas → nucleus accumbens and olfactory tubercle (ventral striatum) → ventral pallidum.
      Serves "limbic" functions, such as motivation, aggression, sexual behavior, and some addictions.
      b. Area 8 (frontal eye fields [FEF]), association areas → prefer caudate. Helps coordinate eye movements and some cognitive functions.
      c. Areas 1, 2, 3, 4, 6 (primary sensorimotor area) → prefer putamen.
      Most intricately involved in coordinating motor movements.
   3. The caudate and putamen are not directly connected to the thalamus. Output is mediated by the globus pallidus.
   4. The output from the BG is not direct. It must first go through the thalamus, then back to the cortex.
   5. The caudate and putamen receive the major input (afferents), and the pallidum sends the major outputs (efferents).
   6. The output from the BG goes mainly to the VA of the thalamus (and also to the VL, and the intralaminar nuclei).
   7. The internal segment of the globus pallidus and pars reticulata of the SN are similar in structure and function (output nuclei). The caudate and putamen are similar in structure and function (input nuclei).
   8. Neurotransmitters:
      a. Cortex to striatum = Glutaminergic/excitatory
      b. Striatum to globus pallidus = GABA-ergic/inhibitory
      c. All outputs from globus pallidus = GABA-ergic/inhibitory
      d. Subthalamic nucleus to globus pallidus = Glutaminergic/excitatory
      e. Striatum to SN = GABA-ergic/inhibitory
      f. SN pars compacta to striatum = Dopaminergic/excitatory
   9. Movement results when the thalamic cells are released from tonic inhibition.
   10. Dopamine inhibits the indirect pathway and facilitates the direct pathway. Both actions serve to facilitate movement.

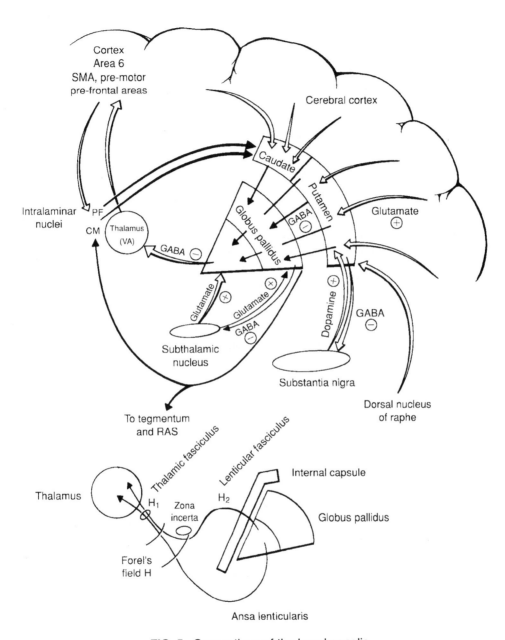

FIG. 5. Connections of the basal ganglia.

B. The Indirect Pathway
  1. The second route by which information can get from the striatum to the globus pallidus, by way of the subthalamic nucleus
  2. There is a two-way connection between the subthalamic nucleus and the globus pallidus. (These two structures are related, both derived from the diencephalon.)
  3. Output from globus pallidus = GABA
  4. Output from subthalamic nucleus = Glutamate

VI. The Pallidothalamic Connections (Fields of Forel and Associated Structures)
  A. Ansa Lenticularis—formed by fibers that come from the ventral part of the medial globus pallidus and sweep around the posterior limb of the internal capsule on their way to the thalamus.
  B. Forel's Field H2 (lenticular fasciculus)—formed by fibers that come from the inner part of the medial globus pallidus and that pass *through* the posterior limb of the internal capsule, around the zona incerta, and on to the thalamus.
  C. Forel's Field H1 (thalamic fasciculus)—the ansa lenticularis and the lenticular fasciculus merge in the fields of Forel (H) to form this bundle of fibers, which then travel on together to the thalamus.
  D. Most of the fibers terminate in the VA nucleus of the thalamus, some to VL and some to the intralaminar nuclei.
  E. The thalamocortical fibers project to area 6 (SMA, premotor, and prefrontal areas).
  F. Zona Incerta—thought to be a rostral continuation of the midbrain reticular formation.

VII. Connections—Summary
  A. The cortex sends fibers to
    1. Caudate and putamen
    2. Substantia nigra
    3. Red nucleus
    4. Subthalamic nucleus
    5. Reticular formation
  B. Afferents to the striatum come from the:
    1. Cortex
    2. Substantia nigra
    3. Others: Intralaminar nuclei (CM, Pf), dorsal raphe nucleus, reticular formation
  C. Efferents from the striatum go to the:
    1. Globus pallidus
    2. Substantia nigra
  D. Globus pallidus receives afferents from the
    1. Striatum
    2. Subthalamic nucleus
    3. *not from the cortex*
  E. Globus pallidus efferents go to the:
    1. Thalamus (direct pathway)
  2. Subthalamic nucleus (indirect pathway)

VIII. Clinical Application—Diseases of the Basal Ganglia
  A. Carbon Monoxide Intoxication
    1. Bilateral necrosis of the globus pallidus

2. Other things that can cause bilateral lesions in the basal ganglia:
   a. Cyanide, ethylene glycol (antifreeze)—both globus pallidus, methanol poisoning (putamen), aminoacidopathies, infarction, Hallervorden-Spatz syndrome, Huntington's disease, Leigh's disease, Wilson's disease, mitochondrial encephalopathies, neoplasms (lymphoma, glioma), multiple system atrophy (MSA)

B. Hallervorden-Spatz Disease
   1. Autosomal recessive (AR), childhood/adolescent onset, insidiously progressive
   2. Clinical indications: stiff gait, toe-walking with arms held stiff and fingers hyperextended, distal wasting, pes cavus, frozen pained expression, speaking through clenched teeth, dystonic and bizarre postures
   3. Caused by increased uptake of iron by the basal ganglia
   4. T2 MRI: striking hypointensity of the medial segment of the globus pallidus, called the "eye-of-the-tiger" sign
   5. Path: Hallmark is a golden-brown discoloration of the medial globus pallidus.

C. Hemiballismus
   1. Most often due to a contralateral lesion of the subthalamic nucleus
   2. Usually vascular etiology

D. Fahr's Disease—Basal ganglia calcification

E. "Status Marmoratus"
   1. Perinatal damage to the striatum; results in glial scars that resemble marble.
   2. Involuntary movements, bizarre postures, spasmodic outbursts of laughing/crying. Intelligence may be normal. (Similar to choreoathetoid cerebral palsy.)

F. Parkinson's Disease

G. Huntington's Disease

H. Wilson's Disease

I. "Status Lacunaris"—arteriosclerotic Parkinsonism

J. Striatonigral Degeneration

CRANIAL NERVES

I. Introduction—Definition of Functional Components
   A. Cranial Nerves (CN)
      1. Special visceral afferent (SVA)—afferent fibers related to special senses (smell and taste) concerned with visceral functions. Cell bodies lie in olfactory epithelium or in sensory ganglia.
      2. Special sensory afferent (SSA)—fibers related to special sense organs of the head (eyes and ears). Cell bodies are located in the retina and sensory ganglia of CN VIII.
      3. Special visceral efferent (SVE)—motor fibers that supply all skeletal muscles derived from the pharyngeal arches. Cell bodies in the brain stem.
   B. Spinal and Cranial Nerves
      1. General somatic afferent (GSA)—fibers carry information from the body wall (e.g., somite-derived structures such as skin, skeletal muscle, joints, oral mucosa) to the central nervous system (CNS). Unipolar cell bodies lie in the spinal ganglia (dorsal root ganglia) and sensory ganglia of the cranial nerves.

2. General visceral afferent (GVA)—fibers carry information from viscera (e.g., heart, vessels, gut) to the CNS. Unipolar cell bodies lie in the dorsal root ganglia and sensory ganglia of the cranial nerves.
3. General somatic efferent (GSE)—motor fibers that supply all skeletal muscles of the body, except those derived from the branchial arches.
4. General visceral efferent (GVE)—autonomic motor fibers with preganglionic cell bodies in the CNS that send axons to peripheral autonomic ganglia. Fibers from postganglionic neurons innervate all smooth muscle, cardiac muscle, and glands throughout the body.

II. Cranial Nerve I—Olfactory Nerve
   A. Function: Smell—SVA
   B. Pathways
      1. Primary sensory neurons in olfactory epithelium → Pass through cribriform plate → Synapse on secondary neurons in the olfactory bulb (mitral and tufted cells) → Tufted cells synapse in the anterior olfactory nucleus and send projections to all olfactory areas, mitral cells send collaterals to the anterior olfactory nucleus and project only to the lateral olfactory area → Olfactory tract → Olfactory trigone → Olfactory stria
   C. Olfactory Stria
      1. Medial—projects to the frontal lobe (medial olfactory area). Mediates emotional response to odors and has connections to the limbic system.
      2. Intermediate—projects to the anterior perforated substance.
      3. Lateral—projects to the lateral olfactory area. The lateral olfactory stria have many important connections:
         a. Lateral Olfactory Stria → Stria Medullaris → Habenula
         b. Lateral Olfactory Stria → pyriform lobe, prepyriform cortex, periamygdaloid area, uncus, insula (primary olfactory cortex) → entorhinal cortex (secondary olfactory cortex)
   D. Definitions
      1. Pyriform lobe—parahippocampal gyrus, uncus, lateral olfactory stria
      2. Prepyriform cortex—entorhinal cortex, uncus, insula, amygdala
      3. Primary olfactory cortex—pryiform lobe and periamygdaloid area
      4. Secondary olfactory cortex—entorhinal cortex
      5. Diagonal band of Broca—connects the medial, intermediate, and lateral olfactory areas
   E. Lesions
      1. Anosmia—lack of smell. Occurs ipsilateral to the lesion and may be due to:
         a. Trauma—olfactory fibers are torn as they traverse the cribriform plate.
         b. Frontal lobe masses—such as tumor, abscess. Due to olfactory tract or olfactory bulb compression.
      2. Hyposmia—decreased smell. Occurs commonly with
         a. Cystic fibrosis
         b. Parkinson's disease
         c. Adrenal insufficiency
      3. Cacosmia—repugnant smells. Can result from

a. Damage to the olfactory area in the temporal lobe

b. Epilepsy—"uncinate fits"

Note: Olfaction is the only special sense that does not go through the thalamus.

III. Cranial Nerve II—Optic Nerve

A. Function: Sight—SSA

B. Anatomy

The retina is composed of three cell layers:

1. Rods and Cones—photoreceptors that convert light waves into electrical impulses. Rods are responsible for night vision and are absent at the fovea. Cones are involved with color vision and acuity and are concentrated at the fovea.

2. Bipolar Cell Layer—also contains supporting cells such as Müller cells, horizontal cells, and amacrine cells. Bipolar cells receive impulses from the photoreceptors (rods and cones).

3. Ganglion Cell Layer—the innermost layer of the retina. Receives impulses from the bipolar cells. Axons from the ganglion cells travel inward on the inner surface of the retina and form the optic nerve.

C. Pathways

1. Visual pathway

Rods/Cones → Bipolar Cells → Ganglion Cells → Optic Nerve → Optic Chiasm (nasal fibers cross and temporal fibers remain uncrossed) → Optic Tracts → Lateral Geniculate Body of Thalamus (most fibers of the optic tract synapse are here but a small number of fibers bypass the lateral geniculate body and synapse instead on intercalated neurons in the midbrain as part of the pupillary light reflex; see next section) → Optic Radiations (Geniculocalcarine Tracts) → Occipital Lobe (Area 17—Primary Visual Cortex)

2. Pupillary Light Reflex

Rods/Cones → Bipolar Cells → Ganglion Cells → Optic Nerve → Optic Chiasm → Optic Tracts → Intercalated neurons, pretectal nuclei in midbrain → Bilateral Edinger–Westphal Nuclei → Ciliary Ganglia (via CN III) → Short Ciliary Nerves → Pupils

D. Important Anatomic Facts

1. The pupillary light reflex bypasses the lateral geniculate body (does not synapse there) and synapses in the midbrain. The pupillary light reflex does not involve the cortex.

2. Nasal fibers from the retina cross at the optic chiasm, whereas temporal fibers remain uncrossed.

3. The lateral geniculate body is somatotopically arranged and is composed of six layers. Layers 2, 3, and 5 receive uncrossed fibers. Layers 1, 4, and 6 receive crossed fibers.

4. Inferior Visual Field → Superior Retina → Parietal Lobe → Upper Lip of Calcarine Fissure in Occipital Cortex. (Therefore a lesion in the parietal lobe will give an inferior quadrantanopia.)

5. Superior Visual Field → Inferior Retina → Temporal Lobe and Meyer's Loop → Lower Lip of Calcarine Fissure in Occipital Cortex. (Therefore a lesion in the *temporal lobe* will give a superior quadrantanopia or *"pie in the sky"* defect.)

6. Wilbrand's knee—Where nasal retinal fibers course slightly anterior in the chiasm before joining the temporal retinal fibers from the contralateral eye. A lesion just anterior to the chiasm can damage these fibers, giving a monocular visual loss in the affected eye plus a temporal field defect in the contralateral eye.

E. Lesions (Fig. 6)

Site of Lesion	Associated Field Defect
1. Retina (glaucoma)	Arcuate defect from increased pressure
2. Optic nerve	Monocular blindness
3. Optic nerve (Traquair)	Monocular hemianopia (ipsilateral)
4. Optic nerve near chiasm (affecting Wilbrand's knee fibers)	Monocular blindness plus contralateral temporal field defect
5. Optic chiasm	Bitemporal hemianopia
6. Optic tract	Homonymous hemianopia (usually noncongruous if incomplete)
7. Lateral geniculate body	Homonymous hemianopia with spared central region (rectangle)
8. Temporal lobe	Superior homonymous quadrantanopia
9. Parietal lobe	Inferior homonymous quadrantanopia
10. Occipital lobe	Variable homonymous hemianopias (Range from total to small homonymous hemianopias, depending on amount of cortex involved. High degree of congruity.) Macular sparing secondary to dual blood supply.

F. Fields
   1. Nasal—50°
   2. Superior—60°
   3. Inferior—70°
   4. Temporal—80°

IV. Cranial Nerve III—Oculomotor Nerve
   A. Function
      1. Motor to extraocular muscles—GSE
      2. Parasympathetics to pupil constrictor muscle—GVE
      3. Proprioception for extraocular muscles—GSA
   B. Pathways
      Nucleus lies at the level of the superior colliculus → the nerve exits the midbrain in the interpeduncular fossa between the midbrain and the pons → passes between the posterior cerebral and superior cerebellar arteries → through the cavernous sinus → through the tendinous ring in the superior orbital fissure → divides into superior and inferior divisions

Superior Division	1. Superior Rectus
	2. Levator Palpebrae
Inferior Division	1. Inferior Rectus
	2. Inferior oblique
	3. Medial rectus
	4. Parasympathetic fibers → ciliary ganglion → short ciliary nerves → iris and ciliary body (pupil constrictors)

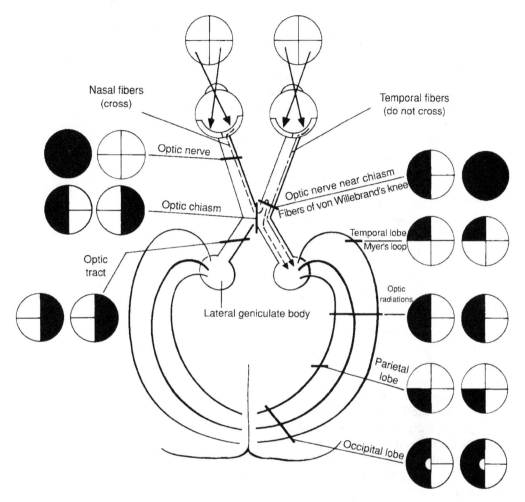

FIG. 6. Visual field defects.

C. Oculomotor Nucleus—A V-shaped complex that lies at the level of the superior colliculus in the midbrain. Made of many subnuclei:

Lateral	0	0 —————	Inferior Rectus
Group	0	0 —————	Inferior Oblique
	0	0 ——	Medial Rectus
Medial	0	0 —————	Contralateral Superior Rectus
Central		0 —————	Bilateral Levators

D. Lesions
   1. Weber's syndrome—Ipsilateral CN III palsy and contralateral weakness. Due to lesion of the midbrain affecting CN III and cerebral peduncle.
   2. Benedikt's syndrome—Ipsilateral CN III palsy and contralateral intention tremor. Due to lesion of midbrain affecting CN III and red nucleus.
   3. Claude's syndrome—Weber's and Benedikt's syndromes
   4. Differential diagnosis of CN III palsy also includes:
      a. Aneurysm—Posterior communicating artery > basilar tip > posterior cerebral artery. Pupil affected in 80% of cases.
      b. Cavernous sinus syndrome
      c. Syphilis
      d. Tuberculosis
      e. Diabetes mellitus—pupil spared in 80% of cases
      f. Temporal lobe herniation
      g. Myasthenia—pupil spared

V. Cranial Nerve IV—Trochlear Nerve
   A. Function
      1. Motor to superior oblique—GSE
      2. Proprioception for superior oblique—GSA
   B. Pathways
      Nucleus at level of inferior colliculus in midbrain tegmentum → axons cross in the superior medullary velum → exits dorsally and passes around brain stem → passes between the posterior cerebral and superior cerebellar arteries (lateral to CN III) → through the cavernous sinus → enters superior orbital fissure (above the tendinous ring) → to superior oblique
   C. Four Unique Features of CN IV
      1. Smallest cranial nerve (approximately 2,400 axons)
      2. Only CN that exits the brain stem on the dorsal aspect
      3. Only CN that crosses (decussates)
      4. Longest intracranial course (approximately 7.5 cm)
   D. Lesions
      1. Head tilts toward the contralateral side (away from the affected eye). Tilting the head to the contralateral side allows the good eye to intort and line up with the bad eye and alleviates diplopia.
      2. The affected eye is deviated higher and extorted.
      3. Myasthenia
      4. Cavernous sinus lesions
      5. Orbital lesions

VI. Cranial Nerve V—Trigeminal Nerve
   A. Function
      1. GSA—Sensation for face, oral mucosa, nasal mucosa, meninges of the anterior and middle cranial fossae, conjunctiva, and proprioception for muscles of mastication
      2. SVE—Motor for muscles derived from the first branchial arch:
         a. Muscles of mastication—temporalis, masseter, medial, and lateral pterygoids

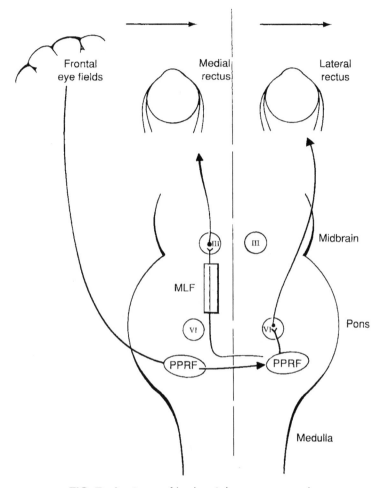

FIG. 7. Anatomy of horizontal eye movements.

    b. Tensors—tensor tympani and tensor veli palatini
    c. Mylohyoid
    d. Anterior belly of digastric
       Note: CN VII supplies the stylohyoid and the posterior belly of the digastric.
B. Anatomic Facts
    1. CN V has three divisions:
       a. V1—Ophthalmic
       b. V2—Maxillary
       c. V3—Mandibular
    2. All three divisions exit the skull via different foramina:
       a. V1—Superior orbital fissure

        b. V2—foramen rotundum

        c. V3—foramen ovale

    3. V1 and V2 pass through the cavernous sinus.

    4. V1 and V2 are purely sensory.

    5. V3 is sensory and motor.

    6. CN V exits the pons as a large sensory root and a small motor root.

    7. The trigeminal ganglion sits in a depression called *Meckel's cave.*

C. Subnuclei (Fig. 8)

    1. Motor nucleus

        a. Lies just medial to the main sensory nucleus in the mid pons.

        b. Axons run with the V3 branch and supply muscles of the first branchial arch
           (see earlier section for list of muscles).

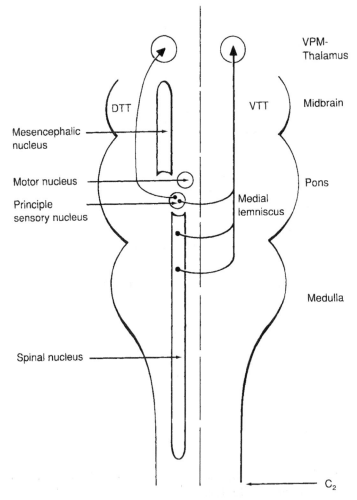

FIG. 8. Cranial nerve V—nuclei and tracts.

2. Sensory nucleus
   a. Largest of all cranial nerve nuclei
   b. Extends from the midbrain to C2
   c. In the medulla it cases a ridge called the *tuber cinereum*.
   d. The sensory nucleus contains three subnuclei:
      (1) Mesencephalic nucleus
         (a) Lies in the midbrain (mesencephalon)
         (b) Contains primary sensory neurons (really a ganglion)
         (c) Is the only exception to the rule that ganglia lie outside the CNS
         (d) Receives *proprioception* and deep pressure from the muscles of mastication
      (2) Pontine trigeminal nucleus (principal sensory nucleus)
         (a) Lies in the mid pons
         (b) Receives touch sensation from the face and is involved in the corneal reflex
      (3) Spinal nucleus
         (a) Runs from the pons to C2
         (b) Carries pain and temperature sensation from the face
D. Main Pathways
   1. Ventral trigeminothalamic tract (VTTT)
      Fibers from the principal sensory and spinal nuclei → cross and join fibers from the medial lemniscus → contralateral VPM nucleus of the thalamus → parietal cortex
   2. Dorsal trigeminothalamic tract (DTTT)
      Fibers from the principal sensory nucleus → ipsilateral VPM → parietal cortex
      Note: DTTT does not cross.
E. Functional Divisions and Pathways
   1. V1—Ophthalmic
      a. Sensation from scalp, conjunctiva, eye/orbit, bridge, ala and apex of nose, frontal and ethmoidal sinuses → to V1 via frontal, nasociliary, and lacrimal nerves → superior orbital fissure → cavernous sinus → trigeminal ganglion → principal sensory and spinal nuclei → DTTT and VTTT → VPM → sensory cortex
      b. Sensation from cornea → V1 → principal sensory nucleus → bilateral CN VII (corneal reflex pathway)
      c. Parasympathetic fibers from CN III → ciliary ganglion → to V1 via short ciliary nerves → pupil
      d. Parasympathetic fibers from CN VII → pterygopalatine ganglion → to V1 via lacrimal nerve → lacrimal gland
   2. V2—Maxillary
      a. Sensation from lower lids, side and vestibule of nose, cheeks, upper teeth and gums, palate → to V2 via zygomatic, infraorbital, and superior alveolar nerves → foramen rotundum → cavernous sinus → trigeminal ganglion → principal sensory and spinal nuclei → DTTT and VTTT → VPM → sensory cortex

  b. Parasympathetic fibers from CN VII → pterygopalatine ganglion → V2 → mucous glands of the nose and sinuses

 3. V3—Mandibular

  a. Sensory from lower jaw, lower teeth and gums, anterior two-thirds of tongue, lower face to the angle of the jaw → to V3 via buccal, lingual, inferior alveolar, mental, and auriculotemporal nerves → foramen ovale → trigeminal ganglion → principal sensory and spinal nuclei → DTTT and VTTT → VPM → sensory cortex

  b. Parasympathetic fibers from CN VII → Submandibular gland → to V3 via lingual nerve → submandibular and sublingual glands

  c. Parasympathetics from CN IX → otic ganglion → to V3 via auriculotemporal nerve → parotid gland

  d. Motor nucleus → trigeminal ganglion → V3 → foramen ovale → muscles of mastication, tensors, mylohyoid, anterior belly of digastric

F. Lesions—cause loss of ipsilateral facial sensation and sometimes jaw weakness.

VII. Cranial Nerve VI—Abducens Nerve

 A. Function

  1. GSE—Motor to lateral rectus muscle

  2. GSA—Prioprioception from lateral rectus muscle

 B. Pathways

 Nucleus at level of pontine tegmentum → emerges from brain stem at level of pontomedullary junction → cavernous sinus → enters the superior orbital fissure through the tendinous ring → lateral rectus muscle

 C. Lesions—cause diplopia on lateral gaze; worse when looking toward side of lesion

  1. Aneurysm—PICA > basilar tip > ICA

  2. Increased intracranial pressure ("false localizing sign")

  3. Skull fracture

  4. Tumor or vascular disease

  5. Multiple sclerosis

  6. Gradenigo syndrome—CN V and VI palsies due to a lesion at the apex of the temporal bone (infection or tumor most common)

  7. Myasthenia

Special Notes Regarding Cranial Nerves II Through VI

 1. Structures that run through the *cavernous sinus*:

  a. Cranial nerves III, IV, V1, V2, and VI

  b. Internal carotid artery

 2. Cranial nerves that course *through the tendinous ring* in the superior orbital fissure:

  a. II, III, VI

 3. Cranial nerves that run *above the tendinous ring* in the superior orbital fissure:

  a. IV and VI

 4. Miscellaneous factoids

  a. The auriculotemporal nerve splits to encircle the middle meningeal artery.

  b. The middle meningeal artery enters the skull through the foramen spinosum.

VIII. Cranial Nerve VII—Facial Nerve (Fig. 9)
  A. Function
    1. GSA—Sensory to external ear, auditory canal, external tympanic membrane
    2. SVA—Taste from anterior two-thirds of tongue
    3. GVE—Lacrimal gland, nasal and palate mucosae, submandibular and sublingual glands
    4. SVE—Motor to muscles of the second branchial arch:
      a. Muscles of facial expression (frontalis, orbicularis oculi, orbicularis oris, buccinator, platysma)
      b. Stapedius
      c. Stylohyoid
      d. Posterior belly of the digastric

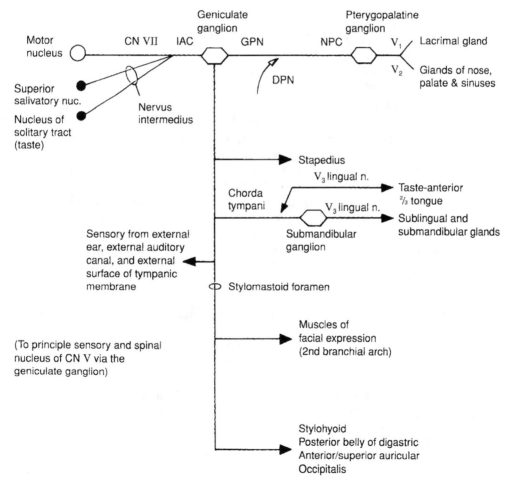

FIG. 9. Cranial nerve VII.

   e. Occipitalis
   f. Anterior and superior auricular
B. Anatomic Facts
   1. The facial nerve nucleus is located in the ventral pons, near the medulla.
   2. The axons emerge from the nucleus and run dorsally toward the floor of the fourth ventricle and loop around the sixth nerve nucleus. This loop of axons forms a bump called the *facial colliculus* on the floor of the fourth ventricle.
   3. CN VII exits the brain stem at the pontomedullary junction, just lateral to CN VI.
   4. CN VII exits the skull via the stylomastoid foramen.
C. Pathways
   Motor cortex → posterior limb of internal capsule (corticobulbar tract) → motor nucleus → CN VII → internal auditory canal → geniculate ganglion → stylomastoid foramen → to muscles of facial expression via five main branches (and to other muscles listed earlier):
   1. Temporal → Frontalis
   2. Zygomatic → Orbicularis Oculi
   3. Buccal → Buccinator
   4. Marginal Mandibular → Orbicularis Oris
   5. Cervical → Platysma
   Parasympathetics from *superior salivatory nucleus* → nervus intermedius/CN VII → internal auditory canal → geniculate ganglion → greater petrosal nerve → nerve of the pterygoid canal → pterygopalatine ganglion → to lacrimal gland (via CN V1) and glands of the nose, palate, and sinuses (via CN V2)
   Parasympathetics from *superior salivatory nucleus* → nervus intermedius/CN VII → internal auditory canal → geniculate ganglion → chorda tympani → submandibular ganglion → to sublingual and submandibular glands (via lingual branch of CN V3)
   Taste for anterior two-thirds of tongue → lingual branch of CN V3 → chorda tympani → CN VII → geniculate ganglion → solitary tract/nucleus
   Sensation/pain from external ear, external tympanic membrane (TM), auditory canal → CN VII → geniculate ganglion → CN V → to principal sensory and spinal nucleus of CN V
D. Lesions
   1. Lower motor neuron lesions—produce ipsilateral weakness of both the upper and lower face. Causes include
      a. Bell's palsy—facial weakness, taste distortion (chorda tympani), hyperacusis (due to loss of sound dampening by stapedius), pain behind the ear. Treat with ocular lubrication/eye patching, prednisone, +/– acyclovir
      b. Ramsay-Hunt syndrome—Herpes zoster infection of geniculate ganglion.
      c. **Note:** Abnormal reinnervation after these lesions may result in synkinetic movements and paradoxical gustolacrimal reflex ("crocodile tears").
   2. Upper motor neuron lesions—produce contralateral weakness of the lower face only. The frontalis is spared because of bilateral innervation to upper facial muscles.
      a. Most common etiology is vascular (stroke).

3. Moebius syndrome—Congenital bilateral CN VI and VII palsies.
IX. Cranial Nerve VIII—Vestibulocochlear Nerve
  A. Function: SSA-Balance
  B. Anatomy of the Vestibular Apparatus
    1. Saccule and utricle
      a. These contain sensory receptors called *macula* that consist of ciliated hair cells covered with a gelatinous mass. $CaCO_3$ crystals (otoliths) are embedded in the gel.
      b. With movement otoliths stimulate the hair cells by bending cilia.
      c. Detects position relative to gravity and linear acceleration (static labyrinth).
    2. Semicircular canals
      a. Three canals sit at right angles to each other.
      b. Each canal is filled with endolymph and terminates in the utricle.
      c. Just before joining the utricle, the canal dilates and forms the *ampulla*. The ampulla contains an area of thickening (the ampullary crest) that houses the gelatinous *cupula*. The cupula contains hair cells that sense movement of endolymph within the canals.
      d. Each hair cell has many stereocilia and a single kinocilium. Movement of the sterocilia toward or away from the kinocilium changes the firing rate of the hair cell.
      e. Detects angular motion (kinetic labyrinth).
  C. Pathways
  Hair cells synapse with primary sensory neurons in the vestibular ganglion (Scarpa's ganglion) → vestibular nerve → internal auditory meatus → vestibular nuclei in the medulla.The vestibular nuclear complex consists of four subnuclei:
    1. Lateral (Deiter's) Vestibular Nucleus—Axons run ipsilaterally down the spinal cord to innervate antigravity (extensor) muscles. Fibers form the lateral vestibulospinal tract.
    2. Inferior Vestibular Nucleus—Fibers enter the inferior cerebellar peduncle to the flocculonodular lobe of the cerebellum.
    3. Medial and Superior Nuclei—Mediate vestibuloocular reflexes.
  Fibers from the vestibular nuclei run through the medial longitudinal fasciculus (MLF):
      a. Ascending MLF
        (1) All four nuclei (mostly medial and superior) contribute.
        (2) Fibers terminate on bilateral CN III, IV, and VI nuclei to maintain visual fixation with head movement.
      b. Descending MLF
        (1) Medial and inferior nuclei contribute.
        (2) Fibers descend to form the **medial vestibulospinal tract,** which influences cervical cord lower motor neurons.
  D. Lesions/Clinical Application
    1. Meniere's disease—overproduction of endolymph. Severe episodic vertigo, vomiting, progressive hearing loss, tinnitus. Affects both vestibular and cochlear divisions of CN VIII.

2. Decerebrate rigidity—due to unopposed excitatory effect of the lateral vestibulospinal tract on antigravity (extensor) muscles.

The **cochlear component** consists of the following:

A. Function: SSA—Hearing

B. Anatomy

   1. The cochlea contains three compartments:
      a. Scala vestibuli
      b. Scala tympani
      c. Scala media (cochlear duct)—contains hair cells with basilar surfaces on the basilar membrane and cilia that are embedded in the tectorial membrane.

   2. The cochlear nucleus has tonotopic organization and is composed of two parts:
      a. Dorsal cochlear nucleus—responsible for high frequencies.
      b. Ventral cochlear nucleus—responsible for low frequencies.

   3. Hair cells along the basilar membrane respond to different sound frequencies.
      a. Base of membrane—cells respond to high frequencies.
      b. Apex of membrane—cells respond to low frequencies.

   4. Spiral ganglion (organ of Corti)—contains primary sensory neurons (bipolar).

   5. Probst's commisure—connections between the two lateral lemniscus tracts.

   6. Sound dampening—provided by the stapedius muscle (supplied by CN VII). A small number of fibers from the superior olive project to bilateral CN VII.

   7. Humans can hear from about 20 to 20,000 Hz.

C. Pathways

Sound waves → tympanic membrane vibrates → malleus, incus, and stapes move → a fluid wave occurs in the cochlea → hair cells in scala media → spiral ganglion (organ of Corti) → cochlear nerve → cochlear nuclei → superior olive → lateral lemniscus → inferior colliculus → medial geniculate → Heschl's gyrus (transverse temporal gyrus, primary auditory cortex, Broca's area 41)

   1. Mnemonic "NCSLIMA" corresponds to the five peaks on the brain stem auditory evoked potential recordings (N is peak #1, C is peak #2, etc.). The entire pathway takes approximately 9 msec
      a. N—Nerve (cochlear)
      b. C—Cochlear nuclei
      c. S—Superior olive
      d. L—Lateral lemniscus
      e. I—Inferior colliculus
      f. M—Medical geniculate
      g. A—Auditory cortex

   2. Other helpful memory tricks
      a. Superior Sight (the superior *colliculus* is involved in vision; the inferior, with hearing)
      b. Medial Music, Lateral Light (the medial *geniculate ganglion* is involved in hearing; the lateral, with vision)

   3. Other things to note
      a. Some fibers from the ventral cochlear nucleus cross in the trapezoid body and ascend in the opposite lateral lemniscus.

      b. There are four pathways that provide bilateral connections
        (1) Dorsal acoustic stria
        (2) Intermediate acoustic stria
        (3) Trapezoid body (fibers come from the ventral cochlear nucleus)
        (4) Probst's commisure (fibers from one lateral lemniscus to the other)
      c. Unilateral lesions above the level of the cochlear nuclei do not cause deafness because of these extensive bilateral connections.
    D. Lesions/Clinical Application
      1. Acoustic neuroma—initially causes tinnitus and deafness. The most common cerebellopontine angle tumor.
      2. Two types of deafness:
        a. Conduction deafness—usually due to disease of the middle ear (otitis media, otosclerosis, glomus tumor).
          (1) Rinne test: bone > air
          (2) Weber test: tone heard best in affected ear
        b. Nerve deafness—due to disease of the cochlear nerve, organ of corti, or central pathways
          (1) Rinne test: air > bone
          (2) Weber test: tone heard best in unaffected ear
X. Cranial Nerve IX—Glossopharyngeal
  A. Function
    1. GVA—Chemoreceptors and baroreceptors, sensation from pharyngeal mucosa and posterior third of tongue
    2. SVA—Taste from posterior third of tongue
    3. GSA—Pain/temperature sensation from postauricular skin, inner surface of tympanic membrane. Proprioception from stylopharyngeus muscle
    4. SVE—Motor to stylopharyngeus muscle
    5. GVE—Parotid gland, mucosa of pharynx, and posterior third of tongue
  B. Pathways

Function	Ganglion	Nucleus
Taste in posterior third of tongue	Inferior IX (petrosal)	Solitary
Sensory posterior third of tongue	Inferior IX (petrosal)	Solitary
Carotid body (chemoreceptor—O2)	Inferior IX (petrosal)	Solitary
Carotid sinus (baroreceptor—BP)	Inferior IX (petrosal)	Solitary
Postauricular skin, inner TM	Superior IX	Spinal nucleus of V
Proprioception (stylopharyngeus)	Superior IX	Mesencephalic nucleus of V
Motor to stylopharyngeus		Ambiguus
Parotid gland	Otic	Inferior salivatory

  C. Anatomic Facts
    1. CN IX exits the skull via the jugular foramen.
    2. CN IX supplies only one muscle, the stylopharyngeus.
    3. The nucleus ambiguus supplies motor fibers to CN IX and X.
  D. Lesions/Clinical Applications
    1. Due to its close association with CN X and XI, there is seldom an isolated lesion of CN IX.

2. The gag reflex becomes absent on the side of the lesion.
3. Glossopharyngeal neuralgia
   a. Paroxysmal and excruciating pain of sudden onset and brief duration
   b. Begins at the tongue base and radiates to the ear.
   c. Triggered by swallowing, chewing, coughing, speaking, or touching the tonsils or posterior pharynx.
   d. May be associated with pharyngeal tumor.
   e. Treat with carbamazepine, phenytoin ± surgery (sectioning the nerve).
XI. Cranial Nerve X—Vagus Nerve
   A. Function
      1. GSA—Sensation from vocal cords, external ear, external auditory canal, and external surface of tympanic membrane
      2. GVA—Visceral sensation from the larynx to the gut
      3. SVE—Motor to all striated muscles of the pharynx, larynx, and palate except stylopharyngeus (CN IX) and tensor veli palatini (CN V3)
      4. GVE—Motor to smooth muscle of the pharynx, larynx, and viscera
   B. Pathways

Function	Ganglion	Nucleus
Sensation—external ear and auditory canal, external surface of TM	Superior X (jugular)	Spinal nucleus of V
Visceral sensation	Inferior X (nodose)	Solitary
Motor to striated muscles	—	Nucleus ambiguus
Motor to smooth muscles	Intramural ganglia in wall of gut muscles: myenteric (Auerbach's) plexus and submucosal (Meissner's) plexus	Dorsal motor nucleus of X

   C. Anatomic Facts
      1. CN X exits the skull via the jugular foramen.
      2. Sensory fibers from below the vocal cords are carried by the recurrent laryngeal nerve. Sensory fibers from above the vocal cords are carried by the internal laryngeal nerve.
      3. In the neck, the vagus runs between the internal jugular vein and internal carotid artery within the carotid sheath.
   D. Lesion/Clinical Applications
      1. Unilateral CN X lesion—produces hoarseness, dysphagia, inability to elevate the soft palate on the affected side (deviation of uvula to unaffected side).
      2. Unilateral lesion of recurrent laryngeal—produces hoarseness (can occur with surgical procedures in the neck, aortic aneurysm, or metastatic disease with enlarged lymph nodes compressing the nerve).
XII. Cranial Nerve XI—Accessory
   A. Function: Motor to sternocleidomastoid and trapezius muscles—SVE
   B. Pathway
      Accessory nucleus from C1 to C5 → CN XI → ascends through the foramen magnum → exits the skull via the jugular foramen → to sternocleidomastoid and trapezius.

C. Lesions/Clinical Applications
    1. Lesions result in ipsilateral shoulder droop, scapula that is rotated down and outward, and weak head turn to the contralateral side.

XIII. Cranial Nerve XII—Hypoglossal
  A. Function
    1. GSE—Motor to tongue muscles (except palatoglossus, which is CN X). Nucleus: Hypoglossal nucleus.
    2. GSA—Prioprioception to tongue muscles (except palatoglossus). Nucleus: mesencephalic nucleus of V.
  B. Pathway
    Nucleus of CN XII in the medulla → axons exit medulla between the olive and the pyramids → CN XII → exits skull via hypoglossal foramen → to tongue muscles
  C. Lesions/Clinical Applications
    1. Upper motor neuron lesion—tongue deviates away from the lesion.
    2. Lower motor neuron lesion—tongue deviates toward side of lesion.

XIV. Cranial Nerves and Associated Foramina

Cranial Nerve	Foramen
Olfactory	Cribriform plate
Optic	Superior orbital fissure
Oculomotor	Superior orbital fissure
Trochlear	Superior orbital fissure
Trigeminal	
V1—Ophthalmic	Superior orbital fissure
V2—Maxillary	Foramen rotundum
V3—Mandibular	Foramen ovale
Abducens	Superior orbital fissure
Facial	Stylomastoid foramen
Vestibulocochlear	Acoustic meatus
Glossopharyngeal	Jugular foramen
Vagus	Jugular foramen
Accessory	Enters: Foramen magnum/Exits: Jugular foramen
Hypoglossal	Hypoglossal foramen

SPINAL CORD ANATOMY AND DISEASES

I. Epidemiology
  A. Approximately 10,000 new cases per year
  B. 200,000 quadriplegics in the United States

II. Anatomy
  A. Embryology
    1. Neural tube is formed from ectoderm during the third and fourth weeks of gestation by invagination of the neural plate.
    2. In the first-trimester fetus, the spinal cord travels the length of the vertebral column, but the column grows longer than the cord, so that in the newborn, the cord ends at the third lumbar vertebra.
    3. In the adult, the cord ends at L1 but spinal roots continue caudally as the cauda equina.

B. Spinal Tracts
  1. Dorsal columns
     a. Light touch, vibration, and proprioception
     b. Travels ipsilaterally in the cord and crosses in the medulla
  2. Spinothalamic tract (anterolateral tract)
     a. Pain and temperature
     b. Crosses immediately (or sometimes first travels up one or two segments) in the cord; therefore contralateral.
  3. Corticospinal tract
     a. Carries motor commands from the brain.
     b. Crosses in the brain stem prior to the spinal cord, so travels ipsilaterally down the cord.
     c. 80% of motor fibers decussate to lateral corticospinal tract; 20% of motor fibers continue ipsilaterally as the medial corticospinal tract.
C. Vascular Supply
  1. Vertebral arteries form one anterior spinal and two posterior spinal arteries and are responsible for the cervical cord.
  2. Segmental arteries from the aorta and internal iliac arteries supply the thoracic and lumbar cord—radicular artery of Adamkiewicz from T10 or T11 supplies nearly two-thirds of the caudal cord.
  3. Segmental branches of the lateral sacral arteries supply the sacral cord.
  4. Segmental branches join and continue as the anterior and posterior spinal arteries.
  5. Anterior spinal artery supplies the anterior two-thirds of cord.
  6. Posterior spinal arteries supply the posterior third.
  7. Vasculature is not prone to atherosclerotic disease, but it may be involved in vasculitis, traumatic emboli, and infarction from dissecting aneurysms or from surgery.
  8. Watershed injuries resulting from hypotension usually occur in the upper thoracic region.
III. Pathology
  A. Immediate
    1. Pericapillary hemorrhages coalesce and enlarge.
    2. Experimental findings: gray matter infarction followed by white matter edema in 4 hours; global infarction 8 hours later with necrosis and paralysis.
  B. Chronic
    1. Gliosis occurs in necrotic areas over months.
    2. May lead to cavitation with syrinx formation (see later section on Etiologies, Degenerative).
IV. Localization
  A. Central nervous (spinal cord) vs. peripheral nervous system
    1. Loss of sensation below a certain level means cord disease, but it can be anywhere above that level because the cord is laminated so that sensory fibers to the legs are on the outside and those to the arms are to the inside. The lower part of the body is affected first even if the lesion is high enough to affect the top, assuming the

problem is working from the outside in (cord compression). Should not get a sensory level with peripheral nervous system disease.

2. Bowel and bladder changes raise suspicion of cord disease.
3. Back pain and point spinal tenderness are the most accurate localizing findings.
4. Weakness is associated with central and peripheral nervous system diseases, but upper motor neuron signs (e.g., hyperreflexia, Babinski sign, increased muscle tone) are seen only with central nervous system disease.

B. Longitudinal Localization
　1. High C-spine
　　a. Usually associated with trauma
　　　(1) Jefferson's fracture: atlas ring burst (diving)
　　　(2) Hangman's fracture: C2 pedicle fracture with subluxation of C2 on C3
　　b. Involves quadriparesis and respiratory failure (phrenic nerve: C3, C4, C5)
　2. Low C-spine
　　a. Biceps weakness localizes to C5 and C6.
　　b. Triceps, wrist extensors, and pronator weakness localizes to C7.
　　c. Hand weakness localizes to C8 through T1.
　　d. Sensory loss over arms
　3. Thoracic spine
　　a. High thoracic spine and low C-spine have sympathetic nervous system involvement, including hypotension, bradycardia, and Horner's syndrome (miosis, ptosis, anhydrosis).
　　b. Sensory level found along the trunk
　　c. Some degree of weakness in the legs
　4. Lumbar spine
　　a. Weakness in the legs
　　b. Sensory changes in the legs and saddle area
　　c. Conus medullaris: lesion of the tip or cone of the spinal cord, giving less pain and weakness but early bowel/bladder involvement
　5. Cauda equina
　　a. Involvement of the spinal roots only with lesions below L1
　　b. Lower motor signs of flaccidity, areflexia and weakness but with bowel/bladder involvement and sensory level in saddle up to L1.

C. Transverse Localization
　1. Anterior cord syndrome
　　a. Involves the spinothalamic and corticospinal tracts, giving paresis and loss of pain below the level
　　b. Usually associated with cord compression, but also can be seen with infarction of the anterior spinal artery
　2. Central cord syndrome
　　a. Cape anesthesia with involvement of pain fibers as they cross the cord in the anterior commisure but sparing dorsal column functions
　　b. Weakness in upper extremities > lower extremities
　　c. Urinary retention

      d. Most commonly seen with neck hyperextension

  3. Posterior cord syndrome

      a. Refers mainly to dorsal columns.

      b. Occurs with vitamin B_{12} deficiency and syphilis.

  4. Brown-Séquard syndrome

      a. Consists of ipsilateral weakness and light touch, proprioceptive and vibratory sensory loss, and contralateral pain and temperature sensory loss.

      b. Occurs with lesion that affects only half of the cord transversely.

V. Etiologies

  A. Mechanical

    1. Cervical spondylosis

      a. Disease found mainly in older men

      b. Caused by a combination of disc bulge, osteophytic spurs on dorsal-vertebral bodies, partial subluxation, and hypertrophy of dorsal spinal ligaments

      c. Plain X-ray films can suggest problem if the spinal canal sagittal diameter is less than 15 mm (normal 16 to 22 in cervical/thoracic).

      d. Findings include a stiff, painful neck, radicular pain/numbness, and hyporeflexia in arms along with spastic paraparesis and ataxia.

    2. Herniated disc disease

      a. Most commonly found in L4/L5 and L5/S1; rarely in thoracic region.

      b. Findings usually include radicular pain and weakness in the legs and, less commonly, upper motor signs suggesting spinal cord involvement.

      c. If no signs of cord compression, may be treated conservatively with pain medications or later with laminectomy/discectomy if this fails.

    3. Trauma

      a. Presentations vary widely with mode and location of injury.

      b. With nonmissile modes, injury mostly with anteroflexion, retroflexion, and neck extension.

      c. Spinal shock may occur and last 1 to 2 weeks: areflexia, atonic bowel/bladder, gastric dilatation, loss of vasomotor control.

      d. Upper motor neuron signs of spasticity and hyperreflexia occur later.

      e. Reduction of compressions is critical in the first few hours to salvage function; steroids also help in the acute setting.

  B. Tumors

    1. Epidural location most common

      a. Mostly metastatic in origin: prostate, breast, or lung cancers; lymphoma and plasma cell dyscrasias

      b. Most common in the thoracic cord

      c. Pain felt first, which is worse at night and in recumbent position and increases with Valsalva maneuvers

      d. Local tenderness along spine

      e. Neural changes occur after several days to weeks.

      f. Treatment

    1. Decadron 100 mg IV, then 20 mg IV q6h

    2. Radiation therapy

3. Surgical decompression
4. Intradural extramedullary location
   a. Usually a meningioma or neurofibroma
   b. Symptoms begin with radicular sensory loss and asymmetric cord syndrome.
   3. Intradural intramedullary location very infrequent
   a. Usually gliomas
   b. Very rarely metastatic: melanoma or lung cancer
C. Epidural Abscess
   1. Associated with furunculosis of the back or scalp and minor back injury, but etiology is usually bacteremia.
   2. Pott's disease with spinal tuberculoma
   3. Nidus of osteomyelitis may be big enough to show cord compression.
   4. Presentation includes fever, mild spinal ache with local tenderness, and later radicular pain.
   5. Treatment includes laminectomy and antibiotics.
D. Inflammation
   1. Most common in the middle to low thoracic spine
   2. Etiologies include collagen/vascular diseases such as lupus; postinfectious demyelination associated with rubella, mumps, and varicella; and multiple sclerosis.
   3. *Arachnoiditis* is inflammation, scarring and fibrous thickening of the arachnoid leading to compression; may be secondary to postoperative changes or, in the past, radiographic dye with myelograms.
E. Infarction
   1. Usually not atherosclerotic, but distant vascular occlusion or aortic disease with thrombosis, dissection, or surgical clamping
   2. Sometimes with microscopic fragments of herniated nucleus pulposus
   3. Arteriovenous malformations may cause ischemia.
      a. Mostly in low thoracic or lumbar regions and in middle-aged men
      b. Fluctuating symptoms with exercise and postural changes
F. Infection
   1. Herpes zoster: radicular pain with dermatomal eruption
   2. Poliomyelitis: destroys anterior horn cells
   3. Retroviruses HTLV-1 (tropical spastic paraparesis) and HIV-1
   4. Neurosyphilis: tabes dorsalis—lancinating pains, dorsal column loss, slapping gait
G. Degenerative
   1. Amyotrophic lateral sclerosis (ALS or Lou Gehrig's disease)
   2. Primary lateral sclerosis
   3. Spinal muscular atrophy
   4. Friedreich's ataxia
   5. Syringomyelia (syrinx)
      a. Cavitation of the central spinal canal
      b. Not truly a degenerative disease, but it can be caused by trauma, tumor, compression with necrosis, or necrotic myelitis, or it can be idiopathic or developmental, as with Arnold-Chiari malformations.

      c. Typically have pain and temperature loss in a cape distribution with muscle wasting and hyporeflexia in the neck, shoulders, and arms.

  H. Metabolic: Subacute Combined Degeneration

     1. Vitamin B_{12} deficiency leading to demyelination of the posterior columns and spreading secondarily to the corticospinal tract

     2. Some peripheral nerve involvement may also occur.

     3. Signs and symptoms include paresthesias, loss of vibratory and position sensation, and weakness and spasticity of the legs.

VI. Management

  A. Acute management as stated earlier usually consists of steroids and decompression emergently if applicable.

  B. Very difficult to reverse damage once it is more than a few hours old

  C. Chronic management is centered around problems developed secondary to immobility.

     1. Decubitus ulcer prevention requires frequent changes in position if patient is immobile.

     2. Subcutaneous heparin may be necessary to prevent deep venous thrombosis and pulmonary emboli.

     3. Gastrointestinal ileus and ulcers are common.

     4. Good bladder hygiene required (frequent Foley changes or in-out catheters) to prevent urinary retention from developing into urinary tract infections.

THE PLEXI AND EXTREMITIES

I. Brachial Plexus (Fig. 10)

  A. Comprised of the anterior primary rami of C5, C6, C7, C8, and T1

  B. Components

     1. Undivided primary rami

     2. Trunks (upper, middle, and lower)

     3. Divisions of the trunks (anterior and posterior)

     4. Cords (lateral, posterior, and medial)

  C. Trunks

     1. Upper—composed of C5, C6, and sometimes C4

     2. Middle—composed of C7

     3. Lower—C8, T1, and sometimes T2

  D. Divisions—fibers reaching the ventral arm travel in the anterior division, and fibers reaching the dorsal arm travel in the posterior division.

  E. Cords

     1. Lateral—derived from the anterior divisions of the upper and middle trunks. It divides into the musculocutaneous nerve and lateral head of the median nerve.

     2. Medial—derived from the anterior division of the lower trunk. It divides into the ulnar nerve, medial cutaneous nerve of the forearm, and the medial head of the median nerve.

     3. Posterior—derived from the posterior divisions of all three trunks. It divides into the axillary, radial, thoracodorsal, and subscapular nerves.

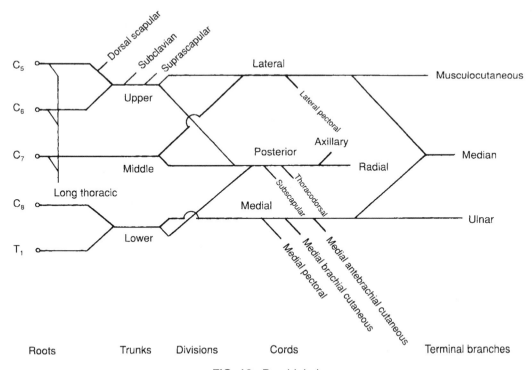

FIG. 10. Brachial plexus.

F. Pre- and Post-fixed Plexus
  1. A pre-fixed plexus is one in which all components are shifted up one spinal level (composed of C4 through C8).
  2. A post-fixed plexus is one in which all components are shifted down one spinal level (composed of C6 through T2).
G. Martin-Gruber Anastomosis
  1. Occurs in 15% to 30% of population
  2. Is a communicating branch from median to ulnar nerve in forearm
  3. Supplies first dorsal interosseous, adductor pollicis, abductor digiti minimi
H. Lesions
  1. Brachial plexus neuritis/Parsonage-Turner syndrome/neuralgic amyotrophy
    a. Etiology: Postinfectious neuritis
    b. S/S: Local pain, weakness, and atrophy of affected muscles
    c. Lab: CSF normal
    d. Course: Partial-to-complete resolution
  2. Erb-Duchenne syndrome/upper radicular syndrome
    a. Location: Lesion of C4, C5, C6, or upper trunk
    b. Etiology: Blow to neck or birth injury

       c. S/S: Waiter's tip arm position

       d. Course: Loss of arm abduction, elbow flexion, supination, lateral arm rotate

   3. Middle radicular syndrome

       a. Etiology: Lesion of C7 or middle trunk

       b. S/S: Loss of radially innervated muscles except brachioradialis and part of triceps. Crutch paralysis

   4. Klumpke syndrome/lower radicular syndrome

       a. Location: Lesion of C8 and T1 (appears to be combined median and ulnar palsy)

       b. Etiology: Occurs after sudden pull of arm or during delivery

       c. S/S: Paralysis of thenar muscles and flexors. Flattened simian hand.

II. Peripheral Nerves of the Upper Extremity

  A. Long Thoracic Nerve

    1. Roots: C5, C6, and C7

    2. Innervates: Serratus anterior

    3. Lesion: Winged scapula

  B. Pectoral Nerves (Anterior Thoracic Nerves)

    1. Medial Pectoral Nerve

      a. Roots: C8 and T1

      b. Innervates: Pectoralis minor and inferior portion of pectoralis major

    2. Lateral Pectoral Nerve

      a. Roots: C5, C6, and C7

      b. Innervates: Pectoralis major

  C. Dorsal Scapular Nerve

    1. Roots: C5

    2. Innervates: Levator scapulae, rhomboid major, and rhomboid minor

  D. Subclavian Nerve

    1. Roots: C5 and C6

    2. Innervates: Subclavius muscle

  E. Suprascapular Nerve

    1. Roots: C5 and C6. Branch of the upper trunk

    2. Innervates: Supraspinatus and infraspinatus

    3. Lesions: Suprascapular-abduction of arm weakness; infraspinatus-external rotation of arm weakness

  F. Thoracodorsal Nerve

    1. Roots: C6, C7, and C8

    2. Innervates: Latissimus dorsi

  G. Subscapular Nerve

    1. Roots: C5 and C6

    2. Innervates: Subscapular and teres major muscles

  H. Axillary Nerve

    1. Roots: C5 and C6

    2. Innervates: Deltoid and teres minor

    3. Lesion: Deltoid weakness and hyperesthesia of lateral shoulder

I. Musculocutaneous Nerve
   1. Roots: C5, C6, and C7
   2. Innervates: Biceps, brachialis, and coracobrachialis
   3. Lesion: Weakness of arm flexion while supinated
J. Median Nerve
   1. Roots: C6 through T1 and portions from all three trunks
   2. Median nerve proper innervates:
      a. Pronator teres
      b. Flexor carpi radialis
      c. Flexor digitorum sublimis
      d. Palmaris longus
      e. Flexor pollicis longus
      f. Flexor digitorum profundus
      g. Abductor pollicis brevis
      h. Opponens pollicis
      i. Flexor pollicis brevis
      j. First and second lumbricals
   3. Anterior interosseous nerve innervates:
      a. Flexor pollicis longus
      b. Flexor digitorum profundus (I, II)
      c. Pronator quadratus
   4. Lesions
      a. Carpal tunnel syndrome
         (1) Epidemiology: Age 40 to 60 years; three times more common in women.
         (2) Etiologies
            (a) Reduced space in the carpal tunnel
               i. Rheumatoid arthritis
               ii. Ganglia cysts
               iii. Exostoses
               iv. Osteophytes
               v. Gout
               vi. Anomalous muscles and tendons
               vii. Congenital tunnel stenosis
            (b) Increased pressure sensitivity
               i. Diabetes mellitus
               ii. Hereditary pressure palsy neuropathy
               iii. Associated cervical radiculopathy
            (c) Miscellaneous
               i. Pregnancy/Lactation
               ii. Hypothyroidism or hyperthyroidism
               iii. Acromegaly
               iv. Amyloidosis
               v. Multiple myeloma
               vi. Chronic renal failure

                vii. Familial carpal tunnel syndrome

              viii. Work-related

                ix. Vitamin B$_6$ deficiency

          (d) Idiopathic

      (3) Symptoms

          (a) Pain and numbness in wrist, hand, thumb, first and second fingers

          (b) Symptoms occur most frequently during sleep.

      (4) Signs

          (a) Tinel's—tingling with wrist percussion

          (b) Phalen's—tingling with wrist flexion

          (c) Thenar atrophy

          (d) Palmar sensory loss in median distribution

          (e) Decreased thumb abduction and opposition

          (f) "Hand of Papal Benediction"

   b. Pronator teres syndrome

      (1) Etiology: Compression of the median nerve by the pronator teres

      (2) Symptom: Pain in anterior forearm worse with exertion and pronation

      (3) Signs: Tinel's positive over pronator teres; mild motor deficit

   c. Anterior interosseous syndrome

 1. Etiology: Anterior interosseous nerve compression by a fibrous sheath

 2. Symptoms: Pain in forearm

 3. Signs: Weakness in flexor pollicis longus, and half of flexor digitorum profundus

K. Ulnar Nerve

   1. Roots: C8 and T1; lower trunk

   2. Innervates:

      a. Flexor carpi ulnaris

      b. Flexor digitorum profundus (III, IV)

      c. Adductor pollicis

      d. Interossei

      e. Third and fourth lumbricals

      f. Flexor pollicis brevis (deep head)

      g. Palmaris brevis

      h. Abductor digiti quinti

      i. Opponens digiti quinti

      j. Flexor digiti quinti

   3. Lesions

      a. Compression at the elbow (ulnar groove or cubital tunnel)

          (1) Loss of wrist flexion and adduction

          (2) Loss of flexion of the third and fourth digits

          (3) Loss of hypothenar (opposition and abduction)

          (4) Loss of thumb adduction

          (5) Loss of finger abduction and adduction

          (6) Atrophy of hypothenar and interosseous muscles

          (7) Sensory loss in the lateral half of the third finger and the fourth finger

        (8) Clawing of the hand
- b. Compression at Guyon's canal: same as compression at the elbow
- c. Physical examination technique: Froment's sign—flexion of thumb to compensate for weak adduction

L. Radial Nerve
1. Roots: C5 to C8; posterior divisions and posterior cord
2. Radial nerve proper innervates:
   - a. Triceps
   - b. Anconeus
   - c. Brachioradialis
   - d. Extensor carpi radialis longus
3. Posterior interosseous nerve (the terminal branch) innervates:
   - a. Extensor carpi radialis brevis
   - b. Supinator
   - c. Extensor digitorum
   - d. Extensor digiti quinti
   - e. Extensor carpi ulnaris
   - f. Abductor pollicis longus
   - g. Extensor pollicis longus
   - h. Extensor pollicis brevis
   - i. Extensor indicis
4. Lesions
   - a. Radial groove compression (Saturday night palsy) signs
     - (1) Weak flexion of forearm (brachioradialis)
     - (2) Wrist/finger drop
     - (3) Preserved finger extension at distal joints
     - (4) Loss of supination
     - (5) Loss of hand adduction
     - (6) Loss of thumb abduction
     - (7) Sensory loss over back of hand, thumb, and the first and second digits
   - b. Axillary compression signs—same as for radial groove compression plus triceps weakness
   - c. Posterior interosseous syndrome/Supinator syndrome signs
     - (1) No sensory loss
     - (2) Finger drop
     - (3) Loss of thumb extension

Muscle—Nerve Relationships in Upper Extremity

Segment	Muscle	Nerve
C5–C6	Biceps brachii	Musculocutaneous
C5–C6	Brachialis	Musculocutaneous and radial
C5–C6	Brachioradialis	Radial
C5–C6	Coracobrachialis	Musculocutaneous
C5–C6	Deltoid	Axillary
C5–C6	Infraspinatus	Suprascapular
C5–C6	Subscapularis	Upper and lower subscapular
C5–C6	Supraspinatus	Suprascapular
C5–C6	Teres major	Lower subscapular
C5–C6	Teres minor	Axillary
C6–C7	Abductor pollicis longus	Deep radial
C6–C7	Extensor carpi radialis brevis	Deep radial
C6–C7	Extensor carpi radialis longus	Radial
C6–C7	Extensor pollicis brevis	Deep radial
C6–C7	Flexor carpi radialis	Median
C6–C7	Palmaris longus	Median
C6–C7	Pronator teres	Median
C6–C7	Supinator	Deep radial
C6–C7	Extensor carpi ulnaris	Deep radial
C6–C7	Extensor digitorum	Deep radial
C6–C7	Extensor indicis	Deep radial
C6–C7	Extensor pollicis longus	Deep radial
C6–C7	Triceps brachii	Radial
C7–C8	Anconeus	Radial
C7–C8	Extensor digiti minimi	Deep radial
C7–C8	Flexor digitorum profundus	Median and ulnar
C7–C8	Flexor digitorum superficialis	Median
C8–T1	Abductor digiti minimi	Deep ulnar
C8–T1	Abductor pollicis brevis	Median
C8–T1	Adductor pollicis	Deep ulnar
C8–T1	Flexor carpi ulnaris	Ulnar
C8–T1	Flexor digiti minimi	Deep ulnar
C8–T1	Flexor pollicis brevis	Median
C8–T1	Flexor pollicis longus	Median
C8–T1	Interossei	Deep ulnar
C8–T1	Lumbricales	Deep ulnar and median
C8–T1	Opponens digiti minimi	Deep ulnar
C8–T1	Opponens pollicis	Median
C8–T1	Palmaris brevis	Superficial ulnar
C8–T1	Pronator quadratus	Median

III. Peripheral Nerves of the Lower Extremity (Fig. 11 and Fig. 12)
    A. Iliohypogastric Nerve
        1. Roots: T12, L1
        2. Innervates: Skin on buttocks and above pubis
    B. Ilioinguinal Nerve
        1. Roots: T12, L1
        2. Innervates: Skin over mons pubis and root of penis
    C. Genitofemoral Nerve

        1. Roots: L1, L2
        2. Innervates: Cremaster
  D. Lateral Femoral Cutaneous Nerve of the Thigh
        1. Roots: L2, L3
        2. Innervates: Skin of the lateral thigh
        3. Lesions
           a. Meralgia paresthetica
             (1) Entrapment of the nerve, resulting in burning paresthesias
             (2) Worsened by obesity, prolonged walking
  E. Obturator
        1. Roots: L2, L3, L4
        2. Innervates
           a. Hip adductors—obturator, gracilis
           b. Skin on medial thigh
        3. Lesions: Injured by fetal head or forceps
  F. Femoral Nerve
        1. Roots: L2, L3, L4
        2. Innervates:
           a. Hip flexors—iliopsoas, sartorius, pectineus
           b. Knee extensors—rectus femoris, vastus (LIM)
           c. Anterior cutaneous nerve of the thigh
           d. Saphenous—skin on medial leg below knee
        3. Lesions
           a. Weak psoas only if femoral nerve injured in the pelvis
           b. Differentiate femoral neuropathy from plexopathy by testing hip adduction.
           c. Differential Diagnosis
             (1) Diabetes
             (2) Tumor
             (3) Surgery
             (4) Trauma
             (5) Polyarteritis nodosa
  G. Superior Gluteal Nerve
        1. Roots: L4, L5, S1
        2. Innervates: Gluteus minimus, gluteus medius
  H. Inferior Gluteal Nerve
        1. Roots: L4, L5, S1, S2
        2. Innervates: Gluteus maximus
  I. Sciatic Nerve
        1. Roots: L4, L5, S1, S2, S3
        2. Innervates:
           a. Knee flexors—biceps femoris, semimembranosis, semitendinosis
           b. Tibial (plantar flexes and inverts)
             (1) Plantar flexors-gastrocnemius, soleus, flexor hallucis longus, flexor digitorum

           (2) Sural—skin on lateral calf ankle and foot
           (3) Foot invertor—posterior tibialis
       c. Common peroneal
           (1) Deep peroneal
               (a) Dorsiflexors—anterior tibialis, extensor hallucis, extensor digitorum
               (b) Skin in the web of the big toe
           (2) Superficial peroneal
               (a) Foot evertors—peroneus longus and brevis
               (b) Skin on the top of the foot
           (3) Cutaneous branch
               (a) Skin on the lateral lower leg
    3. Lesions: Differentiate common peroneal from deep peroneal injuries by foot eversion
  J. Posterior Femoral Cutaneous Nerve (Fig. 13)
    1. Roots: S1, S2, S3
    2. Innervates: Skin on the posterior thigh
  K. Pudendal
    1. Roots: S2, S3, S4
    2. Inferior rectal innervates:
      a. External anal sphincter
      b. S4
    3. Dorsal nerve of the penis/clitoris
    4. Perineal innervates: Scrotum/labia
  L. Sympathetics T1 through L2
  M. Parasympathetics S2 through S4

Summary of Muscle—Nerve Relationships in the Lower Extremity

Segment	Muscle	Nerve
L2–L3	Adductor brevis	Obturator
L2–L3	Adductor longus	Obturator
L2–L3	Gracilis	Obturator
L2–L3	Sartorius	Femoral
L2–L4	Iliacus	Femoral
L2–L4	Psoas	Femoral (nerve to psoas)
L3–L4	Obturator externus	Obturator
L3–L4	Pectineus	Femoral
L3–L4	Quadriceps femoris	Femoral
L3–S1	Adductor magnus	Obturator and sciatic
L4–L5	Tibialis anterior	Deep peroneal
L4–S1	Gluteus medius	Superior gluteal
L4–S1	Gluteus minimus	Superior gluteal
L4–S1	Inferior gemellus	Nerve to quadratus femoris
L4–S1	Lumbricales	Medial and lateral plantar
L4–S1	Plantaris	Tibial
L4–S1	Popliteus	Tibial
L4–S1	Quadratus femoris	Nerve to quadratus femoris
L4–S1	Tensor fascia lata	Superior gluteal
L4–S2	Biceps femoris	Sciatic
L4–S2	Semimembranosis	Sciatic
L4–S2	Semitendinosis	Sciatic
L5–S1	Extensor digitorum longus	Deep peroneal
L5–S1	Extensor hallucis longus	Deep peroneal
L5–S1	Peroneus brevis	Superficial peroneal
L5–S1	Peroneus longus	Peroneal
L5–S1	Tibialis posterior	Tibial
L5–S2	Gluteus maximus	Inferior gluteal
L5–S2	Obturator internus	Nerve to obturator internus
L5–S2	Soleus	Tibial
L5–S2	Superior gemellus	Nerve to obturator internus
L5–S2	Biceps femoris	Sciatic
S1–S2	Abductor digiti minimus	Lateral plantar
S1–S2	Abductor hallucis	Medial plantar
S1–S2	Adductor hallucis	Lateral plantar
S1–S2	Extensor digitorum brevis	Deep peroneal
S1–S2	Extensor hallucis brevis	Deep peroneal
S1–S2	Flexor digiti minimi	Lateral plantar
S1–S2	Flexor digitorum brevis	Medial plantar
S1–S2	Flexor digitorum longus	Tibial
S1–S2	Flexor hallucis brevis	Medial plantar
S1–S2	Flexor hallucis longus	Tibial
S1–S2	Gastrocnemius	Tibial
S1–S2	Interossei	Lateral plantar
S1–S2	Piriformis	Nerve to piriformis
S1–S2	Quadratus plantae	Lateral plantar

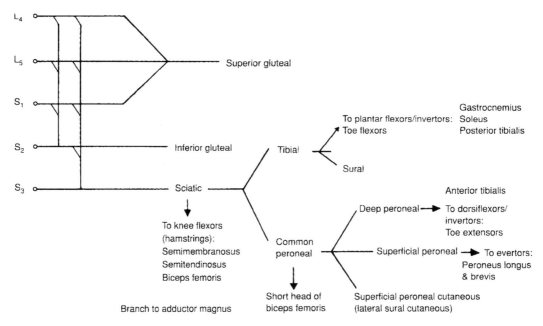

FIG. 11. Lumbosacral plexus.

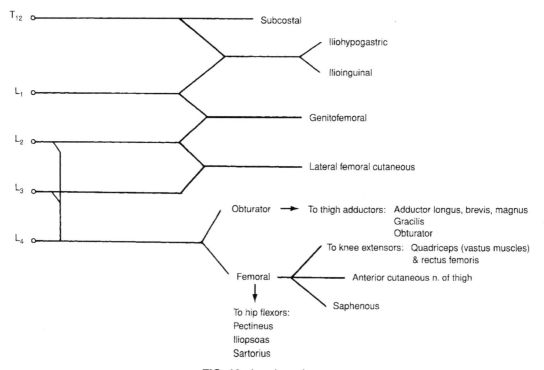

FIG. 12. Lumbar plexus.

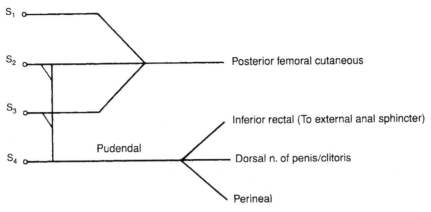

FIG. 13. Sacral plexus.

IV. Bladder
    A. Micturition
        1. Micturition center in pons
        2. Sympathetic innervation T11 through L2
        3. Inhibit detrusor
        4. Activate trigone
    B. Continence
        1. Parasympathetics S2 through S4
           a. Activates detrusor
        2. S2 through S4 voluntary
           a. External urinary sphincter
    C. Treatment
        1. Detrusor areflexia
           a. Intermittent catheterization
           b. Crede method
           c. In-dwelling Foley
           d. Urinary diversion
        2. Detrusor Hyperreflexia
           a. Anticholinergics
           b. Intermittent catheterization
           c. Biofeedback
           d. Electrical stimulation
           e. Augmentation cystoplasty
           f. Denervation procedures
        3. Dyssynergia
           a. Baclofen
        4. Failure to empty
           a. Alpha blockers

5. Failure to store (neurogenic)
   a. Anticholinergics
      Note: Use urodynamics only if absolutely necessary since the testing is extremely uncomfortable.

MUSCLE

I. Anatomy
   A. Muscle Fiber
      1. Muscle is composed of numerous fibers, each consisting of a single cell.
      2. *Sarcolemma*—the cell membrane of the muscle cell. Has an outer polysaccharide coat covered with collagen fibers. This outer surface fuses with tendon fibers at the end of the fiber.
      3. *Sarcoplasm*—muscle cell cytoplasm.
      4. *Sarcoplasmic reticulum*—specialized endoplasmic reticulum in muscle cell.
   B. Myofibrils
      1. Each muscle cell (fiber) contains several hundred to several thousand cylindrical structures called *myofibrils*. These are the contractile units of the cell.
      2. Each myofibril is composed of units called *sarcomeres* strung end-to-end.
         a. Sarcomeres are bounded on each end by proteinaceous disks called *Z-discs*.
         b. Attached to each Z-disc are thin filaments composed mainly of actin.
         c. In between actin filaments are thick filaments composed mainly of myosin.
         d. Each sarcomere contains approximately 1,500 myosin and 3,000 actin filaments.
         e. When viewed under a light microscope, the overlapping actin and myosin filaments result in a series of light and dark bands. These include the I-bands (light, contain only actin), A-bands (dark, contain myosin and overlapping actin), and the H-zone (a light band appearing in the center of the A-band whenever muscle is stretched beyond its resting length).
      3. Each myofibril is enveloped by the sarcoplasmic reticulum, which forms a flattened, sacklike structure surrounding the myofibril.
      4. Tiny invaginations of the sarcolemma called *T-tubules* also interweave among the myofibrils. T-tubules communicate directly with the extracellular space.
   C. Myofilaments
      1. Thin filaments
         a. Composed mainly of actin units polymerized into long chains and woven into a double helix.
         b. *Tropomyosin* is a long filamentous protein that winds around the actin helix, lying in the groove between the two strands.
         c. *Troponin* forms small molecular complexes that are attached to the tropomyosin filament at discrete intervals.
      2. Thick filaments
         a. Thick filaments are made up of about 250 myosin molecules.
         b. Each myosin molecule has two entwined tails and two globular heads. The heads contain an ATPase (hydrolyzing ATP to ADP + Pi).

II. Muscle Contraction

Until the 1950s, muscle contraction was thought to arise from contraction of an individual muscle protein. In 1954, however, the *sliding filament theory* was proposed, stating that muscle contraction is the result of thick and thin filaments sliding over each other, resulting in shortening of the sarcomere.

  A. The Action Potential

    1. ACh from the neuromuscular junction binds to muscle receptors and generates an action potential within the muscle membrane.

    2. The action potential spreads throughout the muscle fiber via the T-tubules. The T-tubule system ensures that all sarcomeres contract nearly simultaneously, so that the shortening of activated sarcomeres is not canceled out by the lengthening of slack sarcomeres.

  B. Role of Calcium

    1. The depolarization of the T-tubule activates voltage-gated channels within the sarcoplasmic reticulum, triggering the release of calcium. Calcium is normally stored within the sarcoplasmic reticulum at concentrations much higher than in the surrounding cytoplasm.

    2. Calcium binds to troponin, producing a conformational change in the actin molecule that exposes a receptor site for the myosin head.

  C. Sliding Mechanism

    1. The myosin head spontaneously binds to the exposed actin site. Adjacent sites on the myosin head bind to a series of adjacent sites on the actin molecule, resulting in rotation of the myosin head.

    2. This rotation pulls the actin filament toward the center of the sarcomere, causing the sarcomere to shorten.

    3. After the myosin head has rotated, the ATPase contained within it hydrolyzes an ATP to ADP. The energy from this reaction dissociates the myosin head from the actin filament, and "cocks" it, restoring it to its original position.

    4. This process of attachment, rotation, and detachment repeats several times, resulting in shortening of the sarcomere and contraction of the muscle.

  D. Relaxation

    1. When depolarization ends, Ca^{++} is pumped back into the sarcoplasmic reticulum, and troponin covers the actin-binding sites.

    2. Myosin can no longer form cross bridges, and the sarcomere returns to its resting length.

III. Energy Sources for Muscle Contraction

  A. ATP can sustain contraction for only a few seconds before intracellular stores are depleted.

  B. Phosphocreatinine also carries a high-energy phosphate bond, which can be used to regenerate ATP. This still only allows a few seconds of contraction.

  C. Glycolysis can supply energy via the breakdown of glucose. Muscles may use either the anaerobic pathway (quick but builds up lactic acid) or the oxidative pathway (slow but can produce low-level contractions for several hours).

IV. Muscle Fiber Types

Muscle fibers are classified into two (or three, depending on nomenclature) types, based on their speed of twitch and metabolic capability.

    A. Fast Fibers (Type II)
        1. Larger cross-sectional areas capable of generating 10 times the strength of slow fibers
        2. Extensive sarcoplasmic reticulum for more rapid calcium release
        3. Large amounts of glycolytic enzymes for rapid release of energy
        4. Less extensive blood supply, since they rely on anaerobic metabolism
        5. Fatigues quickly (on the order of minutes)
        6. Stains dark with alkaline ATPase
    B. Slow Fibers (Type I)
    (Remember IRS-type I, Red, Slow)
        1. Smaller
        2. More extensive vascular supply
        3. Large amounts of mitochondria since they rely on oxidative metabolism
        4. Large amounts of myoglobin (an iron-containing protein within muscle that binds oxygen and stores it until needed)
        5. Fatigues slowly (on the order of hours).
        6. Stains dark with acid ATPase or NADH.
    C. Fast, Fatigue-Resistant Fibers—those with properties that fall between those of the other two fiber types.
  V. Motor Units and Control of Muscle Contraction
    A. A motor neuron, along with all the muscle fibers it innervates, is called a *motor unit*.
    B. Motor units contain varying numbers of muscle fibers, from 10 (extraocular muscles) to 100 (hand muscles) to 2,000 (gastrocnemius). The fewer fibers there are per motor unit, the finer control the CNS has over the muscle.
    C. While each motor neuron may innervate several muscle fibers, each muscle fiber is innervated by only one motor neuron.
    D. Muscle fibers within a single motor unit are all of the same type (i.e., fast or slow). However, muscles are composed of varying mixtures of fast and slow motor units. Eye muscles, for example, are predominately fast, whereas the gastroc is predominately slow.
    E. The CNS controls the amount of contraction via two mechanisms.
        1. Recruitment—the smallest motor neurons are easiest to depolarize and therefore are recruited first. As corticospinal input increases, progressively larger motor neurons are recruited. This is called the *size principle*.
        2. Firing rate—increasing the frequency with which motor units fire results in increased force of contraction secondary to summation of twitches. However, frequency range is limited, from 8 to 25 Hz. Muscles are rarely pushed to tetanus under physiologic conditions.
 VI. Muscle Spindles
  Muscles are endowed with two types of receptors important for motor control. *Muscle spindles* detect changes in muscle length, and the *Golgi tendon organ* (discussed in the next section) measures force.
    A. Anatomy
        1. Muscle spindles are encapsulated structures, ranging from 4 to 10 mm in length. Each spindle has three main components—specialized muscle fibers (called *intra-*

fusal to differentiate them from ordinary muscle fibers, which are called *extra-fusal*), sensory axons that terminate on the muscle fibers, and motor axons that regulate the sensitivity of the spindle. The spindle capsule is thick at the center, tapered at the ends, and filled with gelatinous fluid. The ends of the capsule are attached to the surrounding, much larger, extrafusal fibers, such that when extrafusal fibers stretch, the spindle is stretched, and when they contract, the spindle is shortened. In other words, the spindle is attached *in parallel*.

2. Intrafusal fibers have a noncontractile center with contractile poles at each end. There are three types of intrafusal fibers, each with different sensitivities.
    a. Nuclear chain fibers—slender with nuclei lined up single file.
    b. Nuclear bag fibers—central bulge, with nuclei all clustered in the middle. There are two types of nuclear bag fibers, static and dynamic. Each muscle spindle typically contains two bag fibers—one of each type—and about five chain fibers.
3. Spindle innervation
    a. Sensory—The primary sensory ending consists of a group IA axon, which terminates on all three types of intrafusal fibers, spiraling around the central region. There is also a secondary sensory ending that consists of a group II afferent terminating only on the chain and static bag fibers.
    b. Motor—Gamma motor neuron axons innervate the contractile poles and regulate spindle sensitivity.

B. Function

Recall muscle spindles basically detect changes in muscle length. They can also detect the rate of change in length (i.e., velocity).

1. Stretching of the muscle spindle lengthens the central region of intrafusal muscle fibers. This elongates afferent endings, activating stretch-sensitive channels that depolarize the membrane and generate action potentials. The rate of firing is proportional to the amount of stretch.
    a. Primary sensory endings are highly sensitive to the rate of change in muscle length as well as to the absolute length. They are thus ideal for detecting transient length changes, such as those induced by tendon tap.
    b. Secondary sensory endings are less sensitive to dynamic changes and primarily respond to static length. Thus quick transient inputs, such as tendon tap, have little effect on secondary endings.
2. Regulation of spindle sensitivity with gamma motor neuron
    a. Imagine a muscle contracts and shortens. The intrafusal muscle fibers contained within that muscle also shorten to the point that they buckle. In this position, they are unable to detect muscle stretch, because changes in muscle length do not cause any changes in the length of the central region of the collapsed fiber.
    b. The CNS accounts for this problem using the gamma motor neurons. When these neurons fire, the contractile poles of the muscle spindles shorten, taking up the slack in the spindle. Thus the spindle is once again sensitive to any changes in muscle length.

        c. Gamma motor neurons can also regulate the sensitivity of the spindles by applying a "pre-stretch" on the central region, so that further muscle stretch will result in a higher than usual sensory neuron output.

        d. Gamma motor neurons are usually activated by higher centers simultaneously with the alpha motor neurons going to the larger extrafusal fibers. They can also be activated independently, depending on the level of control required by a particular motor task.

VII. The Stretch Reflex

  A. This is a monosynaptic reflex arc used by the CNS to regulate muscle tone, by neurologists to facilitate diagnosis, and by us to carry large, imposing-looking hammers. The afferent limb consists of muscle spindles and IA axons, and the efferent limb consists of alpha motor neurons plus the associated muscle.

  B. Banging on a tendon with a hammer results in a transient stretch being applied to the muscle fibers. Muscle spindles (especially primary endings) detect this stretch and send a signal via the IA axon to the spinal cord.

  C. The IA axon terminus synapses directly on alpha motor neurons belonging to that particular muscle. These in turn send a signal to the muscle to contract. There is also reciprocal inhibition of the antagonist muscle, via an inhibitory interneuron in the spinal cord.

  D. While stretch reflexes are modulated by input from higher centers, they are not dependent on them. Thus stretch reflexes may be present even in brain death.

VIII. Golgi Tendon Organs (GTOs)

  A. Anatomy

    1. Slender encapsulated structures about 1 mm long and 0.1 mm in diameter. They are typically located at the junction of muscle and tendon and contain a meshwork of collagen fibers intertwined with the endings of an IB afferent.

    2. The GTO is in series with the muscle (in contrast with the muscle spindle, which is in parallel).

  B. Function

    1. Contraction of the muscle results in stretching of the GTO, which in turn stretches the IB afferent endings. These depolarize, resulting in an action potential.

    2. Passive muscle stretch causes little IB firing, but active muscle contraction generates significant amounts. This implies that GTOs are sensitive to muscle force, rather than muscle length.

    3. The IB afferent synapses on an inhibitory interneuron in the spinal cord, which in turn synapses on the alpha motor neuron belonging to the particular muscle. Stimulation of the GTO (e.g., muscle contraction) therefore results in inhibition of the muscle. The GTO is thought to serve a protective role, preventing dangerous levels of tension in the muscle. One example: the clasp knife response in spasticity.

3

Pharmacology

NEUROTRANSMITTERS AND RECEPTORS

I. Acetylcholine
  A. Synthesis: occurs in the nerve terminal.

$$\text{Choline} + \text{AcetylCoA} \xrightarrow{\text{Choline Acetyl Transferase}} \text{Acetylcholine}$$

  This is the rate-limiting step in production of acetylcholine (ACh).
  The supply of choline is the rate-limiting factor in production.
  B. Release: Voltage-dependent Ca channels open with depolarization causing an influx of Ca.
  This results in fusion of the synaptic vesicles and release of neurotransmitter.
  C. Degradation: Occurs in the synaptic cleft.

$$\text{Acetylcholine} \xrightarrow{\text{Acetylcholinesterase}} \text{Choline} + \text{Acetate}$$

  D. Reuptake: Choline is recycled by the presynaptic terminal.
  E. Receptors
     1. Muscarinic (M) receptors (in brain, muscarinic > nicotinic)
        a. All subtypes linked to G-proteins
        b. M 1,3,5 activate phosphytidyl inositide hydroxylase.
        c. M 2,4 inhibits adenyl cyclase.
        d. Muscarinic agonists (cholinergic, parasympathomimetic)
           (1) Bethanechol—bladder (not degraded by esterase), carbechol—gut
           (2) Pilocarpine—eye
           (3) Methacholine
        e. Muscarinic antagonists (anticholinergic)
           (1) Atropine, scopolamine, tricyclic antidepressants
           (2) Pupils dilate, tachycardia, reduced secretions, decreased sweating, increased intraocular pressure.
           (3) May help control tremor and rigidity in Parkinson's disease.
     2. Nicotinic receptors (N1 through N4)
        a. Neuromuscular junction (NMJ) and nerve receptors differ in pharmacology.
        b. Nicotinic antagonists

          (1) Tubocurare—competitive blocker at NMJ causes hypotension by blocking autonomics.

          (2) Succinylcholine—depolarizing blocker

          (3) Atracurium—short half-life at *in vivo* pH

F. Central Nervous System (CNS) Sources

    1. Nucleus basalis of Meynert

    2. Diagonal band of Broca

    3. Caudate

G. Locations

    1. Nicotinic and muscarinic

       a. All preganglionic synapses (sympathetic and parasympathetic)

       b. CNS (M > N)

    2. Muscarinic

       a. All postganglionic parasympathetic

       b. Postganglionic sympathetic at sweat glands. (The rest of the postganglionic sympathetic synapses use epinephrine and/or norepinephrine.)

    3. Nicotinic

       a. NMJ

       b. Adrenal medulla

H. Disease States

    1. Acetylcholine Deficiency

       a. NMJ release blockade (presynaptic disorders)

          (1) Botulinum toxin—blocks presynaptic vesicle mobility.

          (2) Lambert-Eaton syndrome—blocks presynaptic calcium channels.

          (3) Tick paralysis

          (4) Sea snake toxin

       b. NMJ receptor blockade (postsynaptic disorders)

          (1) Myasthenia gravis—ACh receptor antibodies

          (2) Depolarizing blockade—succinylcholine

          (3) Nondepolarizing blockade—curare, procainamide, aminoglycosides

          (4) Alpha bungarotoxin—irreversible ACh receptor blockade

       c. Alzheimer's disease

          (1) Degradation of ACh nuclei in nucleus nasalis

          (2) Basal forebrain atrophy

    2. Acetylcholine Excess

       a. Anticholinesterases (acetylcholinesterase inhibitors)

          (1) Prevent breakdown of ACh at the synaptic cleft and increase amount of ACh available in the cleft. Some examples:

             (a) Pyridostigmine (mestinon)—used in myasthenia gravis

             (b) Physostigmine

             (c) Edrophonium (tensilon)

             (d) Tacrine, donepezil—used in Alzheimer's disease

             (e) Organophosphates, diiopropyl fluorophosphate, sarin, soman—irreversible

      b. Black widow spider venom
        (1) Causes explosive release of ACh
      c. Beta bungarotoxin
        (1) Promotes release of ACh

II. Norepinephrine (NE)
  A. Synthesis

$$\text{L-Tyrosine} \xrightarrow[\text{Hydroxy}]{\text{Tyrosine}} \text{L-DOPA} \xrightarrow[\text{Decarboxy}]{\text{LAA}} \text{Dopamine} \xrightarrow[\text{Hydroxy}]{\text{Beta}} \text{NE}$$

    1. Rate-limiting step is mediated by tyrosine hydroxylase.
    2. NE is a feedback inhibitor of tyrosine hydroxylase.
    3. L-aromatic amino acid (LAA) decarboxylase requires a vitamin B6 cofactor.
    4. Dopamine beta hydroxylase is a copper-containing enzyme and requires oxygen and vitamin C as cofactors.
    5. NE is converted to epinephrine by phenylethanolamine-N-methyl transferase in the adrenal medulla only.

  B. Storage
    1. Dopamine (DA) and NE are transported into the vesicles by a magnesium (Mg) and ATP-dependent process.
    2. Transport into vesicles is inhibited by reserpine and tetrabenazine.
    3. Oxidation of dopamine to NE occurs in the vesicles.
    4. NE is displaced from the vesicles by amphetamines and ephedrine.

  C. Release
    1. Vesicles are released after depolarization results in calcium influx.
    2. Catecholamines in the synaptic cleft then inhibit further vesicle release.
    3. Amphetamines increase release.

  D. Metabolism
    Metabolism of catecholamines occurs more slowly than does ACh metabolism.
    Catechol-O-methyl transferase (COMT) and monoamine oxidase (MAO) are the two major enzymes in catecholamine metabolism.

$$\text{NE} \xrightarrow{\text{COMT}} \text{NM} \xrightarrow{\text{MAO}} \text{MHPG} \xrightarrow[\text{Transferase}]{\text{Sulfo}} \text{MHPG-s}$$

    1. MAO
      a. Found on the outer surface of presynaptic mitochondria and on the postsynaptic cell membrane. MAOb is found primarily in the CNS.
      b. MAOa is blocked by clorgyline and pargyline.
      c. MAOb is blocked by selegiline and pargyline.
    2. COMT
      a. Found only on the postsynaptic cell membrane
      b. COMT is blocked by tropolone.

  E. Reuptake

  1. Reuptake is the primary mode of NE termination.

  2. Reuptake is mediated by Na/ATP channel.

  3. Reuptake is inhibited by cocaine, nortriptyline, amitriptyline, imipramine, and desipramine.

 F. Receptors

  1. All receptors work via G—proteins.

  2. Alpha-1 is most sensitive to epinephrine and blocked by prazosin and clonidine. It is postsynaptic.

  3. Alpha-2 inhibits adenyl cyclase and is inhibited by yohimbine and clonidine. It is presynaptic.

  4. Phentolamine and phenoxybenzamine—block both alpha-1 and alpha-2 receptors.

  5. Labetalol—blocks both alpha and beta receptors.

 G. Location

  1. Locus ceruleus

  2. Hypothalamus

  3. Reticular activating system

III. Dopamine

 A. Synthesis

$$\text{Tyrosine} \xrightarrow[\text{Hydroxylase}]{\text{Tyrosine}} \text{L-DOPA} \xrightarrow[\text{Decarboxylase}]{\text{LAA (B6)}} \text{Dopamine}$$

Tyrosine hydroxylase (TH) mediates the rate-limiting step.

LAA decarboxylase is a vitamin-B6-dependent enzyme.

Dopamine is a feedback inhibitor of TH and of the release of vesicles.

 B. Release: Action potentials cause calcium influx that results in the fusion of vesicles.

 C. Metabolism: After reuptake, presynaptic intraneuronal MAO converts dopamine to DOPAC. Extraneuronal postsynaptic COMT and MAO convert dopamine to homovanillic acid (HVA).

 D. Reuptake: Presynaptic terminals contain high-affinity dopamine transporters.

 E. Receptors

  1. D1,5

   a. Postsynaptic linked to G-protein

   b. Excitatory

   c. Stimulates cAMP

  2. D2,3,4

   a. Presynaptic—inhibitory (high affinity)

   b. Postsynaptic—inhibitory (low affinity)

 F. Dopamine Pathways

  1. Nigrostriatal—substantia nigra to striatum

  2. Tuberoinfundibular

  3. Mesolimbic—ventral tegmentum to limbic areas/nucleus accumbens

  4. Mesocortical—ventral tegmentum to prefrontal cortex

 G. Medications

  1. Antipsychotics
     a. Dopamine blockers (D2). The antipsychotics block the inhibitory D2-receptors with a resultant excitatory effect. D2-receptor affinity correlates with efficacy.
  2. Amphetamines
     a. Increase release and decrease reuptake of dopamine.
  3. MAO inhibitors—antidepressants
     a. Increase dopamine by decreasing metabolism.
     b. Examples: selegiline, pargyline
  4. Cocaine and tricyclic antidepressants
     a. Block reuptake
  5. Reserpine and tetrabenazine
     a. Prevent uptake of dopamine and norepinephrine into vesicles.
H. Model of Parkinson's Disease (MPTP)
  1. MAO converts MPTP to MPP+ (toxic to dopaminergic cells). This is the basis for using selegiline in Parkinson's disease.

IV. Serotonin
 A. Synthesis

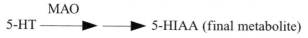

Tryptophan $\xrightarrow[\text{Hydroxylase}]{\text{Tryptophan}}$ 5-Hydroxytryptophan $\xrightarrow[\text{Decarboxyl}]{\text{A.A.}}$ 5-HT

Tryptophan hydroxylase mediates the rate-limiting step.
Increasing the level of L-tryptophan increases the production of 5-hydroxy tryptamine (5-HT).
Amino acid decarboxylase requires a vitamin B6 cofactor.
 B. Storage
  1. 5-HT complexes with proteins, divalent cations, and adenosine diphosphate in granules.
  2. Storage is disrupted by reserpine and tetrabenazine.
 C. Release
  1. Amphetamine and fenfluramine cause the release of 5-HT.
  2. Clomipramine and amitriptyline both increase release and block reuptake of 5-HT.
 D. Metabolism

5-HT $\xrightarrow{\text{MAO}}$ $\longrightarrow$ 5-HIAA (final metabolite)

 E. Reuptake: is the primary mechanism of inactivation; blocked by clomipramine, amitriptyline, sertraline, and fluoxetine.
 F. Receptors
  1. 5-HT1a
     a. Linked to G-protein inhibiting adenyl cyclase
     b. Agonist—buspirone
  2. 5-HT1b/d
     a. Linked to G-protein-inhibiting adenyl cyclase

        b. Both act as autoreceptors.

        c. Agonist—sumatriptan (5-HT1d)

    3. 5-HT1c

        a. Only type 1 receptor that has an antagonist; really more like a 5-HT2

        b. Linked to G-protein activating PLC to increase DAG and IP3

        c. Agonist—alpha-methyl-5-HT, LSD

        d. Antagonist—retanserine, pizotofen, clozapine. **Note:** This is the exception to the no antagonist rule for 5-HT1 receptors.

    4. 5-HT2

        a. Linked to a G-protein activating PLC to increase DAG and IP3

        b. Agonist—alpha-methyl-5-HT, LSD

        c. Antagonists—retanserine, pizotofen, clozapine

    5. 5-HT3

        a. Agonists—2-alpha-5-HT

        b. Antagonists—metoclopramide, cocaine (weak), ondasetron (potent)

  G. CNS Source: midline raphe nuclei

V. Glutamate

  A. Excitatory Amino Acid Neurotransmitter

  B. Receptors

    1. NMDA

        a. Activate mainly calcium channels

        b. Five binding sites alter channel opening

            (1) Glutamate-increase

            (2) Glycine-increase

            (3) Polyamine-increase

            (4) Mg—decrease flow

            (5) Zinc—decrease flow

        c. Glutamate and glycine are required for channel opening.

        d. Voltage-dependent blockers—PCP, ketamine, Mg, MK-801

        e. Voltage-independent blockers—Zinc

        f. Found in hippocampal pyramidal cells

        g. Excitotoxicity theory—Normally the NMDA receptor is blocked by Mg. With enough glutamate binding, the Mg-induced blockade can be overcome and calcium is allowed to enter the cell. This activates intracellular biochemical processes that can lead to cell destruction.

    2. AMPA

        a. Activate mainly sodium channels

        b. Major source of CNS fast excitatory postsynaptic potentials (EPSPs)

        c. Receptor affinity-AMPA > glutamate > Kainate

        d. GluR3 receptor implicated in Rasmussen's encephalitis

    3. Kainate

        a. Receptor affinity-Kainate > Glu > AMPA

    4. APCD—G-protein coupled formation of IP3

    5. L-AP4—G-protein coupled formation of AMP

C. Inactivation
    1. Reuptake is primary mode of termination.

            GAD
    Glutamate ⟶ GABA

    Glutamic acid decarboxylase (GAD) is a vitamin-B6-requiring enzyme.
    B_6-responsive seizures—Decreased B6 can lead to increased glutamate and decreased GABA, and in theory can lead to increased seizures.
    Administration of vitamin B_6 helps some children with seizures.

VI. GABA
    A. Inhibitory Amino Acid Neurotransmitter

            GAD (B6)
    Glutamate ⟶ GABA

    B. Receptors
        1. GABA-a—fast inhibitory postsynaptic potentials (IPSPs). Increase chloride conductance.
            a. Has five binding sites:
                1. Benzodiazepines increase the frequency of Cl channel opening.
                2. Barbiturates prolong the duration of Cl channel opening.
                3. Steroid site
                4. Picrotoxin site—blocker (model for epilepsy)
                5. GABA
            b. Locations—cortex, hippocampus, basal ganglia
        2. GABA-b—slow IPSPs. Increase potassium conductance.
            a. Coupled to G-proteins that use adenyl cyclase as a second messenger
            b. Agonist—baclofen
            c. Antagonist—phaclofen
            d. Location—cerebellum, spinal cord
    C. Inactivation
        1. Reuptake
        2. Enzymatic degradation:

            GABA
    GABA ⟶ Succinic Semialdehyde ⟶ Succinic Acid ⟶ to TCA Cycle
        Transaminase

    D. Inhibitors of GABA Transaminase
        1. Decreased metabolism of GABA leads to increased GABA levels and fewer seizures.
        2. Some antiepileptic drugs have this mechanism:
            a. Valproic acid
            b. Vigabitrin
VII. Glycine
    A. Inhibitory neurotransmitter of the spinal cord

    B. Acts as the neurotransmitter for inhibitory interneurons (Renshaw cells) that inhibit alpha motor neurons in the spinal cord

    C. Blocked by strychnine

    D. Release blocked by tetanus toxin

VIII. Taurine

    A. Inhibitory neurotransmitter

    B. The most abundant neurotransmitter in the body

    C. Stellate cells in the cerebellum use taurine.

    D. Blocked by strychnine

IX. Opioids

    A. Mu Receptor

       1. Agonist—beta endorphin (most potent), morphine

       2. Antagonist—naloxone, naltrexone

       3. Analgesia

    B. Delta Receptor

       1. Agonist—leu-enkephalin (most potent), met-enkephalin

       2. Antagonist—naloxone (weak)

       3. Cardiac effects

    C. Kappa Receptor

       1. Agonists—dynorphins (most potent), prodynorphins (weird names like U69,593)

       2. Antagonist—naloxone (very weak)

       3. Salt and water resorption, analgesia

       4. Different from Mu and Delta in that antagonists cannot reverse morphine withdrawal

X. Substance P

    A. Pain transmission

    B. Release is inhibited by morphine.

    C. Release is calcium dependent.

    D. Capsaicin—depletes substance P.

XI. Axonal Transport

Component	Rate (mm/d)	Structure
Fast transport		
Anterograde	200–400	Neurotransmitters
Mitochondria	50–100	Mitochondria
Retrograde	200–300	Lysosomes
Slow transport		
SCb	2–8	Microfilaments
SCa	0.2–1	Microtubules, neurofilaments

ANTIDEPRESSANTS

I. Depression—General Information

    A. Reactive 60%; major depression 25%; bipolar 15%

    B. Biogenic Amine Hypothesis: NE and serotonin metabolites (MHPG, 5HIAA) are decreased in the CNS in patients with depression.

II. Classification of Antidepressants

Antidepressants

	Anti-ACh	Sedation	Hypotension	Sexual Dysfunction	Comment
TCA					
Amitriptiline	++++	++++	+++		
Clomipramine	++++	++++	++++	++++	Used in OCD
Desipramine	++	++	++	+++	Blocks NE reuptake
Doxepin	++++	++++	++++	+++	
Imipramine	++++	+++	++++	+++	Used for cataplexy
Nortriptyline	++	++	++	+++	
Protriptyline	++++	+	++	+++	
SSRI					
Citalopram	0	+	0	++++	
Fluoxetine	0	0	0	++++	
Fluvoxamine	0	++	0	++++	
Paroxetine	+	+	0	++++	
Sertraline	0	+	0	++++	
MAO					
Phenelzine	++	++	++++	+++	
Irreversible MAOI					
Tranylcypromine	++	0	++++	+++	
Reversible MAOI					
Amoxapine	+	+	+	+++	
Bupropion	0	0	0	0	Seizures
Mirtazapine	++	++	++	++	
Nefazodone	0	+++	0	0	
Trazadone	+	++++	++++	0	
Venlafaxine	0	+	+	+++	

A. Tricyclics (TCAs)
  1. Types—see table.
  2. Mechanism: Blocks reuptake of NE, serotonin
  3. Pharmacokinetics: High protein binding, high lipid solubility
  4. Side effects
    a. CV: postural hypotension (alpha-1 blockade), arrhythmias, and myocardial depression (anticholinergic)
    b. CNS: drowsiness, lethargy, fatigue, confusion, delusions, hallucination (especially in the elderly), lowering of seizure threshold, myoclonus, extrapyramidal symptoms (EPS) (e.g., tardive dyskinesia, tremor, rigidity, akathisia, dystonia)
    c. Anticholinergic: dry mouth, constipation, urinary retention, blurred vision
  5. Uses of the TCAs: depression, chronic pain, enuresis, OCD, cataplexy, narcolepsy, ADHD, panic attacks, irritable bowel syndrome, pseudobulbar palsy
B. Second Generation Antidepressants
  1. Types—see table.
  2. Mechanism
    a. Blocks reuptake of NE, serotonin, and dopamine in various combinations
C. MAO Inhibitors
  1. MAO$_a$ types—see table.

2. MAO_btypes—see table.
3. Mechanism: Blocks oxidative deamination of monoamines.
   NE ⟶ MHPG (MAO_a)
   5HT ⟶ 5HIAA (MAO_a)
   Dopamine ⟶ HVA (MAO_b)
4. Side effects
   a. Common: orthostatic hypotension, mania, agitation
   b. Rare: hypertensive crisis. Can be precipitated by ingestion of foods containing tyramine (wine, cheese, preserved fish). Blockade of MAOa in the intestine does not allow for the inactivation of tyramine and more is absorbed. Must also avoid stimulants, sympathomimetics, TCAs, and L-dopa.
5. Uses: narcolepsy (MAOIs suppress REM sleep), depression, phobias, PTSD, OCD, bulimia.

D. CNS Stimulants: Amphetamines (Ritalin)
   1. Uses: ADHD, narcolepsy
   2. Side effects: withdrawal can cause increased REM sleep, increased appetite, fatigue, and muscle pain.

E. Lithium
   1. Uses: bipolar disorder, mania, cluster headache
   2. Pharmacokinetics: renal excretion, narrow therapeutic window
   3. Side effects
      a. Early: increased WBC, increased TSH
      b. Renal interstitial fibrosis
      c. Do not use in patients with psoriasis
      d. Can cause myoclonus, ataxia, delirium, nystagmus (looks like C-J disease!)
      e. In toxicity, EEG may also look like that seen in C-J disease.
      f. May worsen myasthenia

F. Buspirone (Buspar)—an anxiolytic. Low to moderate potency. Mechanism: Agonist at the 5HT1-a receptor. Unlikely to cause sedation.

ANTIPSYCHOTICS

I. Classification
   A. Phenothiazines
      1. Piperazines: fluphenazine (Prolixin)—high potency; trifluoperazine (Stelazine)—high potency; perphenazine (Trilafon)
      2. Aliphatics: chlorpromazine (Thorazine)
      3. Piperadines: thioridazine (Mellaril)
   B. Thioxanthenes
      1. Thiothixine (Navane)
   C. Butyrophenones
      1. Haloperidol (Haldol)—high potency
   D. Heterocyclics and Others
      1. Molindone (Moban)

2. Loxapine (Loxitane)
3. Pimozide (Orap)—high potency
4. Clozapine (Clozaril)—D3, D4 blockade
5. Risperdone—D3, D4 blockade

Antipsychotic Side Effects

	Extrapyramidal Side Effects	Potency	Orthostasis/Sedation
Haloperidol (Haldol)	+++	+++	+
Fluphenazine (Prolixin)	+++	+++	+
Trifluoperazine (Stelazine)	+++	+++	+
Thiothixine (Navane)	++	++	++
Chlorpromazine (Thorazine)	+	++	++/+++
Thioridazine (Mellaril)	+	+	++/+++
Quetiapine	±		++
Loxapine	+++		+++
Clozaril	±		++
Risperdone	±		++
Olanzapine	±		++

II. General Side Effects
   A. The most potent drugs (Haldol, Prolixin, Stelazine) have more extrapyramidal but fewer anticholinergic side effects.
   B. The least potent drugs (Thorazine, Mellaril) have fewer extrapyramidal but more anticholinergic side effects.
   C. Most work by blocking D2 receptors. Clozaril and Rusperidol block D3 and D4 receptors and reportedly cause less extrapyramidal side effects than the more traditional neuroleptics.
   D. Most common side effects
      1. Neurologic—dystonia, Parkinsonism, akathisia, tardive dyskinesia, neuroleptic malignant syndrome (NMS), decreased seizure threshold (especially with low-potency agents)
      2. Anticholinergic—dry mouth, decreased sweating, impotence, urinary retention, constipation, decreased accommodation (blurred vision), tachycardia
      3. Cardiovascular—orthostatic hypotension/reflex tachycardia (alpha-1 blockade); arrhythmias—quinidine-like with prolonged QT (especially with Mellaril)
      4. Endocrine—amenorrhea, galactorrhea, gynecomastia, change in libido (due to increase in prolactin from blockage of prolactin inhibitory hormone; i.e., dopamine)
      5. Sedation—from histamine blockade
III. Neurologic Side Effects
   A. Acute
      1. Acute Dystonic Reaction
         a. Epidemiology: 2% of patients
         b. Onset—1 to 5 days after beginning treatment
         c. S/S: Usually affects tongue/face/neck/back.
         d. Treatment: Anticholinergics (Benadryl)

B. Early
   1. Parkinsonism
      a. Epidemiology: 20% to 40% of patients
      b. Onset: 5 to 30 days after beginning treatment
      c. S/S: Usually bradykinesia/rigidity, tremor least common. Late variant—perioral "rabbit syndrome," rare, beginning months to years after treatment
      d. Treatment: discontinue neuroleptic, anti-Parkinson's disease drugs
   2. Akathisia
      a. Epidemiology: 20% of patients
      b. Onset: 5 to 60 days after beginning treatment
      c. S/S: Motor restlessness (possible variant of tardive dyskinesia)
      d. Treatment: decrease neuroleptic, propranolol, benzodiazepines (anticholinergics can worsen)
C. Later
   1. Tardive dyskinesia
      a. Epidemiology: 20% of patients. Usually older patients.
      b. Onset: 3 months to years after treatment
      c. S/S: Usually orofacial, choreoathetoid; but can have tardive tics, dystonia, ballism, akathisia, and so on. Can be voluntarily suppressed. Can be temporarily improved by increased dosage of drug. Does not necessarily improve with stopping drug.
      d. Treatment: d/c anticholinergic medications (may worsen), dopamine depletors (reserpine, tetrabenazine), cholinergics
D. Dangerous
   1. Neuroleptic malignant syndrome
      a. Epidemiology: 0.5% to 1% of patients. More males than females (1.4:1). Mortality is 22%.
      b. S/S: All four signs need not be apparent.
         (1) Fever
         (2) Rigidity
         (3) Altered alertness or stupor
         (4) Autonomic instability
         (5) Labs—increased CK, WBC, LFTs, myoglobinuria
      c. Treatment
         (1) d/c neuroleptic and anticholinergic
         (2) Hydration, cooling, telemetry, etc.
         (3) Bromocriptine, dantrolene, ± amantadine
IV. Drug-Specific Side Effects
   A. Chlorpromazine (Thorazine)—Cholestatic jaundice, photosensitive skin reaction
      1. Contraindicated in myasthenia gravis
      2. The most anticholinergic
   B. Thioridazine (Mellaril)—Retinal deposits (retinitis pigmentosa) "browning of vision"; arrhythmias—quinidine-like with prolonged QT interval
   C. Clozapine (Clozaril)—Agranulocytosis (0.5% to 1% incidence); tachycardia, hypersalivation, sedation

V. Uses of Neuroleptics
   A. Schizophrenia/Psychosis
   B. Tourette's syndrome (especially Haldol and Pimozide. Clonidine also used. Ritalin worsens).
   C. Nausea—Blocks dopamine receptors in the chemoreceptor trigger zone.
   D. Sedation/Itching—histamine-blocking effects
   E. Psychosis in PD patients—(Clozapine and Risperdone, because they act on D3,4)
VI. Dopamine Pathways
   A. Nigrostriatal—substantia nigra to striatum
   B. Tuberoinfundibular—arcuate nucleus of hypothalamus to infundibulum (pituitary stalk)
   C. Mesolimbic—ventral tegmentum to limbic system/nucleus accumbens
   D. Mesocortical—ventral tegmentum to prefrontal cortex
VII. Positive/Negative Theory of Schizophrenia
   A. Positive Symptoms: hallucinations, psychosis due to increased dopamine in the mesolimbic pathway
   B. Negative Symptoms: flat affect, decreased motivation due to decreased dopamine in the mesocortical pathway. Atypical agents seem to be more effective for negative symptoms.

Note: Most antipsychotics work by blocking dopamine receptors and work well for the positive symptoms of schizophrenia, but not the negative symptoms.

DRUGS ASSOCIATED WITH NERVOUS SYSTEM DISORDERS

I. **Neuroleptic Malignant Syndrome**
   Neuroleptics
   Atypical neuroleptics
   Miscellaneous:

Amphetamines	Cocaine
Antidepressants	Fenfluramine
Amantidine	Lithium
Levodopa	Metoclopramide
Carbamazepine	Phencyclidine (PCP)

II. **Benign Intracranial Hypertension**

Amiodarone	Lithium
Amphotericin	NSAIDs
Aspirin	Oral contraceptives
Ciprofloxacin	Phenytoin
Corticosteroid withdrawal	Retinoids
Cytosine arabinoside	Sulfonamides
Danazol	Tetracycline
Growth hormone	Vitamin A

III. **Cerebellar Disorders**

Alcohol	Cytosine arabinoside
Antidepressants	Isoniazid

Cyclosporin
Metronidazole
Phenytoin
IV. **Myopathy**
Amiodarone
Chloroquine
Cholesterol-lowering agents
Cimetidine
Colchicine
Corticosteroids
Cyclosporin
Penicillamine
Gold
V. **Myalgias**
ACE inhibitors
Anticholinesterases
Beta agonists
Calcium channel blockers
Carbimazole
Cimetidine
Clofibrate
Colchicine
Corticosteroid withdrawal
VI. **Neuromuscular Transmission Abnormalities**
Anesthetic
  Diazepam
  Halothane
  Ketamine
  Lidocaine
  Methoxyflurane
Antibiotics
  Aminoglycosides
  Ciprofloxacin
  Clindamycin
  Colistimethate
  Colistin
  Penicillin
  Polymyxin B
  Sulfonamide
  Tetracycline
  Vancomycin
Anticonvulsants
  Barbiturates
  Carbamazepine

Lithium
Procainamide
Vaccinations

Growth hormone
Interferon
Ipecac
Labetalol
Phenytoin
Propylthiouracil
Retinoids
Vincristine
Zidovudine

Cytotoxic agents
Danazol
Diuretics
Filgrastatin
Lithium
Penicillamine
Procainamide
Zidovudine

Cardiovascular agents
  Antiarrhythmic agents
  Calcium channel blockers
  Beta blockers
Corticosteroids
Thyroid hormone
Neuromuscular blocking agents
Psychotropic agents
  Chlorpromazine
  Lithium
 Botulinum toxin
Chloroquine
Diuretics
Carnitine
Iodinated contrast media
Ketoprofen
Sodium lactate
Tetanus antitoxin
Artane

Ethosuximide
Phenytoin

VII. **Ototoxicity**

Aminoglycoside antibiotics
Nonaminoglycoside antibiotics
   Ampicillin
   Azithromycin
   Cephalosporins
   Chloramphenicol
   Erythromycin
   Polymyxin
   Sulfonamides
   Vancomycin
Antiinflammatory agents
Antimalarial agents
Antineoplastic agents
   Cisplatin
   Cytosine arabinoside
   Nitrogen mustard

Diuretics
Miscellaneous
   Beta blockers
   Calcium channel blockers
   Carbimazole
   Desferoxamine
   Interferon
   Lidocaine
   Metrizamide
   Oral contraceptives

VIII. **Nystagmus**

Amiodarone
Amitriptyline
Aspirin
Baclofen
Barbiturates
Benzodiazepines
Bupivicaine
Carbamazepine
Cephalosporins
Chloral hydrate
Chloroquine
Chlorpromazine
Cytosine arabinoside
Disulfiram
Fenfluramine
5-fluorouracil

Glutethimide
Ibuprofen
Isoniazid
Ketamine
Lithium
Meperidine
Meprobamate
Metrizamide
Nalidixic acid
Nitrofurantoin
Perhexiline
Phenelzine
Phenytoin
Piperazine
Streptomycin
Valproic acid

IX. **Parkinsonism**

Amiodarone
Amlodipine
Amphotericin
Antineoplastic agents
Calcium channel blockers
Disulfiram
Fluoxetine

Methyl dopa
Methylphenidate
Neuroleptics
Phenelzine
Procaine
Reserpine
Tacrine

Lithium
Manganese
Meperidine

X. **Physiologic Tremor**
Antiepileptic agents
  Lamotrigine
  Valproic acid
Beta agonists
  Caffeine
  Fenfluramine
  Amphetamine
  Ephedrine
Calcium channel blockers
H2 blockers
Levodopa
Lithium

XI. **Myoclonus**
Antidepressants
Carbamazepine
Metoclopramide
Neuroleptics

XII. **Restless Leg Syndrome**
Benzodiazepines
Carbamazepine
Droperidol

XIII. **Tics**
Carbamazepine
Cocaine
Dextroamphetamine

XIV. **Dystonia**
Antihistamines
Baclofen
Bethanechol
Carbamazepine
Chloroquine
Fluoxetine

XV. **Chorea**
Amphetamines
Amoxapine
Anabolic steroids
Anticholinergic agents
Antiepileptic drugs
  Carbamazepine
  Ethosuximide

Vaccinations
Valproic acid

Methyldopa
Metoclopramide
Neuroleptics
Reserpine
Tricyclic antidepressants
Vidarabine
Withdrawal
  Barbiturates
  Benzodiazepines
  Beta blockers
  Opiates

Opioids
Phenytoin
Propafenone

H2 blockers
Levodopa
Psychotropic agents

Methylphenidate
Pemoline
Tricyclic antidepressants

H2 blockers
Levodopa
Metoclopramide
Midazolam
Ondansetron
Phenytoin

Cocaine
Cyclosporin
H2 blockers
Levodopa
Lithium
Methadone
Neuroleptics

Phenobarbital   Oral contraceptives
Phenytoin   Theophylline
Valproic acid   Tricyclic antidepressants
Baclofen

XVI. **Asterixis**

Antiepileptic drugs   Ceftazidime
   Carbamazepine   Methyldopa
   Phenobarbital
   Primidone
   Valproic acid

XVII. **Akathisia**

Antidepressants   Levodopa
Benzodiazepines   Lithium
Buspirone   Neuroleptics
Carbamazepine

XVIII. **Leukoencephalopathy**

Amphotericin   Corticosteroids
Antineoplastic agents   Cyclosporin
   Cisplatin   FK-506
   Cytosine arabinoside   Heroin
   5-fluorouracil   Interferon
   Fludarabine   Interleukin-2
   Mesna
   Methotrexate

4

Central Nervous System Infections

I. Bacterial Meningitis
  A. Etiology varies by age and immune status.

Etiology of Meningitis by Age

Neonate (<1 mo)	Child (1 mo to 15 yr)	Adult (15 yr to 60 yr)	Elderly (>60 yr)
Gram-negative rods (50% to 60%)	H. influenza (50%)	Pneumococcus (50%)	Pneumococcus
Group B streptococcus (30%)	Meningococcus (30%)	Meningococcus (25%)	Gram-negative rods
Listeria (2% to 10%)	Pneumococcus (20%)	Staphylococcus (15%)	Listeria

  Bacteria reach the meninges by hematogenous spread, direct extension from the sinuses or the ears, penetrating trauma, surgery, shunt, ruptured abscess, or sinus tracts. Once the bacteria have crossed the blood-brain barrier, they flourish.
  This results in an aggressive immune response.
  B. Clinical Presentation
    1. Symptoms include fever, headache, photophobia, seizures, nausea, vomiting, altered consciousness, and neck stiffness.
    2. In children, vomiting, irritability, and seizures are most common.
    3. In the elderly, low-grade fever and altered consciousness predominate.
    4. Signs include meningismus, positive Kernig's sign, positive Brudzinski's sign.
    5. Petechial rashes suggest meningococcal meningitis (palpable purpura).
  C. Diagnostic Procedures
    1. CBC, CT head, LP, blood cultures, serum and CSF antigen studies
  D. Treatment
    1. Begin treatment immediately.
    2. Waiting for test results results in increased morbidity and mortality risk.
    3. Ceftriaxone 2 g q12h or cefotaxime 2 g q4h.
    4. Add ampicillin for suspected listeria (< 3 mo or >50 yr).
    5. Add vancomycin if staphylococcus is suspected.
    6. Add aminoglycosides if Gram-negative rods are suspected.
    7. Dexamethasone 15 mg/kg/d should be used in children.
    8. Rifampin prophylaxis should be given to those exposed to meningococcus.
    9. Add acyclovir for herpes coverage.
  E. Complications
    1. Stroke—usually secondary to thrombophlebitis

2. Hydrocephalus—secondary to occlusion of arachnoid villi or adhesions between meninges and brain
3. Cranial nerve dysfunction
4. Seizures
5. Disseminated intravascular coagulation (DIC)—most common with meningococcus and Gram-negative rods
6. Syndrome of inappropriate antidiuretic hormone secretion (SIADH)
7. Abscess or subdural empyema
8. Ventriculitis—usually in neonates

II. Subdural Empyema
   A. A subdural empyema is a pyogenic exudate in the subdural space.
      1. Subdural empyemas are typically secondary to direct extension from sinuses, osteomyelitis, brain abscess, or neurosurgical procedures.
   B. Clinical Presentation
      1. Symptoms include headache, fever, nausea, vomiting, and altered mental status.
      2. Signs are usually focal (aphasia, hemiplegia), including focal seizures.
   C. Diagnostic Procedures
      1. CT Head.
      2. Do not LP—risk of herniation.
   D. Treatment
      1. Surgical drainage is required.
      2. Appropriate antibiotic coverage

III. Brain Abscess
   A. A brain abscess is a localized area of pyogenic exudate in the brain parenchyma. Brain abscesses arise from hematogenous spread, direct extension from sinuses or otitis media (the most common cause), trauma, or rarely, meningitis.
   B. Clinical Presentation
   Symptoms include headache, nausea, vomiting, fever, altered mental status, and progressive neurologic deficits. In many cases, the patient has a progressive neurologic deficit with no signs or symptoms of infection. Physical examination often reveals focal neurologic deficits and evidence of increased intracerebral pressure (papilledema).
   C. Diagnostic Procedures
      1. Do not LP—may rupture abscess, resulting in ventriculitis or arachnoiditis.
      2. Head CT with and without contrast shows an enhancing lesion at the gray/white junction.
   D. Treatment
      1. Superficial abscesses should be surgically drained.
      2. Drainage is followed by IV antibiotics (PenG + flagyl + cephalosporin).
      3. Decadron should be used in lesions with appreciable mass effect.

IV. Viral Meningitis
   A. Viral meningitis is frequently referred to as *aseptic meningitis.*
   B. May have a wide variety of etiologies, including enterovirus (coxsackie, echo, polio), paramyxovirus (mumps), herpesvirus (Epstein-Barr, cytomegalovirus, herpes simplex), and human immunodeficiency virus (HIV). Nonviral causes of aseptic meningitis in-

clude partially treated bacterial meningitis, tuberculosis, Lyme, syphilis, amoeba, fungus, rickettsia, sarcoid, subarachnoid hemorrhage (SAH), systemic lupus erythematosus, and demyelinating diseases.

C. Clinical Presentation
  1. Viral meningitis is often preceded by a flu-like illness.
  2. Symptoms include headache, fever, seizures, nausea, vomiting, and stiff neck.
  3. Signs include positive Kernig's and Brudzinski's signs.
D. Diagnostic Testing
  1. LP reveals abnormal CSF with slightly increased glucose and increased protein.
  2. There is a CSF pleocytosis (initially, neutrophils, followed by lymphocytes).
  3. Viral cultures and polymerase chain reaction (PCR) are only occasionally positive.
E. Treatment
  1. Supportive

ATYPICAL BACTERIAL INFECTIONS

I. Tuberculosis
  A. Etiology: *Mycobacterium tuberculosis*
  B. Incidence: Risk factors include HIV and alcohol (ETOH).
  C. Disease (neurologic)
    1. Basilar meningitis with multiple cranial neuropathies
    2. Tubercle formation
    3. Parenchymal invasion
  D. Pathology
    1. Basilar meningitis with lower cranial nerve palsies
    2. Caseating granulomas
    3. CSF-acid-fast bacilli (AFB) positive occasionally, very low glucose
  E. Treatment: Three-drug antitubercular therapy
II. Leprosy
  A. Etiology: *Mycobacterium leprae*
  B. Incidence: Transmitted by prolonged direct contact
  C. Disease (neurologic)
    1. Cutaneous and peripheral nerve lesions
    2. Infected nerve nodules
    3. Repeated attacks of neuralgic pain precede anesthesia
  D. Pathology
    1. Affected nerves are nodular and thickened.
    2. Bacilli are present in the perineurium.
    3. 33% have false-positive rapid plasma reagin (RPR).
  E. Treatment: Dapsone, rifampin, and clofazimine for 2 years
III. Mycoplasma
  A. Etiology: *Mycoplasma pneumoniae*
  B. Incidence: Respiratory aerial transmission
  C. Disease (neurologic)

   1. Meningitis
   2. Encephalitis
   3. Transverse myelitis
   4. Acute cerebellar ataxia
   5. Postinfectious leukoencephalitis
   D. Pathology
   1. CSF—Normal glucose and protein. Neutrophils and monocytes.
   2. Cold agglutinins positive in 50%
   3. Cultures usually negative
   4. Antimycoplasma antibodies usually become positive.
   E. Treatment: Erythromycin, azithromycin
IV. Legionella
   A. Etiology: *Legionella pneumophila*
   B. Incidence: Epidemic. Contaminated air, water, or soil.
   C. Disease (neurologic)
   1. Acute encephalomyelitis
   2. Acute cerebellar ataxia
   3. Chorea
   4. Peripheral neuropathy
   D. Pathology: Myoglobinuria. Antibodies become positive.
   E. Treatment: Erythromycin IV for 14 to 21 days, azithromycin

SPIROCHETE INFECTIONS

 I. Syphilis
   A. Etiology: *Treponema pallidum*
   B. Incidence: Increasing with HIV infection
   C. Transmission: Sexual
   D. Disease
   1. "The Great Pretender"
   2. Spirochetes invade the CSF within 3 to 8 months.
   3. Meningitis occurs in 25%, occasionally becoming chronic.
   4. Granuloma or gumma formation—focal signs.
   5. Stroke secondary to endarteritis
   6. Tabes Dorsalis
      a. Dorsal roots, dorsal columns, brain stem
   7. Optic Neuritis
   8. General paresis of the insane
   E. Pathology
   1. CSF—mononuclear and lymphocytic infiltrate VDRL positive.
      Increased protein.
      Increased IgG index.
   2. MHA-TP, fluorescent treponemal antibody absorption (FTA-ABS) positive.
      VDRL/RPR may be negative in tertiary syphilis.

F. Treatment
  1. Penicillin-G (PCN-G) 4 million units IV q4h.
  2. CSF at 6 wk, 3 mo, 6 mo, 12 mo, and 24 mo
II. Lyme
  A. Etiology: *Borrelia burgdorferi*
  B. Incidence: Early summer transmission most common
  C. Transmission: Ixodid nymph tick vector
  D. Disease
    1. Erythema chronicum migrans
    2. Headache
    3. Myalgia
    4. Meningismus
    5. Cranial nerve palsies—Bell's palsy most common
    6. Mononeuritis multiplex
    7. Demyelinating disease
  E. Pathology: CSF—oligoclonal bands (OCB) positive, PCR positive
  F. Treatment: Azithromycin, ceftriaxone

VIRAL DISEASES

I. Poliomyelitis
  A. Etiology: Enterovirus (picorna virus); polio, coxsackie, echovirus
  B. Incidence: Rare in United States with widespread use of the vaccine
  C. Transmission: Fecal-oral
  D. Disease: Broad spectrum of disease
    1. Mild flu-like illness in 95% with no central nervous system (CNS) involvement.
    2. Nonparalytic poliomyelitis
      a. Flu-like illness
      b. Muscle pain (hamstrings)
      c. Back pain
      d. Aseptic meningitis
      e. May or may not progress to paralytic poliomyelitis
    3. Paralytic poliomyelitis
      a. Rapid limb and bulbar weakness
      b. Fasciculations
      c. Reflexes are initially brisk but are eventually lost.
      d. Most patients recover completely.
      e. Some have residual weakness (atrophied limb).
      f. Bulbar function recovers completely.
      g. Mortality rate is 5% to 10%.
  E. Pathology
    1. Neuronophagia
    2. Immune response in the thalamus, hypothalamus, CN motor nuclei, anterior horn, cerebellar nuclei

       3. Cowdry B inclusions in the anterior horn cells

       4. Coxsackie and echovirus can be isolated from the CSF.

   F. Treatment: Supportive. Vaccination with Salk (IM), Sabin (PO)

II. Herpes Zoster [Varicella Zoster (VZV), Shingles]

   A. Etiology: Varicella zoster

   B. Incidence: 5/1,000 and increases with increasing age. Increases with immunosuppression.

   C. Transmission: spontaneous reactivation of latent VZV.

   D. Disease

       1. T5 to T10 dermatomes most common (66%)

       2. Radicular pain with a vesicular eruption in the dermatome

       3. The eruption may follow the onset of pain by several days.

       4. Ramsay Hunt syndrome is a lower seventh nerve palsy associated with vesicular eruption in the auditory canal.

   E. Pathology

       1. CSF pleocytosis and increased protein

       2. Inflammatory cells in the dorsal root ganglion

       3. Tzanck prep positive—multinucleated giant cells

   F. Treatment

       1. Acyclovir 800 mg five times per day for 7 days

       2. Acyclovir shortens the duration of illness.

       3. Acyclovir decreases postherpetic neuralgia.

       4. Zoster ophthalmica—IV acyclovir

       5. Pain management with gabapentin or topical lidocaine.

III. Herpes Encephalitis

   A. Etiology: Herpes simplex type I in adults; herpes simplex type II in neonates.

   B. Incidence: Approximately 2,000 cases per year in the United States

   C. Transmission: Sporadic

       1. Associated with cold sores in adults

       2. In infants, associated with maternal genital herpes infection.

   D. Disease

       1. Often preceded by a flu-like illness

       2. Fever, malaise, nausea, vomiting

       3. Limbic (temporal and cingulate) and orbitofrontal hemorrhagic meningoencephalitis

       4. Seizures are common.

       5. Memory loss

       6. Behavioral changes

       7. Hallucinations—olfactory, gustatory

       8. Klüver-Bucy syndrome

       9. 50% fatal or severe sequelae

     10. Sequelae—amnesia, seizures, dementia, aphasia

   E. Pathology:

       1. CSF—lymphocytic pleocytosis, RBCs, and xanthochromia

2. PCR is more reliable than culture.
3. EEG—temporal spikes at 2 to 3 Hz or periodic lateralized epileptiform discharges (PLEDs)
4. CT and MRI may reveal limbic or orbitofrontal meningoencephalitis.
5. Cowdry A inclusions
    F. Treatment: Acyclovir 10 mg/kg q8 hours for 14 days
IV. Human Immunodeficiency Virus
    A. Etiology: HIV
    B. Incidence: Common
    C. Transmission: Sexual, body fluids
    D. Disease
        1. Acute
            a. Mono-like illness
            b. Aseptic meningitis usually at seroconversion
                (1) Occurs in 5% to 10% of patients.
                (2) HIV ab test often negative, but p24 ag PCR positive
                (3) Cranial nerves V, VII, VIII often involved
                (4) CSF pleocytosis with 20 to 300 mononuclear cells
            c. Guillain-Barré syndrome
            d. Bell's palsy
        2. Chronic
            a. HIV dementia / AIDS dementia complex
                (1) Most common neurologic syndrome of acquired immunodeficiency syndrome (AIDS)
                (2) Occurs in 75%+ of patients.
                (3) Subcortical dementia
                    (a) Slowness (psychomotor retardation)
                    (b) Short-term memory loss
                    (c) Decreased concentration
                    (d) Apathy
                    (e) Forgetfulness
                    (f) No signs of cortical dementia (eg, aphasia)
                (4) Prominent physiologic tremor
                (5) MRI often shows patchy white matter abnormalities.
                (6) Pathology
                    (a) Perivascular cuffing
                    (b) Multinucleated giant cells
                    (c) Myelin pallor
                    (d) Mild neuronal dropout
                    (e) Frontal lobes predominantly involved
            b. Opportunistic infections
                (1) Toxoplasmosis
                    (a) Occurs in 5% to 15% of AIDS patients
                    (b) Occurs most commonly with CD4 100—500

        (c) Enhancing/ring-enhancing lesion with edema on CT or MRI

        (d) Treat with pyramethamine, clindamycin, or azithromycin.

        (e) If no response, consider CNS lymphoma.

    (2) Progressive multifocal leukoencephalopathy (PML)

    (3) Cryptococcal meningitis

    (4) CMV encephalitis

        (a) Typically occurs with very low CD4 counts (< 50)

        (b) Rapidly progressive dementia

        (c) Treat with gancyclovir or foscarnet (if ANC < 500)

    (5) Herpes zoster

    (6) Tuberculosis

    (7) Syphilis

c. Tumors

    (1) Primary CNS lymphoma (B cell)

        (a) Occurs in 2% of AIDS patients

        (b) Occurs most commonly with CD4 < 100

        (c) Thallium SPECT scan may show hot spots.

        (d) Brain irradiation may extend survival 3 to 6 months.

        (e) Steroids "melt" lesions, making diagnosis difficult.

    (2) Lymphomatous meningitis

    (3) Kaposi's sarcoma

        (a) Rarely involves the CNS.

d. Vacuolar myelopathy

    (1) Occurs in 20% of patients

    (2) Spastic paraparesis, sensory ataxia, and incontinence

    (3) Posterior and lateral column demyelination

        (a) Looks like subacute combined degeneration.

e. Neuropathy

    (1) Chronic inflammatory demyelinating polyneuropathy (CIDP)—usually lumbosacral

    (2) Mononeuropathy multiplex

    (3) Polyradiculopathy—usually CMV mediated

    (4) Distal polyneuropathy—most common

        (a) HIV

        (b) Low-dose ddI—sensory neuropathy

        (c) High-dose ddI—painful rapid progression

        (d) Isoniazid (INH)

        (e) ddC, d4T, 3TC—painful sensory neuropathy

f. Stroke—vasculitis

g. Seizures

h. Myopathy

    (1) Polymyositis—steroids may help

    (2) AZT-induced with ragged red fibers

        (a) AZT is toxic to mitochondria.

(b) Resolves when AZT is discontinued
(3) Nemaline rod-like myopathy

Neurologic Complications of HIV

	Early (CD4 >500)	Late (CD4 < 500)
Infections	Aseptic meningitis	Opportunistic diseases
Encephalopathy	Depressive pseudodementia	HIV dementia
	Neurosyphilis	CMV encephalopathy
Neuropathy	Guillain-Barré syndrome	HIV neuropathy
	Bell's palsy	Toxic neuropathy
	CIDP	Mononeuritis multiplex
	Cranial neuropathy	
	Entrapment neuropathy	
Myopathy	Polymyositis	Polymyositis
		Toxic myopathy (AZT)
Myelopathy	HTLV-I	Vacuolar myelopathy
	Epidural abscess	Lumbosacral myeloradiculopathy
		Toxoplasma myelitis

V. Tropical Spastic Paraparesis
  A. Etiology: HTLV-I
  B. Incidence: Female-to-male ratio is 3:1. Most common in Caribbean and Japan.
  C. Transmission: Sexual, body fluids
  D. Disease: Spastic paraparesis
  E. Pathology: 1 of 4 antibody-positive patients has disease.
  F. Treatment: Supportive
VI. St. Louis Encephalitis, Eastern Equine Encephalitis
  A. Etiology: Arbovirus
  B. Incidence: Epidemic
    1. St. Louis encephalitis is more common.
    2. Eastern equine encephalitis is least common.
  C. Transmission: Mosquito-borne virus
  D. Disease: Eastern equine encephalitis is the most rapidly fatal.
  E. Pathology: Inflammation, neuronophagia, cowdry A inclusions
  F. Treatment: Supportive
VII. Rabies
  A. Etiology: Rhabdovirus
  B. Incidence: Sporadic
  C. Transmission: Bite from a rabid animal (skunk, bat, raccoon, dog)
  D. Disease: Long latent period (20 to 60 days)
    1. Virus spreads retrograde along nerves to the CNS.
    2. Prodrome of headache, fever, malaise, anxiety
    3. Dysphagia (foaming at the mouth)
    4. Hydrophobia (laryngeal spasm when swallowing liquids)
    5. Seizures
    6. Death

    E. Pathology: Negri bodies (eosinophilic intracytoplasmic inclusions) in pyramidal cells and cerebellar Purkinje cells
        1. Babes nodules—focal microglial nodules
    F. Treatment
        1. Clean wound with soap and water.
        2. Human rabies immunoglobulin
        3. Human diploid cell vaccine on days 1, 3, 7, 14, 28
        4. The disease is fatal once clinical signs appear.
VIII. Subacute Sclerosing Panencephalitis
    A. Etiology: Measles (rubeola). Measles usually before age 2 years.
    B. Incidence: Less than 1/1,000,000
    C. Disease
        1. Initially, poor school performance, temper, language difficulties
        2. Later, intellectual decline, seizures, myoclonus, ataxia
        3. Decortication
        4. Death in 1 to 3 years
    D. Pathology
        1. Patchy demyelination and gliosis
        2. Intranuclear eosinophilic inclusions (tubules)
        3. CSF has increased IgG and measles antibodies.
        4. EEG shows periodic sharp wave complexes (like burst suppression).
    E. Treatment: Intrathecal alpha interferon may be of benefit.
  IX. Progressive Multifocal Leukoencephalopathy (PML)
    A. Etiology: Papovavirus (JC virus and SV-40 virus)
    B. Incidence
        1. Most common in AIDS patients
        2. Rarely in Hodgkin's and leukemia (CLL)
    C. Disease
        1. Progressive hemiparesis
        2. Visual loss
        3. Dementia
        4. 80% die in 9 months.
    D. Pathology
        1. Multifocal demyelination (begins occipital)
        2. Bizarre astrocytes
        3. Oligodendrocytes contain eosinophilic intranuclear inclusions.
        4. MRI—no enhancement
    E. Treatment: Cytarabine 2 mg/kg/d for 5 days each month. Supportive care.

FUNGAL INFECTIONS

  I. Cryptococcus
    A. Incidence
        1. Most common CNS fungal infection

       2. Usually occurs in immunocompromised patients.
- B. Disease
  1. Chronic meningitis, altered mental status
  2. Increased intracranial pressure
- C. Pathology
  1. Chronic meningitis
  2. Focal granulomas
  3. CSF—India ink positive
     - a. Crypto Ag positive (may be negative from prozone effect at high titers)
     - b. Organisms without a capsule are usually India ink negative.
- D. Treatment: Amphotericin B or fluconazole

II. Mucormycosis
- A. Incidence: Usually occurs in diabetic patients.
- B. Disease
  1. Sinusitis or orbital cellulitis
  2. Strokes secondary to thrombosis
  3. Meningoencephalitis
- C. Pathology: Broad hyphae invading blood vessel walls
- D. Treatment
  1. Amphotericin B
  2. Surgical debridement
  3. Itraconazole

III. Aspergillosis
- A. Incidence: Most common in patients with chronic sinusitis
- B. Disease
  1. Chronic sinusitis
  2. Osteomyelitis
  3. Compressed cranial nerves
  4. Brain abscess
- C. Pathology
  1. Septated hyphae
  2. Brain abscess—fungus ball
- D. Treatment
  1. Amphotericin B
  2. Resection
  3. Itraconazole

IV. Coccidioidomycosis
- A. Incidence: Endemic in southwestern United States
- B. Disease
  1. Usually benign
  2. May cause chronic meningitis
- C. Pathology: Nonbudding spherules
- D. Treatment: Amphotericin B

V. Candidiasis

A. Incidence: Severely ill, immunocompromised patients
B. Disease: Microabscesses
C. Pathology: Blood culture positive in many cases
D. Treatment: Amphotericin B, Fluconazole

PRION DISEASES

I. Creutzfeldt-Jakob Disease
   A. Etiology: Prion
   B. Incidence: 1/1,000,000, sporadic, 15% familial. Has been associated with corneal transplants, depth electrodes, pooled growth hormone (GH).
   C. Disease
      1. Insomnia early
      2. Prominent hallucinations and paranoia
      3. Early-onset dementia—Heidenheim dementia
      4. Stimulus myoclonus—increased startle
      5. Pyramidal and extrapyramidal signs
      6. Seizures
      7. 90% die in 1 year.
   D. Pathology: Vacuolization in the cortex and basal ganglia
      1. EEG: Periodic sharp waves, 1 to 2 Hz high voltage. Periodic sharp waves appear in 80% by 12th week. Evolves into diffuse slowing.
      2. Imaging: CT normal in 80%. MRI increased T2 signal in basal ganglia and thalamus.
   E. Treatment: Supportive. Prion killed by 1 hour of autoclaving or bleach.
II. Gerstmann-Straussler Disease
   A. Etiology: autosomal dominant prion disease
   B. Incidence: Rare
   C. Disease: Lengthy disease course of 2 to 10 years
      1. Insomnia
      2. Euphoria
      3. Pyramidal signs
      4. Supranuclear gaze palsy
   D. Pathology: Atrophy, amyloid plaques (large without surrounding neurites)
      1. EEG rarely shows periodic spikes but frequent slowing.
      2. Imaging
         a. Cerebellar atrophy
         b. MRI decreased T2 signal in basal ganglia (iron)
   E. Treatment: Supportive
III. Kuru
   A. Etiology: Cannibalism-related prion disease. Affects Fore tribespeople in New Guinea.
   B. Disease
      1. Progresses over months to years
      2. Pain in legs

3. Loss of facial motor control
4. Euphoria
5. Late dementia
C. Pathology: Neuronal loss in cortex and cerebellum. Amyloid Kuru plaques in cerebellum.

IV. Fatal Familial Insomnia
A. Etiology: Autosomal dominant prion disease
B. Disease: Insomnia, agitation, ataxia, dysarthria, dysautonomia, memory loss
C. Pathology: Degeneration of the thalamus (VA and MD subnuclei)

PARASITIC DISEASES

I. Naegleria Fowlerii Meningoencephalitis (PAM)
A. Etiology: Amoeba (*Naegleria Fowlerii*)
B. Incidence: Rare. History of swimming in freshwater lakes.
C. Disease
1. Rapidly progressive hemorrhagic meningoencephalitis
2. Amoebae reach the CNS through the cribriform plate.
3. Usually fatal
D. Pathology
1. Hemorrhagic meningoencephalitis
2. Organisms seen in CSF on wet mount
E. Treatment: Amphotericin B and rifampin

II. Toxoplasmosis
A. Etiology: *Toxoplasma gondii*, small intracellular parasite
B. Incidence: Usually in immunocompromised patients (HIV)
C. Disease: Usually brain abscesses. Rarely encephalitis.
D. Pathology
1. Encysted organisms and focal necrosis
2. CT and MRI show ring-enhancing lesions.
3. Congenital toxoplasmosis causes periventricular calcifications.
E. Treatment
1. Pyrimethamine and sulfadiazine and folinic acid
2. Brain biopsy if no improvement to rule out CNS lymphoma

III. Trichinosis
A. Etiology: *Trichinella spiralis* (intestinal nematode)
B. Incidence: History of eating undercooked pork
C. Disease
1. Malaise
2. Weakness
3. Usually self-limited polymyositis involving cranial muscles and heart
4. Decreased DTRs secondary to muscle invasion
5. Meningitis may occur.
D. Pathology

       1. Encapsulated organisms may be seen in CNS and muscle.
   E. Treatment: Thiabendazole
IV. Cysticercosis
   A. Etiology: *Taenia solium* (pork tapeworm)
   B. Incidence: Leading cause of epilepsy in Central America
   C. Disease: Seizures are the most common sequela.
   D. Pathology
       1. Calcified larval cysts
       2. CT often shows multiple cerebral calcified cysts.
       3. Migrating intraventricular cyst is pathognomonic.
   E. Treatment: Praziquantel and steroids

CSF Abnormalities in Infectious Disease

	Pressure (cm H$_2$O)	WBC	Cell Type	Protein	Glucose	Culture	Miscellaneous
Bacterial meningitis	Increased	Up to 100,000	Neutrophils	100–500	<40	+	Increased LDH & lactic acid
Viral meningitis	Normal	Increased	Lymphs/monos	Slightly increased	Normal	—	
Herpes encephalitis	Increased	10–500	Lymphs	Increased	Normal	+	PCR
SSPE		Few	Lymphs	Increased		—	+OCB, increased IgG
Post Rubella encephalitis		Slightly increased	Lymphs	Moderately increased		—	Increased IgG, +OCB, +Rubella titer
TB meningitis	Increased	50–500	Lymphs	100–200	<40	AFB+	
Mycoplasma	Normal	Normal	Lymphs	Increased	Normal	—	Antibody +
Subdural empyema	Increased	50–1,000	Neutrophils	75–300	Normal	±	
Epidural abcess	Normal	20–100	Neutrophils/lymphs	Slightly increased	Normal	±	
Brain abcess	Large increase late	20–300	Neutrophils	<100	Normal	±	
Sarcoid		10–200	Lymphs	Increased	Normal/ decreased	Sterile	+ACE, +IgG, increased ESR
Neurosyphilis		200–300	Lymphs/plasma cells/monos	40–200	Normal		+VDRL, +FTA, +IgG
Lyme	Normal	Up to 3,000	Lymphs	Up to 400	Normal		+OCB
Fungal meningitis	Increased	<1,000	Lymphs	Increased	Decreased	+	Antigens
Spinal abcess	Dynamic block	<100	Lymphs/neutrophils	100–400	Normal	±	
Postinfectious myelitis		20–200	Lymphs	Normal/increased	Normal	—	

ACE, angiotensin converting enzyme; ESR, erythrocyte sedimentation rate; FTA, a treponemal antibody test; IgG, immunoglobulin G; LDH, lactate dehydrogenase; OCB, oligoclonal bands; PCR, polymerase chain reactions; SSPE, subacute sclerosing panencephalitis; WBC, white blood cell.

5

Metabolic Disorders

GLYCOGEN STORAGE DISEASES (GSD)

I. Acid Maltase Deficiency (AMD) (also known as Pompe's Disease)
   A. Infantile
      1. Onset—weeks
      2. Clinical features
         a. Floppy baby, generalized and bulbar weakness
         b. Macroglossia
         c. Cardiomegaly
         d. Hepatomegaly
         e. Death by age 2 years
   B. Adult AMD
      1. Onset: 20s to 30s age group
      2. Clinical presentation
         a. Respiratory weakness > limb-girdle weakness
         b. Intracranial aneurysms secondary to glycogen in vessels
   C. Lab
      1. Normal ischemic exercise test
      2. Increased creatine kinase (CK)
   D. EMG: Myopathy, electrical myotonia without clinical myotonia
   E. Inheritance: Autosomal recessive (AR)
   F. Path: Vacuolar myopathy. Accumulation of PAS-positive material in lysosomes
II. Muscle Phosphorylase Deficiency (McArdle's Disease) GSD Type V
   A. Onset
      1. Childhood with exercise intolerance
      2. Adults with cramps
   B. Clinical Presentation
      1. Premature fatigue, weakness
      2. Myalgias
      3. Cramps
      4. Symptoms resolve with rest
      5. Acute muscle necrosis
      6. Myoglobinuria (dark urine following exercise)
      7. Fixed weakness occurs in one-third of patients.
   C. Lab

           1. Positive ischemic exercise test (no rise in serum lactate after ischemic exercise)
           2. CK elevated in 90%
           3. Myoglobinuria in 50%
    D. EMG: usually normal, may have second-wind phenomenon
    E. Inheritance: AR
    F. Path
           1. Subsarcolemmal glycogen deposits (blebs) that are PAS positive.
           2. Intermyofibrillar vacuoles
           3. Immunohistochemical stains show absent staining for phosphorylase.
III. Muscle Phosphofructokinase Deficiency (Tauri's Disease) GSD Type VII
    A. Onset: Childhood
    B. Clinical Presentation
           1. Premature fatigue, weakness, stiffness induced by exercise
           2. Myalgias
           3. Cramps
           4. Symptoms resolve with rest.
    C. Lab
           1. Positive ischemic exercise test
           2. CK elevated
           3. Mild hemolysis
    D. EMG: Normal, myopathic, or irritative
    E. Inheritance: AR
    F. Path
           1. Subsarcolemmal glycogen deposits (blebs)
           2. Intermyofibrillar vacuoles
           3. Immunohistochemical stains show absent phosphofructokinase staining.
IV. Lafora's Disease
    A. Onset: Childhood
    B. Clinical Presentation
           1. Epilepsy
           2. Myoclonus
           3. Dementia
           4. Death by age 25 years
    C. Inheritance: AR
    D. Path: Basophilic, PAS-positive intracytoplasmic inclusions
V. Glycogen Storage Disease Quick Reference Table

Type	Eponym	Defect	Involved tissue	Special features
I	Von Gierke's	Glucose-6-phosphatase	Liver, kidney	Hypoglycemic seizures
II	Pompe's	Acid maltase	Generalized	Floppy baby
III	Forbe's	Debranching enzyme	Generalized	
IV		Transglucosidase	Generalized	
V	McArdle's	Muscle phosphorylase	Muscle	Cramps, weakness
VI		Liver phosphorylase	Liver, WBC	Hypoglycemia
VII	Tarui's	Phosphofructokinase	Muscle, RBC	Cramps, weakness
VIII		Phosphorylase kinase	Liver	

AMINO ACID METABOLISM

I. Amino Acidemias
   A. Types
      1. Proprionic acidemia
      2. Methylmalonic acidemia
      3. Multiple carboxylase deficiency
      4. Isovaleric acidemia
      5. 3-Oxothiolase deficiency
   B. General Characteristics (common to all acidemias)
      1. Onset: infancy
      2. Clinical presentation
         a. Vomiting
         b. Anorexia
         c. Lethargy
         d. Ketoacidosis
         e. Dehydration
         f. Hyperammonemia
         g. Neutropenia
         h. Failure to thrive
         i. Hypomyelination
         j. Seizures
         k. Mental retardation
         l. Coma
         m. Death
      3. Inheritance: AR
      4. Lab
         a. Hyperammonemia
         b. Hyperglycinemia
         c. Urine and serum organic acids
   C. Specific Characteristics
      1. Biotinidase deficiency—ataxia, optic and auditory degeneration, paraplegia, seizures
      2. Proprionic acidemia—hypotonia, seizures, myoclonus
      3. Methylmalonic acidemia—basal ganglia strokes, spasticity, dystonia, chorea
   D. Treatment
      1. Multiple carboxylase deficiency—biotin 10 mg/d
      2. Methylmalonic acidemia—vitamin B_{12}
      3. Isovaleric acidemia—oral glycine supplements
II. Glutaric Aciduria Type I
   A. Onset: Infancy
   B. Clinical Presentation
      1. Spasticity
      2. Dystonia
      3. Choreoathetosis

    4. Opisthotonos

    5. Developmental delay

    6. Macrocephaly

  C. Lab: Urine and serum organic acids; enzyme assay

  D. Imaging: Atrophy. Gliosis in caudate and putamen; caudate atrophy.

  E. Inheritance: AR

  F. Treatment

    1. Low-protein diet

    2. Carnitine supplements

    3. Riboflavin supplements

III. Gamma Hydroxybutyric Aciduria

  A. Onset: Infancy (rare)

  B. Clinical Presentation

    1. Hypotonia

    2. Seizures

    3. Mental retardation

  C. Inheritance: AR

  D. Treatment: Anticonvulsants

IV. Phenylketonuria (PKU)

  A. Defect

    1. PKU—decreased phenylalanine hydroxylase (conversion of phenylalanine to tyrosine)

    2. Malignant PKU (stiff baby variant)—dihydropterin reductase (biopterin) deficiency

  B. Onset: Infancy

  C. Clinical Presentation

    1. Normal at birth; symptoms appear after baby is exposed to phenylalanine in diet.

    2. Mental retardation

    3. Fair skin

    4. Blue eyes

    5. Blonde hair

    6. Hyperreflexia

    7. Hyperkinetic activity

    8. Photosensitivity

    9. Rash

    10. Seizures

    11. Musty body odor

  D. Lab

    1. Phenylalanine screen positive if phenylalanine level >20 mg/dL

      a. Check level at birth and at 2 weeks of age.

      b. Obtain biopterin screen if phenylalanine levels are high.

    2. Tyrosine is low.

  E. Electroencephalogram (EEG)

    1. Untreated: Paroxysmal; hypsarrhythmia

      2. Treated: Normal
  F. Imaging: Decreased metabolism in the caudate and putamen; atrophy
  G. Inheritance
      1. PKU: AR chromosome 12
      2. Malignant PKU: AR chromosome 4
  H. Treatment
      1. Low phenylalanine diet
      2. Biopterin for malignant PKU (poor prognosis)
V. Nonketotic Hyperglycinemia
  A. Onset: Neonate
  B. Clinical Presentation
      1. Hiccups
      2. Respiratory arrest
      3. Coma
      4. Seizures
      5. Microcephaly
      6. Hypotonia leading to hypertonia
      7. Death is common in the neonatal period.
  C. Lab—CSF glycine: Serum glycine > 0.10 ammonia units umol/L
  D. EEG: Burst suppression; hypsarrhythmia; focal epileptiform discharges
  E. Imaging: Atrophy; hypomyelination
  F. Treatment: Anticonvulsants
VI. Urea Cycle Defects
  A. Specific Defects
      1. Ornithine transcarbamylase deficiency
        a. Most common
        b. X-linked recessive
      2. Carbamoyl phosphate synthetase deficiency
        a. Most severe
        b. Autosomal recessive
      3. Arginosuccinic acid synthase deficiency (citrullinemia)
        a. Autosomal recessive
      4. Arginosuccinase deficiency
        a. Autosomal recessive, chromosome 9
  B. General Characteristics (common to all urea cycle defects)
      1. Onset: Neonate
      2. Clinical presentation
        a. Coma
        b. Seizures
        c. Hypotonia
        d. Respiratory arrest
        e. Occasional hemorrhages
        f. Vomiting
        g. Death without treatment

   h. Normal with early treatment
  3. Lab
   a. Serum ammonia > 500 glycine units umol/L
   b. Serum amino acids (increased glutamine)
  4. Imaging: Cerebral edema; occasional hemorrhage
  5. Path
   a. Cerebral edema
   b. Alzheimer's type II cells
   c. Decreased myelination
   d. Neuronal loss
  6. Treatment
   a. Hemodialysis to decrease ammonia
   b. Dietary restriction of nitrogen (low-protein diet)
   c. Avoid valproate for seizures, as this drug increases ammonia.

VII. Hartnup Disease—Amino Acid Transport Defect
 A. Onset: Infancy
 B. Clinical Presentation
  1. Variable
  2. Failure to thrive
  3. Photosensitive rash
  4. Intermittent ataxia
  5. Nystagmus
  6. Tremor
 C. Lab: Neutral amino acids with low serum tryptophan
 D. Defect: Defective Na-dependent neutral amino acid transport in the small intestine and renal tubules leading to increased fecal and urinary amino acid excretion
 E. Treatment
  1. High-protein diet
  2. Nicotinic acid supplements (niacin)
  3. General improvement with age

VIII. Lowe's Syndrome (Oculocerebrorenal Syndrome)
 A. Onset: Neonate
 B. Clinical Presentation
  1. Mental retardation and developmental delay
  2. Glaucoma
  3. Cataracts
  4. Myopathy
  5. Pendular nystagmus
  6. Punctate cortical lens opacities may be only sign in heterozygote female carriers.
  7. Death from renal failure
 C. Inheritance: X-linked recessive
 D. Path: Loss of central and peripheral myelinated fibers
 E. Defect: Thought to be caused by a membrane transport defect

IX. Maple Syrup Urine Disease

    A. Onset: Neonate

    B. Clinical Presentation

        1. Hypertonic

        2. Opisthotonos

        3. Fluctuating ophthalmoplegia that correlates with serum leucine levels

        4. Clonus

        5. Generalized seizures

        6. Developmental delay

        7. Patient eventually becomes flaccid and areflexic.

        8. Coma

    C. Lab: Elevated leucine, isoleucine, and valine on serum amino acid screen. Positive 2,4-dinitrophenylhydrazine (DNPH) urine test. Characteristic urine odor.

    D. Imaging: Cerebral edema greatest in cerebellar deep white matter and brain stem

    E. Path: White matter cystic degeneration; gliosis

    F. Defect: Alpha-ketoacid dehydrogenase deficiency resulting in abnormal oxidative decarboxylation and accumulation of branched-chain amino acids

    G. Prognosis: May have normal IQ if treated within 5 days.

    H. Inheritance: AR

    I. Treatment

        1. Thiamine supplementation

        2. Dietary restriction of branched-chain amino acids

X. Homocystinuria

    A. Onset: Variable

    B. Clinical Presentation

        1. Marfanoid habitus

        2. Cod fish vertebra (biconcave)

        3. Eye anomalies

            a. 90% have ectopia lentis (lens displaced downward).

            b. Myopia

            c. Glaucoma

            d. Optic atrophy

        4. CNS

            a. Mental retardation

            b. Seizures

            c. Behavior disorders

            d. Stroke (beginning at age 5 to 9 months)

    C. Lab

        1. Increased homocysteine on serum and urine amino acids

        2. Positive methionine challenge test

    D. Path: Intimal thickening and fibrosis of blood vessels leading to arterial and venous thrombosis

    E. Defect: Cystathionine beta synthase deficiency resulting in accumulation of homocysteine and methionine. There is also impaired methylation of homocysteine to methionine from enzyme deficiency or cofactor B12 deficiency.

F. Inheritance: AR, chromosome 21
G. Treatment
   1. Restrict dietary methionine.
   2. Pyridoxine supplements
   3. Vitamin B12 supplements
   4. Cysteine supplements

PURINE METABOLISM

I. Lesch-Nyhan Syndrome
   A. Onset: Age 6 months
   B. Clinical Presentation
      1. Crystalluria
      2. Developmental delay
      3. Choreoathetosis
      4. Dystonia
      5. Opisthotonos
      6. Hyperreflexia
      7. Mental retardation
      8. Self-mutilating behavior
   C. Lab: Hyperuricemia
   D. Defect: Hypoxanthine-guanine phosphoribosyl transferase deficiency
   E. Inheritance: X-linked recessive
   F. Treatment
      1. Allopurinol 20 mg/kg/d (blocks uric acid synthesis)
      2. Physical restraint
      3. L-5-hydroxytryptophan + L-dopa
      4. Fluphenazine (may help decrease self-mutilating behavior)

LIPOPROTEIN METABOLISM

I. Abetalipoproteinemia (Bassen-Kornzweig Disease)
   A. Clinical Presentation
      1. Neurologic symptoms begin by age 12 years.
      2. Fat malabsorption with diarrhea and steatorrhea
      3. Acanthocytosis
      4. Retinopathy
      5. Vitamin A, D, E, and K deficiency
      6. Neuropathy with decreased reflexes, proprioception, and sensation
      7. Progressive ataxia
      8. Positive Romberg
      9. Decreased night vision (retinitis pigmentosa)
      10. Weakness
   B. Lab

    1. Acanthocytosis
    2. Absent beta-lipoproteins (chylomicrons, LDL, VLDL)
    3. Decreased triglycerides and cholesterol
    4. Low vitamin A, D, E, and K levels (fat-soluble vitamins)
    5. Increased PT
  C. Nerve Conduction Velocity (NCV): Slowed conduction
  D. Path
    1. Loss of large myelinated fibers
    2. Spinocerebellar and posterior column degeneration
  E. Defect: Decreased posttranslational processing of apolipoprotein B
  F. Inheritance: AR
  G. Treatment
    1. Dietary restriction of triglycerides
    2. Vitamin E supplements
II. Tangier's Disease
  A. Clinical Presentation
    1. Large orange tonsils
    2. Lymphadenopathy
    3. Splenomegaly
    4. Corneal infiltrates
    5. Relapsing multiple mononeuropathies
    6. Loss of pain and temperature sensation
    7. Peripheral neuropathy in 50% with demyelinating sensory, sensorimotor, or motor neuropathy
  B. Lab
    1. Decreased total cholesterol and LDL
    2. Triglycerides normal or increased
    3. Very low HDL
  C. Path
    1. Lipid droplets in Schwann cells and in reticular endothelial system (RES) of other cells
    2. Neuropathy: demyelination/remyelination
    3. Syringomyelia: like syndrome with axonal degeneration
  D. Defect: Alpha-lipoprotein deficiency
  E. Inheritance: AR
  F. Treatment: None
III. Cerebrotendinous Xanthomatosis
  A. Clinical Presentation
    1. Dementia
    2. Ataxia
    3. Seizures
    4. Paresis
    5. Peripheral neuropathy
    6. Juvenile cataracts

      7. Xanthoma
      8. Atherosclerosis
      9. Mental retardation
   B. Lab: Increased cholestanol
   C. NCV: Slowing
   D. Imaging
      1. MRI: Diffuse hypomyelination
      2. CT: Diffuse hypomyelination with hyperdensities in the cerebellum
   E. Path: Extensive demyelination greatest in the cerebellum and brain stem
   F. Defect: Absent chenodeoxycholic acid (bile acid)
   G. Inheritance: AR
   H. Treatment: Chenodeoxycholic acid 750 mg/d

PORPHYRIA

  I. Subtypes include Acute Intermittent Porphyria, Hereditary Coproporphyria, Variegate Porphyria
 II. General Characteristics
   A. Clinical Presentations: See chart
   B. Lab
      1. Elevated porphobilinogen (PBG) in urine
      2. Quantitative aminolevulinic acid (ALA), PBG, and porphyrins in urine and feces
   C. Path: Patchy demyelination and axonal degeneration
   D. Differential Diagnosis: Guillain-Barré syndrome, lead intoxication, hereditary tyrosinemia
   E. Treatment
      1. Pain: Analgesics, morphine, chlorpromazine
      2. Hyponatremia: Normal saline (NS) + diuretics
      3. Seizures: Valium
      4. Dextrose: 400 g/d
      5. Hematin: 1.5 to 2 mg/kg IV

Porphyria Symptoms and Signs

Symptom	Frequency (%)	Sign	Frequency (%)
Abdominal pain	95	Tachycardia	80
Extremity pain	50	Dark urine	74
Back pain	29	Motor deficit	60
Chest pain	12	Proximal limbs	48
Nausea and vomiting	43	Generalized	42
Constipation	48	Distal limbs	10
Diarrhea	43	Altered mentation	40
		Hypertension	36
		Sensory deficit	26
		Seizure	20

Medications in Porphyria

	Dangerous	Probably Safe
Anticonvulsants		
	Barbiturates	Bromides
	Carbamazepine	Diazepam
	Clonazepam	Magnesium sulfate
	Ethosuximide	
	Phenytoin	
	Primidone	
	Valproic acid	
Hypnotics		
	Barbiturates	Chloral hydrate
	Chlordiazepoxide	Chlorpromazine
	Ethchlorvynol	Diphenhydramine
	Glutethimide	Lithium
	Meprobamate	Lorazepam
	Methyprylon	Meclizine
		Trifluoperazine
Other		
	Alpha-methyldopa	ACTH
	Danazol	Allopurinol
	Ergots	Aminoglycosides
	Estrogens	Aspirin
	Griseofulvin	Codeine
	Imipramine	Colchicine
	Pentazocine	Furosemide
	Pyrazinamide	Ibuprofen
		Insulin
		Meperidine
		Morphine
		Naproxen
		Penicillin
		Warfarin

METAL METABOLISM

I. Wilson's Disease (Hepatolenticular Degeneration)
- A. Etiology: ATPase Deficiency
- B. Clinical Presentation
  1. Onset typically between ages 11 and 25 years
  2. Cirrhosis
  3. Tremor (wing-beating)
  4. Rigidity, dystonia, chorea
  5. Kayser-Fleischer rings (present in 100% of neurologic Wilson's disease patients)
  6. Seizures
  7. Psychosis
- C. Lab
  1. Ceruloplasmin (low or absent in 96% of cases)

        2. Kayser-Fleischer rings present in 100% of neurologic Wilson's cases

        3. Aminoaciduria

    D. Imaging

        1. Caudate and putamen atrophy

    E. Path

        1. Brick-red basal ganglia

        2. Spongy degeneration of the putamen

        3. Alzheimer's astrocytes

        4. Neuronal dropout and axonal degeneration

    F. Inheritance: AR, chromosome 13

    G. Treatment

        1. Copper-poor diet

        2. Sulfide 20 mg tid

        3. Penicillamine 500 to 1,000 mg tid

        4. L-dopa for dystonia

II. Kinky Hair Disease (Menkes' Disease)

    A. Etiology: Copper ATPase Deficiency

    B. Clinical Presentation

        1. Incidence: 1:250,000 live births

        2. Hypothermia

        3. Poor feeding

        4. Seizures

        5. Hypotonia

        6. Cherubic face

        7. Colorless friable kinky hair

        8. Hydronephrosis

    C. Lab

        1. Serial ceruloplasmin levels (falling)

    D. Imaging

        1. Atrophy; focal encephalomalacia

        2. Subdural hematomas

    E. EEG: Hypsarrhythmia

    F. Path

        1. Focal cortical degeneration

        2. Prominent cerebellar neuronal dropout

        3. "Weeping willow" dendritic processes

        4. Increased numbers of mitochondria

    G. Treatment

        1. Copper histidine may be of some benefit

Mucopolysaccharidoses

	Inheritance	Mental Retardation	Dwarf	Corneal Clouding	Other Features
Hurler	AR	+	+	+	Cord compression Retinopathy Zebra bodies
Hunter	X-linked	±	+	±	Nodular skin lesions Progressive deafness Hydrocephalus Cardiac disease
Sanfilippo	AR	+	±	+	Organomegaly Hirsutism Ataxia Dysostosis multiplex Seizures Hearing loss
Morquio	AR	−	+	±	Cord compression
Scheie	AR	−	−	+	Claw hands Retinal degeneration Carpal tunnel syndrome
Maroteaux-Lamy	AR	−	+	+	Hydrocephalus Valvular heart disease Carpal tunnel syndrome
Sly	AR	+	+	±	Hydrocephalus

SPHINGOLIPIDOSES

I. GM-2 Gangliosidosis
  A. Tay-Sachs Disease
    1. Defect: Hexosaminidase A absent and hexosaminidase B increased
    2. Inheritance: AR, chromosome 15
    3. Clinical presentation
      a. Normal development for first 4 to 6 months
      b. Myoclonic jerks
      c. Macular cherry-red spot
      d. Floppy baby
      e. Hyperreflexic
      f. Seizures
      g. Decortication
      h. Macrocephaly
      i. Death by age 3 years
    4. Path
      a. Ballooned neurons
      b. Lamellated lysosomes
    5. Treatment: None
  B. Sandhoff's Disease
    1. Defect: Hexosaminidase A-deficient and hexosaminidase B-deficient
    2. Inheritance: AR, chromosome 5
    3. Clinical presentation: Similar to Tay-Sachs

4. Path: Similar to Tay-Sachs
5. Treatment: None

II. Fabry's Disease
   A. Defect: Alpha-galactosidase A deficiency
   B. Inheritance: X-linked recessive
   C. Clinical Presentation
      1. Symptoms begin in childhood.
      2. Lancinating pains in the limbs
      3. Anhydrosis
      4. Unexplained fever
      5. Angiokeratoma (buttocks, groin)
      6. Renal failure
      7. Stroke
      8. Peripheral neuropathy
   D. Path
      1. Glycolipid storage in blood vessels
      2. Foam cells
   E. Treatment
      1. Phenytoin for pain
      2. Renal transplant for renal failure

III. Gaucher Disease
   A. Defect: Glucocerebroside beta glucosidase deficiency
   B. Inheritance: AR, chromosome 1
   C. Clinical Presentation
      1. Infantile
         a. Developmental regression
         b. Stridor
         c. Poor feeding
         d. Seizures
         e. Spasticity followed by flaccidity
         f. Macular cherry-red spot
         g. Death by age 2 years
      2. Juvenile
         a. Onset in childhood
         b. Dementia
         c. Seizures
         d. Incoordination
         e. Tics
         f. Splenomegaly
      3. Adult
         a. Splenomegaly
         b. Thrombocytopenia
   D. Path
      1. Gaucher cells in bone marrow

IV. Niemann-Pick Disease
   A. Defect: Sphingomyelinase deficiency
   B. Inheritance: AR type C localized to chromosome 18
   C. Clinical Presentation
      1. Infantile: Type A
         a. Developmental regression
         b. Hepatomegaly
         c. Dementia
         d. Hypotonia
         e. Macular cherry-red spot
         f. Death by age 2 years
      2. Juvenile: Type C
         a. Normal infancy
         b. Progressive dementia
         c. Seizures
         d. Spasticity
         e. Vertical gaze paresis
         f. Ataxia
   D. Path
      1. Mulberry cells
      2. Sea-blue histiocytes in Type C

Cutaneous Abnormalities of Metabolic Diseases

Increased pigmentation	Adrenoleukodystrophy
Telangiectasias	Ataxia–telangiectasia
Perioral eruption	Multiple carboxylase deficiency
Absent adipose tissue	Cockayne syndrome
Angiokeratomas	Fabry's disease
	Sialidosis
Xanthomas	Cerebrotendinous xanthomatosis
Ichthyosis	Refsum's disease
Abnormal body/urine odor	
Musty	Phenylketonuria
Maple syrup	Maple syrup urine disease
Sweaty feet	Isovaleric acidemia
	Glutaric acidemia type II
Cat urine	Multiple carboxylase deficiency
Hair abnormalities	
Alopecia	Multiple carboxylase deficiency
	Incontentia pigmenti
Kinky hair	Menkes' kinky hair disease
	Multiple carboxylase deficiency
	Giant axonal neuropathy

Unusual facies
  Coarse   Hunter's/Hurler's diseases
                               GM-1 gangliosidosis
  Slight coarsening   Sanfilippo disease
                               Sialidosis II
Ocular abnormalities
  Cataracts   Galactosemia
                               Cerebrotendinous xanthomatosis
                               Homocystinuria
                               Cockayne's syndrome
  Corneal clouding   Hurler's disease
                               Hunter's disease
                               Morquio's disease
                               Maroteaux-Lamy disease
                               Sialidosis type II
  Cherry-red spot   Tay-Sachs disease
                               Sandhoff's disease
                               GM-1 gangliosidosis
                               Niemann-Pick disease
                               Infantile Gaucher's disease
                               Sialidosis
                               Farber's disease
                               Metachromatic leukodystrophy

WHITE MATTER DISEASES

  I. Metachromatic Leukodystrophy
    A. Defect—Arylsulfatase A deficiency
    B. Inheritance—AR, chromosome 22
    C. Clinical
        1. Normal at birth
        2. Symptoms start at 12—18 months
        3. Weakness
        4. Ataxia
        5. Progressive dementia
        6. Optic atrophy
        7. Abnormal BAEP
        8. Seizures are rare
        9. Cherry-red spot
       10. Schizophrenic symptoms in adult onset
       11. Peripheral neuropathy
       12. Decreased reflexes
    D. Lab
        1. Elevated CSF protein

       2. Positive urine sulfatide test

  E. Imaging

       1. Diffuse demyelination (occurring from frontal to occipital)

       2. Spared subcortical U-fibers

  F. Path

       1. Metachromatic bodies

       2. Diffuse demyelination

  G. Treatment

       1. Bone-marrow transplant slows progression

II. Krabbe's Disease (Globoid Cell Leukodystrophy)

  A. Defect: Galactosyl-ceramide beta galactosidase

  B. Inheritance: AR, chromosome 14

  C. Clinical Presentation

       1. Normal at birth; symptoms start at 3 to 6 months.

       2. Irritable (crabby) baby

       3. Fevers

       4. Seizures

       5. Spasticity followed by hypotonia

       6. Mental retardation

       7. Absent deep-tendon reflexes

       8. Optic atrophy

       9. Peripheral neuropathy

      10. Death by age 2 years

  D. Lab: Elevated CSF protein

  E. NCV: Slow

  F. Imaging

       1. Demyelination

       2. Edematous white matter

       3. Increased signal in thalamus on CT

  G. Path

       1. Globoid cells with PAS positive granules in spleen, marrow, and brain

       2. Demyelination (central and peripheral)

III. Adrenoleukodystrophy (Sudanophilic Cerebral Sclerosis)

  A. Defect: Peroxisomal fatty acid beta oxidation

  B. Inheritance: X-linked recessive

  C. Clinical Presentation

       1. Symptoms start at age 5 to 8 years

       2. Bronze skin pigmentation

       3. Behavioral changes

       4. Dementia

       5. Optic atrophy

       6. Seizures

       7. Adrenal insufficiency

       8. Spastic paraplegia

       9. Hypogonadism
     10. Peripheral neuropathy
  D. Lab
    1. Elevated CSF protein
    2. Elevated CSF white cells
    3. Decreased cortisol in some cases
    4. Increased very-long-chain fatty acids
  E. Imaging
    1. Demyelination (occipital to frontal)
  F. Path
    1. Demyelination
    2. Spares subcortical U-fibers
    3. Sudanophilic lipid inclusions in macrophages and Schwann cells

IV. Pelizaeus-Merzbacher Disease (Tigroid Leukodystrophy)
  A. Defect: Impaired myelin formation
  B. Inheritance: X-linked recessive
  C. Clinical presentation
    1. Onset at or before age 3 months
    2. Infantile trembling eye movements
    3. Developmental delay
    4. Optic atrophy
    5. Spasticity
    6. Ataxia
    7. Pancerebellar syndrome
    8. Involuntary movements
  D. Lab: Normal CSF protein
  E. NCV: Normal
  F. Imaging
    1. Ventricular dilatation
    2. Demyelination
    3. Cerebellar atrophy
  G. Path
    1. Demyelination
    2. No sparing of subcortical U-fibers
    3. Weigert's myelin stain—thin white matter with black dots (Tigroid)
    4. Remaining oligodendroglia have inclusions.

V. Canavan's Disease
  A. Defect: Aspartoacylase deficiency
  B. Inheritance: AR
  C. Clinical Presentation
    1. Symptoms begin at age 2 to 4 months
    2. Developmental delay
    3. Hypotonia progressing to spasticity
    4. Megalencephaly

    5. Optic atrophy

  D. Lab: CSF normal

  E. NCV: Normal

  F. Imaging

    1. Demyelination

    2. Cystic white matter

  G. Path

    1. Cystic white matter degeneration

    2. Intramyelinic vacuolization

VI. Alexander's Disease

  A. Defect: Unknown

  B. Inheritance: Unknown

  C. Clinical Presentation

    1. Symptoms start in the first year of life.

    2. Loss of milestones

    3. Spasticity

    4. Megalencephaly

    5. Seizures

  D. Lab: Normal

  E. Imaging: Predominantly frontal demyelination

  F. Path

    1. Rosenthal fibers (hyaline, eosinophilic, argyrophilic) usually subpial/ependymal

    2. Demyelination

VII. Zellweger's Syndrome

  A. Defect: Abnormal very-long-chain fatty acid metabolism

  B. Inheritance: AR

  C. Clinical Presentation

    1. Manifests at birth

    2. Intrauterine growth retardation

    3. Developmental delay

    4. Limb contractures

    5. Hepatomegaly

    6. Floppy baby

    7. Abnormal facies

  D. Lab

    1. Elevated bilirubin

    2. Elevated serum iron

    3. Elevated CSF protein

    4. Elevated very-long-chain fatty acids

  E. Imaging/Path

    1. Demyelination

    2. Atrophy

    3. Neuronal migration defects

VIII. Peripheral nerve involvement is found in the following diseases:

   A. Metachromatic Leukodystrophy
   B. Krabbe's disease
   C. Canavan's disease
   D. Adrenoleukodystrophy
IX. White Matter Disease Summary Table

Disease	Genetics	Etiology	CSF	Special Features
Metachromatic leukodystophy	AR chromosome 22	Arylsulfatase A deficiency	Increased protein	Frontal demyelinates first
Krabbe's	AR chromosome 14	Beta galactosidase deficiency	Increased protein	MRI thalamus hyperintensities
Adrenoleukodystrophy	X-recessive	Decreased beta oxidation of long-chain fatty acids	Increased protein and WBCs	Occipital demyelinates first; sudanophilic
Pelizaeus Merzbacher	X-recessive	Abnormal myelin formation	Normal protein	Roving eyes; tigroid
Canavan's	AR	Aspartoacytylase deficiency		Cystic degeneration; big head
Alexander's	Unknown	Unknown		Rosenthal fibers; big head

ALCOHOL

  I. Minor Withdrawal/Alcoholic Hallucinosis
    A. Begins after several hours
    B. Resolves after 48 hours
    C. Symptoms
       1. Hyperandrenergic
          a. Tremor
          b. Sweating
          c. Tachycardia
          d. Hypertension
       2. Headache
       3. Anxiety
       4. Agitation
       5. Depression
       6. Insomnia
       7. Transient hallucinations (visual, tactile, and auditory)
    D. Treatment
       1. Benzodiazepines
       2. Barbiturates
 II. Seizures
    A. Usually occur between 12 and 48 hours after last drink
    B. Clinical
       1. Generalized tonic-clonic seizure
       2. Usually single seizure

C. Evaluation
   1. CT head: usually negative with a normal neurologic exam
D. Treatment
   1. No long-term anticonvulsant therapy
   2. Benzodiazepines
   3. Barbiturates
   4. Carbamazepine and valproic acid may be effective acutely.
III. Delirium Tremens
   A. Usually begins 48 to 96 hours after last drink.
   B. Clinical presentation
      1. Hyperandrenergic
      2. Delirium
      3. Persistent hallucinations
      4. Hyperpyrexia
      5. Violent behavior
   C. Treatment
      1. Benzodiazepines
      2. Barbiturates
      3. Clonidine
      4. Beta blockers
      5. Carbamazepine
      6. Hydration
IV. Benzodiazepines

	Oral Absorption	Elimination	Dosage
Chlordiazepoxide	Intermediate	Slow 100 mg	
Diazepam	Rapid	Slow	20 mg
Lorazepam	Intermediate	Intermediate	4 mg
Oxazepam	Slow	Rapid	120 mg

V. Wernicke-Korsakoff Syndrome
   A. Wernicke
      1. Dementia in 90% of cases
      2. Lethargy
      3. Apathy
      4. Amnesia
      5. Ophthalmoparesis
      6. Gait ataxia in 80% of cases
      7. Autonomic signs
   B. Korsakoff
      1. Dementia
      2. Confabulation that gradually disappears
      3. Amnesia (anterograde and retrograde)
   C. EEG: Diffuse slowing
   D. Path

      1. Neuronal dropout
      2. Axonal degeneration
      3. Demyelination
      4. Prominent blood vessels
      5. Gliosis
      6. Affected areas include:
         a. Thalamus (dorsomedial nucleus and medial pulvinar)
         b. Hypothalamus (mamillary bodies)
         c. Midbrain (oculomotor nucleus and periacqueductal area)
         d. Pons (abducens nucleus and medial vestibular nucleus)
         e. Cerebellum
   E. Treatment: Thiamine 100 mg/d for 3 days (minimum)
      1. Ophthalmoparesis resolves in 65% of cases.
      2. Ataxia resolves in 50% of cases.
      3. Amnesia resolves in less than 20% of cases.
      4. Treated mortality rate is 10%.
VI. Alcoholic Cerebellar Degeneration
   A. Clinical Presentation
      1. Truncal ataxia
      2. Arm ataxia is less prominent.
      3. Nystagmus and dysarthria are rare.
   B. Path
      1. Neuronal loss and gliosis in all three cerebellar layers
      2. Superior vermis most affected
      3. Secondary degeneration of the inferior olive and deep cerebellar nuclei
   C. Imaging: Vermian atrophy
VII. Alcoholic Polyneuropathy
   A. Etiology: Most likely secondary to vitamin B deficiency
   B. Clinical Presentation
      1. Occurs in 20% of alcoholics
      2. Insidious onset
      3. Impaired vibratory sense initially
      4. Distal paresthesias and lancinating pain (calves and soles)
      5. Loss of reflexes
      6. Weakness may be severe.
      7. Peripheral nerve pressure palsies are common.
      8. Postural hypotension
   B. Path: Axonal degeneration with concomitant demyelination
VIII. Marchiafava-Bignami Disease
   A. Clinical Presentation
      1. Insidious cerebral dysfunction
      2. Dementia
      3. Depression
      4. Apathy

        5. Delusions

        6. Slowly progressive with death in 3 to 6 years

   B. Path

        1. Necrosis of the central zone of the corpus callosum

        2. No inflammation

        3. Distinct foci coalesce to form a confluent area

        4. Symmetric demyelination and necrosis may also occur in:

           a. Anterior commisure

           b. Posterior commisure

           c. Centrum semiovale

           d. Subcortical white matter

           e. Long association bundles

           f. Middle cerebellar peduncle

   C. Imaging: Corpus callosum necrosis and symmetric demyelination

   D. Treatment: None

IX. Central Pontine Myelinolysis

   A. Etiology: Rapid correction of hyponatremia

   B. Clinical Presentation

        1. Behavioral abnormalities

        2. Ophthalmoparesis

        3. Quadriplegia

        4. Hyperreflexia

        5. Bulbar and pseudobulbar palsy

        6. Seizures

        7. Coma

        8. Death usually occurs within days.

   C. Path

        1. Demyelination of the basis pontis

        2. Extrapontine demyelination occurs in 10% of cases.

   D. Imaging: Demyelination of the basis pontis

   E. Brain stem auditory evoked potential (BAEP): Prolongs I through V and III through V latencies

   F. Treatment: none

6

Demyelinating Diseases

MULTIPLE SCLEROSIS

I. Epidemiology
  A. Onset: Females aged 20 to 35 years; males aged 35 to 45 years
  B. Female:male ratio is 2:1.
  C. Most common in Caucasians.
  D. First-degree relatives have a 10- to 20-fold greater risk.
  E. Residence for the first 15 years of life determines risk.
II. Etiology
  A. Unknown
  B. Genetic Factors: HLA DR2, A3, B7, DQW1, b1, a1
  C. Environmental Factors
III. Pathology
  A. Plaques—areas of demyelination
    1. Usually occur in deep white matter.
    2. Usually occur near ventricles, corpus callosum, optic nerve.
    3. May occur in spinal cord, gray matter, and brain stem.
  B. Acute
    1. Demyelination
    2. Sparing of axons
    3. Perivascular infiltrate with lymphocytes, macrophages, and plasma cells near the leading edge of demyelination
    4. Perivascular edema
    5. Activated astrocytes and hyperplastic oligodendroglia at border
  C. Chronic
    1. Oligodendrocytes disappear
    2. Axonal degeneration
    3. Astrocytic hypertrophy and hyperplasia—sclerosis
IV. Presentation

Symptom	Affected patients (%)
Weakness	26
Sensory change	25
Optic neuritis	21
Ataxia	14
Urinary function change	14
Other	10

V. Clinical Course

Course	Affected Patients (%)
Benign	30
Neurologic dysfunction	60
Malignant	10
Relapsing remitting	35
Relapsing progressive	45
Chronic progressive	20

VI. Prognosis
    A. Better prognosis for females, predominantly sensory disease, less residual after relapse
    B. Worse prognosis for males, multifocal disease, progressive disease
    C. Kurtzke's Five-Year Rule: Minimal dysfunction at 5 years correlates with minimal dysfunction at 15 years.

VII. Diagnosis
    A. Schumacher's Criteria
        1. Two separate CNS lesions
        2. Two separate attacks or 6 months progression
        3. Objective findings on examination
        4. White matter disease
        5. Age 10 to 50 years (usually)
        6. No other disease that explains the constellation of signs and symptoms
    B. Laboratory and imaging serve as confirmatory tests.
    C. Poser Committee for the Diagnosis of Multiple Sclerosis

Category	Relapses	No. of Lesions (Clinical/Paraclinical)	CSF (OCB/IgG)
Clinically definite	2	(1–2/0–1)	NA
Laboratory supported definite	1–2	(1–2/0–1)	+
Clinically probable	1–2	(1–2/0–1)	—
Laboratory supported probable	2	(0/0)	+

VIII. Physical Examination
    A. Signs and symptoms typically develop over hours to days.
    B. Signs and symptoms are highly variable based on the lesions.
    C. Optic Neuritis
        1. Red, swollen optic disc followed by disc pallor
        2. Decreased visual acuity, central scotoma, red desaturation
        3. Marcus-Gunn pupil (afferent pupillary defect)
    D. Paresis
    E. Spasticity (especially in chronic disease)
    F. Ataxia
    G. Fatigue
    H. Heat Sensitivity (Uhthoff's sign)
    I. Depression

    J. Euphoria

    K. Trigeminal Neuralgia

    L. Lhermitte's Sign

    M. Tonic Spasms

    N. Diplopia

    O. Pain (often dysesthetic)

    P. Bladder Dysfunction

        1. Uninhibited neurogenic bladder—frequent urination

        2. Flaccid neurogenic bladder—urinary retention

    Q. Bowel dysfunction

    R. Sexual dysfunction

    S. Hyperactive reflexes

IX. Imaging

    A. MRI: proton density, T2, FLAIR

        1. MRI is abnormal in 85% to 97% of definite MS cases.

        2. MRI is abnormal in 60% to 85% of suspected MS cases.

        3. Abnormalities

            a. Multiple periventricular white matter lesions

            b. Frequent ventricular capping

            c. Ovoid-shaped lesions that are <5 mm (Dawson's fingers)

            d. Corpus callosum thinning or scalloping in 93% of cases

            e. Atrophy in chronic disease

            f. Enhancement with active lesions

X. Cerebrospinal Fluid (CSF)

    A. Opening pressure is normal.

    B. WBC usually <20 lymphs, >50 to 100 rare.

    C. Protein mildly elevated at 50 to 60, >100 rare.

    D. Myelin basic protein is high for first 2 weeks of exacerbation.

    E. CSF oligoclonal bands are elevated in 90% of definite MS cases.

    F. IgG synthesis rate is >3 in 80% to 90% of MS cases.

    G. IgG index (also known as Tourtellott's formula): (CSF IgG/serum IgG)/(CSF albumin/ serum albumin)

        1. Index is >0.7 in 90% of MS cases.

        2. First abnormality seen in CSF

    H. Myelin basic protein increased to 4 ng/mL in 80% of cases.

XI. Evoked Potentials

    A. Visual Evoked Potential (VEP)

        1. Often remain abnormal years after optic neuritis

        2. Prolonged in 40% of possible MS cases, 60% of probable MS cases, and 85% of definite MS cases

    B. Somatosensory Evoked Potential (SSEP)

        1. Prolonged in 50% of possible MS cases, 70% of probable MS cases, and 80% of definite MS cases

    C. Brain Stem Auditory Evoked Potential (BAEP)

1. Prolonged in 30% of possible MS cases, 40% of probable MS cases, and 70% of definite MS cases

XII. Treatment

  A. Immune modulation

    1. "Slam and Taper"—High-dose steroids followed by slow taper

      a. Reduces duration and severity of exacerbations

      b. Does not change the outcome or frequency

      c. Methylprednisolone 500 mg bid for 5d

      d. Prednisone taper

        (1) 60 mg qd for 7d, then

        (2) 60 mg qod for 7d, then

        (3) 40 mg qod for 7d, then

        (4) 20 mg qod for 7d, then

        (5) Stop

      e. H_2 blocker ulcer prophylaxis

      f. Follow blood sugar.

      g. Monitor for signs and symptoms of infection.

      h. Check urinalysis and urine culture and sensitivity on each patient.

    2. Interferons

      a. Interferon beta-1b (Betaseron)

        (1) Reduces the number and severity of exacerbations

        (2) Reduces lesion load on MRI

        (3) Dosage: 8 million units SQ qod

        (4) Site: Rotate anterior thigh, buttock, abdomen.

        (5) Premedicate: Tylenol 650 mg 4 hours before, at, and after injection

        (6) Labs: CBC, LFTs every 3 months

        (7) Precautions: Contraception

        (8) Side Effects

          (a) Local skin reaction with inflammation, thickening, and necrosis

          (b) Flu-like symptoms usually in first 2 weeks

          (c) Fatigue

          (d) Decreased white blood cell count (WBC), platelets, hematocrit

          (e) Increased GGT, GOT > alkaline phosphatase

          (f) Depression

      b. Interferon beta-1a (Avonex)

        (1) Slows accumulation of physical disability and decreases frequency of exacerbations

        (2) Dosage: 30 mg IM q week

        (3) Lab: CBC, platelets, fluid balance profile at least q 6 months

        (4) Precautions: Pregnancy, seizures, cardiac disease, depression

        (5) Side Effects

          (a) Flu-like symptoms (61%)

          (b) Injection site reactions

          (c) Myalgias

        (d) Fever, chills
        (e) Headache
        (f) Depression
        (g) Bronchospasm
        (h) Anxiety
  c. Glatiramer acetate (Copaxone/Copolymer-1)
    (1) Reduces frequency of relapses
    (2) Dosage: 20 mg SQ qd
    (3) Labs: Routine monitoring usually unnecessary
    (4) Side Effects
        (a) Injection site reactions
        (b) Immediate postinjection reaction (10%)
        (c) Transient chest pain (26%)
        (d) Anxiety
        (e) Arthralgias
        (f) Asthenia
        (g) Vasodilatation
        (h) Hypertonia
3. Other immunomodulators undergoing study
  a. Azathioprine
  b. Methotrexate
  c. Cyclophosphamide
  d. Cyclosporin
  e. Linomide (cardiotoxicity and myocardial ischemia)
  f. Sulfasalazine
  g. Leustatin
4. Mitoxantrone
  a. Indicated for reducing neurologic disability in patients with secondary progressive MS.
  b. Dosage: 12 mg/m^2 given as a 15-minute IV infusion every 3 months with a maximum lifetime dose of 140 mg/m^2.
  c. Monitoring:
    (1) Cardiac ECHO for alteration in LVEF.
    (2) Liver function tests prior to each treatment
    (3) CBC prior to each treatment
    (4) Fluid balance profile prior to each treatment
  d. Side effects
    (1) Nausea
    (2) Alopecia
    (3) Menstrual disorders
    (4) Upper respiratory infections
    (5) Urinary tract infection
    (6) Arrhythmia
    (7) Leukopenia

B. Symptomatic Treatment
1. Spasticity
a. Baclofen—start at 10 mg qhs and titrate
b. Benzodiazepines
c. Dantrolene—25 mg qd and titrate
d. Intrathecal baclofen pump if refractory
e. Botulinum toxin injections
f. Tizanidine (Zanaflex)
2. Fatigue
a. Amantadine—100 mg qd bid
b. Pemoline—18.75 mg qd short term
c. 3,4 DAP and 4 AP investigational
d. Modafinil 200 mg qAM or bid.
3. Depression
a. Desipramine—25 mg qhs and titrate
b. Sertraline—50 mg qd and titrate
4. Trigeminal neuralgia
a. Carbamazepine—200 mg qd and titrate
b. Baclofen
c. Phenytoin
d. Rhizotomy
5. Paroxysmal disorders
a. Carbamazepine—pain
b. Hydroxyzine—itching
6. Pain
a. Amitriptyline—25 mg qhs and titrate
b. Carbamazepine—200 mg qd and titrate
7. Uninhibited neurogenic bladder (anticholinergics)
a. Propantheline—15 mg qid and titrate
b. Oxybutynin—5 mg bid and titrate
c. Catheterization
8. Neurogenic bladder (cholinergics)
a. Bethanechol
b. Baclofen
c. Catheterization
XIII. Differential Diagnosis
A. MS Variants
1. Devic's syndrome (transverse myelitis and optic neuritis)
2. Malignant MS (Marburg disease)
B. Other Disorders in the Differential Diagnosis
1. Acute disseminated encephalomyelitis (ADEM)
2. Optic neuritis
3. Acute transverse myelitis
4. Elsberg sacral radiculopathy (sexual and bladder dysfunction)

5. Devic's syndrome
6. Vitamin B_{12} deficiency
7. Rheumatoid arthritis (collagen vascular disease)
8. Sarcoid
9. Human T-cell lymphotrophic virus (HTLV-I) (tropical spastic paraparesis)
10. Adult-onset adrenoleukodystrophy
11. Primary lateral sclerosis
12. Lyme disease
13. HIV
14. Sjögren's disease
15. Systemic lupus erythematosis
16. Progressive multifocal leukoencephalopathy
17. Behçet's syndrome

7

Cerebrovascular Diseases

TRANSIENT ISCHEMIC ATTACK (TIA)

I. Epidemiology
  - A. Risk of stroke after TIA
    1. 4% to 8% in first month
    2. 12% in first year
    3. 24% to 29% in first 5 years
  - B. TIAs occur before:
    1. 25% to 50% of atherothrombotic infarcts
    2. 10% to 30% cardioembolic infarcts
    3. 10% to 15% lacunar infarcts
II. Clinical Features
  - A. Abrupt Onset
  - B. Lasts 5 to 20 minutes (less than 24 hours by definition)
    1. TIAs lasting longer than 1 hour are often associated with small areas of infarction.

STROKE

I. Epidemiology
  - A. More than 500,000 strokes occur per year.
  - B. Third leading cause of death in the United States
  - C. 25% occur in people under age 65 years.
II. Cerebral Blood Flow (CBF)
  - A. 50 mL/100 g/min normal
  - B. 20 mL/100 g/min change in electrophysiologic activity
  - C. 10 mL/100 g/min irreversible ischemia
  - D. Increasing CBF increases collateral blood flow.
  - E. Oxygen delivery equals the cerebral blood flow multiplied by the blood oxygen content.
    1. $DO_2 = CBF \times CaO_2$
III. Stroke Subtypes
  - A. Atherothromboembolic
    1. Clinical criteria
      a. Sudden, gradual, stepwise, or fluctuating
      b. Absence of a cardioembolic source
      c. Prior TIA in the same vascular distribution

  d. Concurrent coronary or peripheral artery disease

 2. Imaging

  a. CT: Bland or hemorrhagic infarct

   (1) Possible hyperdense artery

  b. MRI: Bland or hemorrhagic infarct

   (1) Possible absent flow void

  c. Carotid U/S: Stenosis > 50% or ulcer > 2 mm

  d. Arteriography: Stenosis > 50% or ulcer > 2 mm

  e. Transcranial Doppler (TCD): Normal, collateralization, or absent flow

B. Cardioembolic

 1. Clinical criteria

  a. Sudden onset but may be stepwise/progressive

  b. High Risk—Atrial fibrillation, prosthetic valve, left ventricular thrombus, left atrial thrombus, dilated cardial myopathy, sick sinus syndrome, myocardial infarction (MI) in prior 4 weeks

  c. Moderate Risk—Congestive heart failure (CHF), atrial flutter, mitral valve prolapse, atrial septal defect, PFO, bioprosthetic valve, ventricular hypokinesis, myocardial infarction between 4 and 6 weeks

  d. Recent TIA/stroke in other vascular territories

  e. Evidence of systemic embolization

 2. Imaging

  a. CT: Bland or hemorrhagic infarct

   (1) Possible hyperdense artery

  b. MRI: Bland or hemorrhagic infarct

   (1) Possible absent flow void

  c. Carotid U/S: Various; stenosis typically < 50%

  d. Arteriography: May show occlusion of a vessel.

  e. TEE: May show thrombotic etiology.

  f. TCD: Normal, absent flow, or distal occlusion

C. Lacunar

 1. Clinical criteria

  a. Abrupt or gradual onset

  b. H/O hypertension or diabetes mellitus

  c. No cortical findings

  d. Compatible with a lacunar syndrome

  e. No evidence of embolic sources

 2. Imaging

  a. CT: Infarct < 1.5 cm

  b. MRI: Infarct < 1.5 cm

  c. TCD: Normal or unrevealing

  Note: Description of a stroke by etiology and vascular distribution provides the most meaningful information about the stroke. The dichotomy between cortical and subcortical is not always clear. These terms are, however, frequently used.

Cortical—Stroke involves the cerebral hemispheric gray matter and often involves the underlying white matter. Cortical deficits are dependent on the vessel involved.

Middle cerebral artery—Contralateral hemiparesis and sensory loss (greater in the upper extremity and face), homonymous hemianopia, aphasia/aprosodia, gaze abnormalities, extinction, astereognosis, apraxia

Anterior cerebral artery—Contralateral hemiparesis and sensory loss (greater in the lower extremity), disconnection syndromes, behavior disturbances (abulia, akinetic mutism)

Posterior cerebral artery—Contralateral homonymous hemianopia with macular sparing preserved optokinetic nystagmus (OKN), cortical blindness, disconnection syndrome

Subcortical—Stroke involves the white matter as well as basal ganglia and brain stem nuclei. Cortical signs such as aphasia are typically absent.

Lacunar Syndromes
1. Pure sensory
   a. Ventral posterior thalamus
   b. Contralateral sensory loss
2. Pure motor
   a. Posterior limb internal capsule, cerebral peduncle, pons, or hemispheric white matter
   b. Contralateral weakness
3. Ataxic hemiparesis
   a. Basis pontis but localizes poorly
   b. Contralateral weakness and ataxia
4. Dysarthria clumsy hand syndrome
   a. Genu of the internal capsule
   b. Contralateral clumsy hand and dysarthria
5. Thalamic dementia
   a. Thalamus
   b. Subcortical dementia
6. Sensorimotor
   a. Thalamus and internal capsule
   b. Contralateral sensory loss and weakness
7. Hemiballismus
   a. Subthalamic nucleus
   b. Contralateral hemiballismus
8. Status lacunaris
   a. Multiple widespread lacunes
   b. Parkinsonism, dementia
9. Claude's syndrome
   a. Midbrain tegmentum, red nucleus, cranial nerve (CN) III
   b. Ipsilateral CN III palsy
   c. Contralateral ataxia, tremor

10. Benedikt's syndrome
    a. Midbrain tegmentum, red nucleus, CN III, cerebral peduncle
    b. Ipsilateral CN III palsy
    c. Contralateral ataxia, tremor, and weakness
11. Weber's syndrome
    a. Ventral midbrain, CN III, cerebral peduncle
    b. Ipsilateral CN III palsy
    c. Contralateral weakness
12. Parinaud's syndrome
    a. Dorsorostral midbrain and posterior commisure
    b. Paralysis of upgaze, convergence-retraction nystagmus, lid retraction, and light near dissociation
13. Nothnagel's syndrome
    a. Dorsal midbrain, brachium conjunctivum, CN III, medial longitudinal fasciculus (MLF)
    b. Ipsilateral ataxia, CN III palsy, and vertical gaze palsy
14. Raymond-Cestan syndrome
    a. Mid pons, middle cerebellar peduncle, corticospinal tract
    b. Ipsilateral ataxia
    c. Contralateral weakness
15. One-and-a-half syndrome
    a. Paramedian pontine reticular formation (PPRF) or CN VI and MLF
    b. Ipsilateral horizontal gaze palsy
    c. Contralateral intranuclear ophthalmoplegia (INO)
16. Foville's syndrome
    a. PPRF, CN VI, CN VII, corticospinal tract
    b. Ipsilateral horizontal gaze palsy, CN VII palsy
    c. Contralateral weakness, sensory loss, intranuclear ophthalmoplegia (INO)
17. Millard-Gubler syndrome
    a. Ventral pons, CN VI and VII fascicles corticospinal tracts
    b. Ipsilateral CN VI and CN VII palsy
    c. Contralateral weakness
18. Raymond's syndrome
    a. Ventral pons, CN VI fascicles, and corticospinal tract
    b. Ipsilateral CN VI palsy
    c. Contralateral weakness
19. Babinski-Nageotte syndrome
    a. Dorsolateral pontomedullary junction
    b. Ipsilateral ataxia, facial sensory loss, Horner's syndrome
    c. Contralateral weakness, sensory loss in the body vertigo, vomiting, and nystagmus
20. Wallenberg's syndrome
    a. Dorsolateral medulla, restiform body, CN V, IX, and X

        b. Ipsilateral ataxia, Horner's syndrome, facial sensory loss
        c. Contralateral loss of pain and temperature
  21. Cestan-Chenais syndrome
        a. Lateral medulla
        b. Ipsilateral ataxia, Horner's syndrome, facial sensory loss
        c. Contralateral hemibody sensory loss and weakness
  22. Avellis's syndrome
        a. Lateral medulla, CN IX, CN X, lateral spinothalamic tracts
        b. Ipsilateral paralysis soft palate, vocal cords, posterior pharynx
        c. Contralateral hemiparesis and sensory loss
  23. Vernet's syndrome
        a. Lateral medulla, CN IX, X, and XI
        b. Ipsilateral paralysis palate, sternocleidomastoid (SCM), decreased taste posterior tongue
        c. Contralateral hemiparesis
  24. Jackson's syndrome
        a. Lateral medulla, CN IX, X, XI, and XII
        b. Ipsilateral paralysis palate, vocal cords, SCM, tongue
        c. Contralateral weakness and sensory loss
  25. Preolivary
        a. Anterior medulla, CN XII, pyramid
        b. Ipsilateral tongue weakness
        c. Contralateral hemiparesis

Bulbar vs. Pseudobulbar Signs

	Bulbar	Pseudobulbar
Tongue		
Size	Atrophy	Normal
Movement	Decreased	Slow
Fasciculation	Present	Absent
Speech	Flaccid	Spastic
Face	Weak	Weak
Emotional lability	Absent	Present
Jaw jerk	Absent	Present
Gag	Absent	Hyperactive
Extraocular movements	Decreased	Decreased

IV. Cortical Localization
  A. Occipital Lobe
    1. Mesial—visual defects, agnosia, and hallucinations
      a. Alexia without agraphia (dominant Broca's area)
      b. Anton's syndrome (bilateral—denial of blindness)
    2. Lateral—alexia with agraphia, impaired OKN, impaired ipsilateral scanning
  B. Parietal Lobe
    1. Postcentral—contralateral sensory loss and tactile extinct

2. Mesial—transcortical sensory aphasia/aprosodia
3. Lateral
    a. Dominant (Gerstmann's syndrome)
        (1) Finger agnosia, acalculia, R/L confusion, alexia (supramarginal), alexia with agraphia (angular), and ideational apraxia
    b. Nondominant—anosognosia, autopropognosia, neglect, constructional apraxia, dressing apraxia
C. Parieto-occipital Bilateral
    1. Balint's syndrome—visual simultagnosia (unable to appreciate the meaning of the whole), apraxia of gaze, optic ataxia, altitudinal neglect, decreased visual attention
D. Occipito-temporal
    1. Polyopsia (seeing a single target as many)
    2. Palinopsia (persistence of image after removal of object)
    3. Visual alloesthesia (field transposition)
E. Temporal Lobe
    1. Bilateral anterior poles (Klüver-Bucy syndrome) docility, hyperoral, hypersexual, hypomobile, hypermetamorphosis, visual agnosia
    2. Inferomedial (hippocampus/amygdala)—amnesia
    3. Inferolateral
        a. Dominant—transcortical sensory aphasia, anomia
        b. Nondominant—comprehensive aprosodia
    4. Superolateral
        a. Dominant—pure word deafness, sensory aphasia
        b. Nondominant—sensory amusia, sensory aprosodia
        c. Bilateral—auditory agnosia
F. Temporal Lobe Aura
    1. Mesial—epigastric, fear, déjà-vu, micropsia
    2. Lateral—hallucination, receptive aphasia, vertigo
G. Frontal Lobe
    1. Mesial (cingulate gyrus)—akinesia, perseveration, transcortical motor aphasia
    2. Lateral—impaired contralateral saccades, pure agraphia, motor aphasia
    3. Frontal pole—blunted affect, impotence, speech apraxia, impaired goal-oriented behavior
    4. Nondominant orbitofrontal—anxiety, depression
    5. Dominant dorsofrontal—anger, hostility
V. Aphasia

	Repetition	Fluency	Comprehension	Naming
Broca	−	−	+	−
Wernicke	−	+	−	−
Conduction	−	+	+	±
Transcortical motor	+	−	+	−
Transcortical sensory	+	+	−	−
Mixed transcortical	+	−	−	−
Global	−	−	−	−

VI. Vascular Distributions
  A. Posterior Cerebral Artery
    1. Mesencephalic perforating artery
      a. Tectum
      b. Cerebral peduncles
    2. Posterior thalamoperforating artery
      a. Hypothalamus
      b. Subthalamus
      c. Midline and medial thalamic nuclei
    3. Posterior medial choroidal artery
      a. Quadrigeminal plate
      b. Pineal gland
      c. Choroid plexus
      d. Medial dorsal nucleus of the thalamus
    4. Posterior lateral choroidal artery
      a. Choroid plexus
      b. Fornix
      c. Medial dorsal nucleus of the thalamus
      d. Pulvinar
      e. Part of the lateral geniculate body
  B. Anterior Choroidal Artery
    1. Proximal
      a. Optic tract
      b. Genu of the internal capsule
      c. Medial globus pallidus
    2. Lateral
      a. Piriform cortex
      b. Uncus
      c. Hippocampus
      d. Dentate
      e. Tail of the caudate nucleus
    3. Medial
      a. Cerebral peduncle
      b. Substantia nigra
      c. VA nucleus of the thalamus
      d. VL nucleus of the thalamus
      e. Red nucleus
    4. Distal
      a. Lateral geniculate body
      b. Posterior limb of the internal capsule
      c. Origin of the optic radiations
  C. Anterior Cerebral Artery
    1. Recurrent artery of Heubner
      a. Head of the caudate nucleus

    b. Putamen
    c. Anterior limb of the internal capsule
  D. Middle Cerebral Artery
    1. Medial lenticulostriate arteries
        a. Lateral segment of the globus pallidus
    2. Lateral lenticulostriate arteries
        a. Putamen
        b. Superior internal capsule
        c. Caudate
        d. Corona radiata
VII. Stroke in the Young Adult
  A. Epidemiology
    1. Incidence—0.6/100,000 for age 0 to 14 years; 3/100,000 for age < 35 years; 20/100,000 for age 35 to 44 years
  B. Atherosclerosis, vasculopathy, and embolism account for 70% of these cases.
  C. Etiology
    1. Vascular dissection (trauma, strangulation, arthritis)
    2. Moyamoya disease (large vessel occlusions)
    3. Fibromuscular dysplasia
    4. Vasculitis
        a. Infectious
        b. Necrotizing
            (1) PAN, Wegener's syndrome, Churg-Strauss syndrome, lymphomatosis
        c. Collagen vascular disease
            (1) SLE, RA, Sjögren's disease, scleroderma
        d. Systemic disease
            (1) Behçet's disease, sarcoid, ulcerative colitis
        e. Giant-cell arteritis
            (1) Takayasu's syndrome, temporal
        f. Hypersensitivity (drug, chemical)
        g. Neoplastic
        h. Primary CNS vasculitis
    5. Migraine (diagnosis of exclusion)
    6. Cardiac embolism
    7. Hypercoaguable state (primary)
        a. ATIII deficiency
        b. Protein C deficiency
        c. Protein S deficiency
        e. Dysfibrinogenemia
        f. Factor XII deficiency
        g. Antiphospholipid antibodies
        h. Fibrinolytic abnormalities
        i. Activated protein C resistance, Factor V Leiden mutation (gene on 1 q 23)
        j. Hyperhomocysteinemia (gene on 1 q 36)

      k. CADASIL (gene on 19 p13)—recurrent subcortical infarcts with spared U fibers

    8. Hypercoaguable state (secondary)
      a. Malignancy
      b. Pregnancy
      c. Oral contraceptives
      d. Disseminated intravascular coagulation
      e. Nephrotic syndrome

    9. Platelet abnormalities
      a. Myeloproliferative disease
      b. Diabetes mellitus
      c. Heparin-induced thrombocytopenia

   10. Rheology
      a. Homocystinuria (cystathione synthase deficiency)
      b. Polycythemia vera
      c. Sickle cell disease
      d. Thrombotic thrombocytopenia purpura

   11. Hyperlipidemia
   12. Connective-tissue disease (Ehlers-Danlos syndrome, Menkes' syndrome, homocystinuria)
   13. Organic acidemia
   14. Mitochondrial myopathy (MELAS)
   15. Fabry's disease (alpha-galactosidase A deficiency)
   16. Vasospasm (cocaine)

VIII. Evaluation
  A. Imaging
    1. CT head without contrast
    2. MRI/MRA
      a. Diffusion weighted images may identify ischemic lesions within minutes of symptom onset.
      b. Diffusion perfusion imaging may identify a mismatch (continued perfusion).
    3. Carotid ultrasound
    4. Transcranial Doppler
    5. Transesophageal echocardiogram or transthoracic echocardiogram
    6. Cerebral angiography
  B. EKG
  C. Chest X-ray
  D. Initial laboratory testing
    1. CBC, chem 20, PT, PTT, cholesterol, triglycerides, RPR, beta HCG
    2. Cardiac enzymes, urine drug screen
  E. Further laboratory testing
    1. Vasculitis—RA, ANA, C-reactive protein, ESR, complement (C3, C4, CH50), P-ANCA, C-ANCA, Scl-70, anticentromere antibody, ACE level, immunoglobulins, cryoglobulins, Coomb's test, Schirmer test, CSF

2. Hypercoaguable—Serum viscosity; fibrinogen; ATIII; protein C; protein S; bleeding time; SPEP; HIV; factor V Leiden mutation; factors VII, VIII, IX, X, XI, XII, XIII; thrombin time; fibrin degradation products; sickle prep; antiphospholipid antibodies

IX. Treatment
   A. Vitals q4h
   B. Neurologic checks q4h
   C. Daily weight
   D. Strict input/output q4h
   E. NPO for first 24 hours
   F. Bedrest for first 24 hours
   G. Fluid Balance Profile (FBP) qAM
   H. Oxygen
   I. IV NS bolus 15 mL/kg, then 100 mL/hr (unless CHF, pulmonary edema)
   J. Hypertension (treat for SBP > 220 or DBP > 130)
      1. Nitropaste
      2. Labetolol
      3. ACE inhibitors
      4. Nitroprusside
      5. Avoid calcium channel blockers
   K. Temperature
      1. Treat fever with Tylenol
      2. Evaluate for etiology (pneumonia, UTI, etc.)
   L. Cerebral Edema (greatest at 72 to 96 hours after infarct)
      1. 25% albumin 100 mL and Lasix 20 mg q6h
      2. Hyperventilate for an emergency only
   M. Anticoagulation
      1. Heparin
         a. Criteria for use (not definitively proven beneficial)
            (1) Small-to-moderate size infarct
            (2) Initial head CT without hemorrhage
            (3) Diastolic blood pressure controlled
            (4) Patient not stuporous
            (5) No major contraindications to anticoagulation
            (6) Continue heparin with hemorrhagic conversion if no clinical deterioration.
         b. Protocol
            (1) No bolus
            (2) Start at 18 units per kilogram
            (3) Check PTT q6h
            (4) Adjust per protocol for PTT 55 to 75
      2. Coumadin
         a. Maintain INR 2 to 3
         b. Dietary education for vitamin K diet
         c. Medic alert bracelet

3. Aspirin
   a. Inhibits platelet aggregation by blocking cyclooxygenase
   b. Dosage: 81 to 650 mg/d
   c. Onset: 1 hour
   d. Maximum effect: 2 hours
   e. Side effects: GI
4. Ticlopidine (Ticlid)
   a. Inhibits platelet aggregation by ADP and PAF
   b. Dosage: 250 mg bid with meals
   c. Onset: 4 days
   d. Maximum effect: 8 to 11 days
   e. Side effects: Neutropenia, GI
   f. Laboratory: Follow CBC q 2 weeks for 3 months.
5. Clopidogrel (Plavix)
   a. Inhibits platelet aggregation by ADP receptor antagonism.
   b. Dosage 75 mg qd
   c. Maximum effect in 5 days
6. Aspirin + dipyridamole extended release (Aggrenox)
   a. Inhibits platelets by cyclooxygenase inhibition and phosphodiesterase inhibition.
   b. Dosage 1 capsule (25 mg aspirin + 200 mg dipyridamole extended release BID)
   c. Common side effects include headache, GI upset, and bleeding.
7. Tissue plasminogen activator (t-PA)
   a. Acute management for ischemic stroke presenting within 3 hours of symptom onset
   b. Inclusion criteria: ischemic stroke onset within 3 hours, age > 18 years.
   c. Exclusion criteria: rapid improvement, seizure at stroke onset, recent surgery or head injury, recent hemorrhage, heparin, PT >15, INR > 1.7, platelets < 100,000, glucose < 50, > 400, DBP > 110, SBP > 185
   d. Dosage: 0.9 mg/kg (max 90 kg). 10% given as a bolus and the remaining 90% given as an infusion over 1 hour.

N. Revascularization
   1. Carotid stenosis > 70%
   2. Responsible Lesion
      a. Ulcer, flap, etc., in an appropriate vessel
   3. Endovascular treatment with stent placement

O. Treatment Studies
   1. Asymptomatic Carotid Artery Stenosis (ACAS)
      a. Carotid endarterectomy for asymptomatic stenosis > 60%
      b. Surgical group has 5% chance of ipsilateral stroke in 5 years; surgical complication rate is 2.4%.
      c. Medical group has 11% chance of ipsilateral stroke in 5 years.
   2. North American Symptomatic Carotid Endarterectomy Trial (NASCET)

      a. Carotid endarterectomy for symptomatic stenosis greater than 70%
      b. Surgical group has 9% chance of ipsilateral stroke in 2 years.
      c. Medical group has 26% chance of ipsilateral stroke in 2 years.
          (1) Complication rate higher for ages > 75 years, hypertension, CAD
          (2) Relative risk reduction is 70%.
          (3) Absolute reduction of 9% per year
    3. Chinese Aspirin in Stroke Trial (CAST)
      a. Large trial involving patients presenting with stroke being treated with aspirin
      b. 14% reduction in death rate when treated with aspirin
      c. Small but definite benefit in morbidity and mortality risks

HEMORRHAGE

  I. Etiology
    A. Hypertension
    B. Aneurysm
    C. Amyloid Angiopathy
    D. Mycotic Aneurysm
    E. Arteriovenous Malformation (AVM)
    F. Cavernous Hemangioma
    G. Telangiectasia
    H. Trauma
    I. Germinal Matrix (in newborns)
 II. Location of Hypertensive Hemorrhages
    A. Putamen (50%)
    B. Thalamus (10%)
    C. Cerebellum (10%)
    D. Lobar (10%)
    E. Globus Pallidus (10%)
    F. Other (10%)
III. Subdural Hematoma
    A. Torn Bridging Veins
    B. Lens Shaped
IV. Epidural Hematoma
    A. Torn Meningeal Artery
    B. Biconvex Shape
 V. Subarachnoid Hemorrhage
    A. 5% of all strokes (30,000 per year)
    B. SAH occurs most frequently between ages 40 and 60 years
    C. 12% of patients die prior to treatment
    D. 50% have permanent disability
    E. Causes of SAH
      1. Sacular aneurysms cause 80%
      2. Trauma
      3. AVM

    4. Vessel dissection

    5. Mycotic aneurysm

    6. Vasculitis

    7. Sickle cell disease

    8. Anticoagulation

    9. Neoplasm

F. Hunt and Hess Scale

		Mortality (%)
I	Asymptomatic or mild headache	1
II	Moderate headache or oculomotor palsy	5
III	Confused, drowsy, or mild focal signs	19
IV	Stupor	42
V	Coma	77

G. Symptoms

    1. "Worst headache of my life," "thunderclap"

    2. syncope

    3. seizures

    4. nausea/vomiting

H. Aneurysm clipping should be considered for

    1. Aneurysm with SAH

    2. Aneurysm > 7 mm

I. Complications

    1. Vasospasm—monitor with serial TCD

    2. Hydrocephalus—consider shunt, occurs in 15%

    3. Seizures, occurs in 10%

    4. Rebleeding

J. Treatment

    1. Hydration

    2. partial BP antoregulation

    3. Nimodipine 60 mg PO q4h

K. CT is approximately 85% sensitive in SAH.

VI. Radiology

A. Severe anemia may decrease the intensity of blood on CT.

B. Blood well defined and hyperdense for days 1 through 10, then less well defined days 3 through 20, and isodense after 15 to 20 days.

MRI Findings in Hemorrhage

MRI	T1	T2
Acute (3h–3d)	Iso/Hypo	Iso/Hypo
Subacute (3d–7d)	Hyper	Hypo
Subacute (>7d)	Hyper	Hyper
Chronic		
Hemosiderin	Hypo	Hypo
Resorbed	Hypo	Hyper

8

Neuro-Oncology

CENTRAL NERVOUS SYSTEM TUMORS AND NEUROPATHOLOGY

I. Introduction
   A. Location of Central Nervous System (CNS) Tumors
      1. Intracranial
         a. Supratentorial
         b. Infratentorial
      2. Intraspinal
         a. Extradural (e.g., epidural metastases, bone tumors)
         b. Intradural
            (1) Intramedullary (e.g., ependymomas, astrocytomas, glioblastomas)
            (2) Extramedullary (e.g., schwannomas, meningiomas)
   B. 70% of tumors in children are found in the posterior fossa (e.g., cerebellar medulloblastomas, cerebellar astrocytomas, and fourth ventricle ependymomas).
   C. 70% of tumors in adults are found in the cerebral hemispheres (e.g., astrocytomas, glioblastomas, metastases, meningiomas).
   D. Histogenesis of CNS Cells
      1. The brain and spinal cord develop from the neural tube.
      2. The neural tube is composed of neuroepithelium, which gives rise to all neurons and microglial cells (astrocytes, oligodendrocytes, ependymal cell, and epithelial cells of the choroid plexus).
      3. The mesenchyme gives rise to the microglial cells.
   E. Abnormal cellular proliferation (neoplasia) results from the following:
      1. Loss of tumor suppressor genes

Examples:	Gene	Chromosome	Associated Tumor
	P53	17 p13.1	Glioblastoma
	CDKN2	9 p21	Glioblastoma
	RB1	13 q14	Retinoblastoma
	NF1	17 q11.2	Pilocytic astrocytoma
	NF2	22 q12	Schwannoma/meningioma
	MEN1	11 q13	Pituitary adenoma

      2. Activation of protooncogenes (which encode for growth factors, growth factor receptors, and regulators of gene expression)

Examples:	Gene	Chromosome	Mechanism
	EGFR	7 p12	Amplification/rearrangement
	C-*myc*, N-*myc*	8 q24, 2 p23&24	Amplification
	H-*ras*, N-*ras*	11 p15, 1 p13	Overexpansion/point mutation

II. Grading Systems for Astrocytic Tumors
  A. Kernohan: based on cellularity, mitoses, pleomorphism, vascularity, and necrosis
    1. Grade I: Increased cellularity
    2. Grade II: Greater cellularity than grade I plus pleomorphism
    3. Grade III: Greater cellularity and pleomorphism than grade II plus vascular proliferation
    4. Grade IV: All the above plus necrosis and pseudopallisading
  B. Three-tiered: Also based on cellularity, mitosis, pleomorphism, vascularity, and necrosis
    1. I. Astrocytoma
    2. II. Anaplastic astrocytoma
    3. III. Glioblastoma multiforme (GBM)—necrosis present
  C. World Health Organization (WHO) Classification—1993
    1. Grade I: Pilocytic astrocytoma, subependymal giant-cell astrocytoma
    2. Grade II: Low-grade astrocytoma—hypercellularity, nuclear atypia
    3. Grade III: Anaplastic astrocytoma—mitosis, endothelial proliferation
    4. Grade IV: GBM—necrosis
III. Glial Tumors
  A. Pilocytic Astrocytoma
    1. Epidemiology: Mainly children and adolescents. Can be seen in neurofibromatosis.
    2. Clinical features: Cerebellar lesions produce symptoms secondary to obstruction of cerebrospinal fluid (CSF) flow (hydrocephalus) or cerebellar dysfunction.
    3. Location: Cerebellum (children)
        a. Brain stem, optic nerve, thalamus, hypothalamus (young adults)
    4. Radiology: Cyst with mural nodule that enhances on MRI
    5. Pathology: Rosenthal fibers (opaque, homogenous, eosinophilic bodies); long, slender "hairlike" cells (hence the name *pilocytic*); eosinophilic granular bodies
    6. Treatment: Surgically curable if gross resection possible. Also sensitive to chemotherapy (preferred in children) and X-ray therapy.
    7. Prognosis: Greater than 90% 10-year survival for cerebellar lesions after total resection
  B. Subependymal Giant-Cell Astrocytoma
    1. Epidemiology: Nearly always associated with tuberous sclerosis
    2. Clinical features: Produces symptoms by obstructing CSF flow at the foramen of Monro.
    3. Location: Wall of lateral ventricle
    4. Radiology: Intraventricular enhancing mass on MRI
    5. Pathology: Giant astrocytes without significant anaplasia
    6. Treatment: Surgical debulking for obstructive symptoms
    7. Prognosis: Slow growing and benign, rare malignant degeneration
  C. Pleomorphic Xanthoastrocytoma
    1. Epidemiology: Most common in second decade of life
    2. Clinical features: Frequently long history of seizures

3. Location: Predilection for superficial temporal lobes
4. Radiology: Superficial meningocerebral nodule often associated with a cyst
5. Pathology: Lipid-laden astrocytes, extreme pleomorphism, cellular atypia, multinucleated giant cells. NO NECROSIS (often mistaken for GBM)
6. Treatment: Surgical resection
7. Prognosis: Good with resection. Occasional recurrence, rare malignant degeneration

D. Low-grade Astrocytoma
   1. Epidemiology: 25% to 30% of all cerebral gliomas. Chiefly in young adults, ages 30 to 50 years.
   2. Clinical features: Seizures are more common than functional deficits that depend on location.
   3. Location: Most commonly cerebral hemispheres (adults), but may also occur in the cerebellum, hypothalamus, optic nerve/chiasm, and brain stem (children)
   4. Radiology: Low density on CT *without* enhancement. Low density on T1-weighted and high density on T2-weighted MRI images (also without enhancement)
   5. Pathology: Hypercellular, well-differentiated astrocytes; can be cystic; may be fibrillary (most common) or protoplasmic
   6. Treatment: Surgical resection ± x-ray therapy (XRT) for hemispheric lesions
   7. Prognosis: Median survival, 5 to 6 years with treatment

E. Anaplastic Astrocytoma
   1. Epidemiology: Chiefly in adults ages 30 to 50 years (as with low-grade astrocytoma)
   2. Clinical features: Dependent on location
   3. Location: Most commonly cerebral hemispheres (adults), but may occur in the cerebellum, hypothalamus, optic nerve/chiasm, and brain stem (children)
   4. Radiology: Enhancement usually present, but of variable degree
   5. Pathology: Endothelial proliferation, mitosis, nuclear atypia, hyperchromatic nuclei
      a. No necrosis. Gemistocytic subtype frequently (80%) transforms into GBM.
   6. Treatment: Surgical resection, XRT, chemotherapy
   7. Prognosis: 50% 2-year survival rate. Frequent transformation into GBM.
      a. Mean survival is 18 to 36 months.

F. Glioblastoma Multiforme (GBM)
   1. Epidemiology: Peak age 45 to 55 years. Male-to-female ratio is 2:1. Comprises 20% of all intracranial tumors, 50% to 55% of all cerebral gliomas.
   2. Clinical features: Focal neurologic deficits common and dependent on location
   3. Location: Predominantly cerebral hemispheres (particularly frontal and temporal lobes), but possible occurrence in brain stem, cerebellum, and spinal cord
   4. Radiology: Ringlike/annular enhancement around central necrosis on CT and MRI with vasogenic edema. Frequently tracks along white matter pathways. When it tracks along the corpus callosum into other hemisphere, this is known as "Butterfly" GBM.
   5. Pathology

      a. Gross: Poorly demarcated variegated lesion with areas of necrosis and hemorrhage.

      b. Micro: Pseudopallisading around areas of necrosis and endothelial proliferation are hallmarks. May look "glomeruloid" because it makes its own blood supply.

   6. Treatment: Surgical debulking, XRT, chemotherapy

   7. Prognosis: Poor, mean survival 6 months without treatment and 1 year with treatment. Age is the most important prognostic indicator, with worse survival in the elderly.

G. Oligodendroglioma

   1. Epidemiology: Ages 30 to 50 years. Comprises 5% of intracranial gliomas.

   2. Clinical features: Frequently long history of seizures

   3. Location: Cerebral hemispheres (frontal and temporal lobes most common)

   4. Radiology: Calcification in 50% to 90%; minimal edema and enhancement (may have wispy "chicken wire" enhancement).

   5. Pathology

      a. Gross: Tracks along white matter

      b. Micro: "Fried-egg" cells (artifact of fixation), delicate vessels (most common primary tumor to bleed) and calcification, geometric patterns, round nuclei with stippled chromatin

        (1) Variants

           (a) "Intraventricular oligo"—really a neuronal cell tumor and should be called a central neurocytoma (see section on neuronal-cell tumors).

           (b) Mixed oligoastrocytoma—Oligodendroglial and astrocytic components both occur in significant or roughly equal amounts.

           (c) Anaplastic oligodendroglioma—Increased mitotic rate and pleomorphism. May transform into GBM. Responds to chemotherapy.

   6. Treatment: Surgical resection and chemotherapy (usually good response to chemotherapy)

   7. Prognosis: Median survival, 5 years

H. Ependymoma

   1. Epidemiology: Most frequent in childhood and adolescence, peak age 10 to 15 years

      a. Comprise 6% of intracranial gliomas, 60% of spinal cord gliomas

      b. Most common spinal cord glioma

   2. Clinical features: Symptoms secondary to obstruction of CSF flow

   3. Location: Infratentorial in 60% of cases, supratentorial in 40%. Most frequently in region of fourth ventricle; also common in the lumbosacral spinal cord and filum terminale.

   4. Radiology: Intraventricular mass with contrast enhancement and frequent calcification. Obstructive hydrocephalus may be seen.

   5. Pathology

      a. Gross: Well circumscribed, grown by local extension; may spread in the CSF pathways.

      b. Micro: Ependymal tubules, perivascular pseudorosettes

(1) Variant

(a) Subependymoma—intraventricular, benign; also causes symptoms from obstruction of CSF flow.

6. Treatment: Surgical resection followed by XRT ± full spinal axis radiation
7. Prognosis: 87% 5-year survival rate after resection

I. Gliomatosis Cerebri

1. Epidemiology: Peak incidence in first and second decades of age; range, 6 to 60 years of age
2. Clinical features: Impairment of intellect, headache, seizures, and papilledema are common.
3. Location: Diffusely infiltrating without discrete tumor mass. Arises deep (in thalamus and basal ganglia) and grows along scaffolding of normal brain.
4. Radiology: Homogeneous, hypodensities, loss of gray/white junction, swollen hemispheres on CT. Diffuse increase in T2 signal on MRI. Enhances minimally if at all.
5. Pathology
   a. Gross: Diffusely enlarged brain
   b. Micro: Extensive gray and white matter infiltration by undifferentiated cells with foci of neoplastic astrocytes. Generally falls into the anaplastic astrocytoma subcategory.
6. Treatment: None proven effective
7. Prognosis: Poor; survival is months to years.

IV. Primitive Neuroectodermal Tumors (PNET)—"small blue cell tumors" resembling germinal matrix. Identified by the suffix *blastoma,* with the exception of GBM.

A. Medulloblastoma

1. Epidemiology: Most common PNET. Occurs in first decade of life with a second peak in the 20- to 30-year age category. Accounts for about one-third of all pediatric posterior fossa tumors.
2. Clinical features: Present with cerebellar dysfunction and symptoms secondary to obstruction of CSF flow.
3. Location: Predilection for midline cerebellum (inferior vermis). Tends to infiltrate the cerebellar hemispheres and spread within the neuraxis via CSF pathways ("drop mets").
4. Radiology: Contrast enhancing, rare calcification
5. Pathology: Homer-Wright rosettes (sheets of cells forming rosettes around a central area filled with neuritic processes). These can be seen in any PNET.
   a. Variants
      (1) Desmoplastic—abundant reticulin, more lateral in the cerebellar hemispheres, older children, better prognosis
      (2) Medullomyoblastoma—very rare, contains immature muscle cells, very malignant.
6. Treatment: Surgical resection followed by craniospinal XRT (quite sensitive) ± chemotherapy
7. Prognosis: More than 50% 5-year survival rate with treatment. Recurrence, CSF seeding, and distant metastases are not uncommon.

B. Retinoblastoma
   1. Epidemiology: Children less than 3 years of age. Is the most common potentially fatal intraocular neoplasm of childhood. Sporadic (60%) or autosomal dominant (40%). Hereditary form tends to be bilateral with early onset. Increased incidence with chromosome 13 deletion (deletion of Rb suppressor gene).
   2. Clinical features: Presenting symptoms include leukocoria (white pupil), squint (strabismus), red and painful eye, and secondary glaucoma.
   3. Location: Eye, with intracranial extension via optic nerve. Bone marrow is common site of blood-borne mets.
      a. "Trilateral tumor" = bilateral retinoblastomas + pineoblastoma
   4. Pathology: Homer-Wright rosettes and Flexner-Wintersteiner rosettes (sheets of cells forming rosettes around an empty lumen—recall that Homer-Wright rosettes have neuritic processes filling this central area).
   5. Treatment: Surgical resection
   6. Prognosis: High survival rate (90%) with early treatment
C. Neuroblastoma
   1. Epidemiology: First decade of life; two-thirds of cases occur before the age of 5 years.
   2. Clinical features: Can present with myoclonic encephalopathy neuroblastoma syndrome = opsoclonus, myoclonus, and encephalopathy. May be idiopathic or secondary to an occult neuroblastoma.
   3. Location: Most commonly arises from the sympathetic chain. Cerebral form is uncommon.
   4. Radiology: Large, discrete, contrast-enhancing lesions with calcification and cysts
   5. Pathology: Homer-Wright rosettes, dense sheets of tumor cells. May secrete dopamine and catecholamines, which can be measured in urine (VMA, HVA). Amplification of n-*myc* oncogene present in more than one-third of cases, and degree of amplification correlates with advanced stage and poor prognosis.
   6. Treatment: Surgical resection with tumor bed XRT ± full neuraxis radiation
   7. Prognosis: Recurrence is frequent.
D. Esthesioblastoma—Olfactory Neuroblastoma
   1. Epidemiology: Bimodal age distribution with larger peak in late adulthood
   2. Location: Olfactory neuroepithelium with involvement of the cribriform plate
   3. Radiology: Enhancing, dumbbell-shaped mass centered on the cribriform plate
   4. Pathology: Rare Homer-Wright rosettes, rare olfactory rosettes
   5. Treatment: Surgical resection
   6. Prognosis: Favorable with total resection
E. Pineoblastoma
   1. Epidemiology: Occurs most commonly in children.
   2. Clinical features: May present with Parinaud's syndrome (see section on pineal region tumors).
   3. Location: Pineal gland with frequent leptomeningeal metastasis (drop mets)
   4. Radiology: Contrast-enhancing pineal region mass

5. Pathology: Resembles medulloblastomas and shares their degree of malignancy as well as their tendency to spread in the leptomeninges. May form "flourettes."
6. Treatment: Surgical resection
7. Prognosis: Rapid recurrence with wide dissemination

F. Ependymoblastoma
  1. Epidemiology: First 5 years of life
  2. Location: Most commonly cerebrum with frequent craniospinal metastasis
  3. Radiology: Large, discrete, contrast-enhancing deep lesion
  4. Pathology: Ependymoblastic rosettes in fields of undifferentiated cells
  5. Treatment: Surgical resection ± XRT ± chemotherapy
  6. Prognosis: Death within 1 year of surgery

V. Tumors of the Nerve Sheath and Meninges
  A. Schwannoma (Neurilemmoma)
    1. Epidemiology: Usually solitary but frequently bilateral in neurofibromatosis type II
    2. Clinical features: Hearing loss is a common initial symptom.
    3. Location: Most common on CN VIII (acoustic schwannoma) in the cerebellopontine (CP) angle, but may occur wherever Schwann cells are present (other cranial nerves, spinal nerve roots, peripheral nerve trunks).

  Note: The most common CP angle tumor is an acoustic schwannoma.

    4. Radiology: Intradural, extraaxial, contrast-enhancing mass (usually in the CP angle). If spinal, may extend through the intervertebral foramen, resulting in an hourglass or dumbbell appearance.
    5. Pathology: Antoni A (dense, fibrillary) and Antoni B (loose, reticulated) tissue. Verocay bodies (stacked nuclei alternating with fibrillar zones). Arise at the periphery of the nerve (displace but do not invade).
    6. Treatment: Surgical resection
    7. Prognosis: Usually cured with surgery; malignant degeneration very rare in the CNS but more common in the PNS

  B. Neurofibroma
    1. Epidemiology: Almost always associated with neurofibromatosis (NF) type I; almost always multiple
    2. Location: Most involve dorsal spinal nerve roots; cranial nerve involvement very rare.
    3. Radiology: Widening of the neural foramina with pedicle erosion
    4. Pathology: Hyperplasia of Schwann cells and fibrous elements of the nerve; axons incorporated into the tumor.
    5. Treatment: Palliative surgical decompression as needed
    6. Prognosis: Additional lesions tend to arise. In NF-I, malignant degeneration may occur (malignant peripheral nerve sheath tumor).

  C. Meningioma
    1. Epidemiology: Adults ages 20 to 60 years; strong female predominance (especially with spinal lesions). Comprise 15% of all intracranial tumors, 25% of intraspinal tumors.

        a. Associated with partial or complete deletion of chromosome 22

        b. Increased incidence in patients with breast cancer; may be associated with progesterone receptors.

      Note: NF-II is also associated with chromosome 22 and meningiomas.

    2. Clinical features: Headaches and seizures most frequent presenting symptoms

    3. Location: Extraaxial (i.e., indent but do not invade)

        a. Intracranial: Over convexities—50% of cases; falx/skull base—40%; posterior fossa—10%

        b. Intraspinal: Most common in thoracic segment

    4. Radiology: Dural tail sign, homogenous enhancement

    5. Pathology

        a. Gross: Well-circumscribed, indents but does not invade underlying brain.

        b. Micro: Whorled pattern, psammoma bodies; arise from the arachnoid cap cells of the dura; intranuclear pseudoinclusions; epithelial membrane Ag+.

    6. Treatment: Surgical resection

    7. Prognosis: Good; malignant degeneration uncommon

VI. Neuronal Cell Tumors

  A. Gangliocytoma/Ganglioglioma

    1. Epidemiology: Children/young adults, first two decades of life most common

    2. Clinical features: Seizures frequent

    3. Location: Temporal lobe favored site

    4. Radiology: May be cystic with mural nodule. Cyst margins enhance; calcification common.

    5. Pathology

        a. *Ganglioglioma*: Display two types of neoplastic cells—neuronal and astrocytic.

        b. *Gangliocytoma*: Neoplastic neuronal cells only

    6. Treatment: Surgical resection

    7. Prognosis: Cured with surgery

  B. Central Neurocytoma

    1. Epidemiology: Rare

    2. Clinical features: Hydrocephalus

    3. Location: Intraventricular; formerly called *intraventricular oligodendroglioma*; usually in the body of the lateral ventricle, attached to the septum pellucidum.

    4. Radiology: Appear heterogenous with multiple cysts, calcium, and occasional hemorrhage; contrast enhancement is variable but usually less extensive than gliomas.

    5. Pathology: Composed of small, uniform, well-differentiated neuronal cells

    6. Treatment: Surgical resection

    7. Prognosis: Good with resection; recurrence rare

VII. Pituitary Tumors

  A. Pituitary adenoma

    1. Epidemiology: By far the most common neoplasm of the pituitary

    2. Clinical features: Produce endocrine symptoms early if hormonally active. Present with compressive symptoms late (headaches, visual loss) if they are nonsecretory.

Hemorrhage or infarct of the tumor may produce *pituitary apoplexy* (abrupt headache, visual loss, diplopia, drowsiness, confusion, coma).
3. Location: Sella
4. Radiology: MRI may reveal microadenoma (<10 mm in diameter) or larger compressive lesion. May grow up into the suprasellar space ("Michellin man" appearance) and may invade the cavernous sinus. Primary suprasellar masses usually do not grow *down* through the diaphragm.
5. Pathology: Can be classified by hormonal products.
   a. *Prolactinoma*: Most common subtype. Most often occurs as a microadenoma in young females. Larger ones (usually functionally silent) occur more often in males. Produce symptoms from primary hypersecretion or stalk effect (flow of prolactin inhibitory factor/dopamine is impeded). Symptoms are amenorrhea and galactorrhea in females and decreased libido and impotence in males.
   b. *Growth-hormone (GH) secreting*: Results in acromegaly.
   c. *Adrenocorticotropic hormone (ACTH)–secreting*: Results in Cushing's disease.
   d. *Thyroid-stimulating hormone (TSH)–secreting*: Rare, usually secondary to primary thyroid myxedema
   e. *Follicle-stimulating hormone luteinizing hormone (FSHLH)–secreting*
   f. *Nonsecreting*: 20% of all pituitary tumors. Present with compressive symptoms.
6. Treatment
   a. Prolactinoma: Bromocriptine ± transsphenoidal resection
   b. GH: Transsphenoidal resection ± octreotide
   c. Others: Transsphenoidal resection
7. Prognosis: 70% to 90% remission rate 1 year after resection
VIII. Pineal Region Tumors
   A. Germinoma
      1. Epidemiology: Most common tumor of the pineal gland (50%). Peak incidence is in the second decade, predominantly males (ages 20 to 40 years).
   Note: Germ-cell tumors are the most common tumors of the pineal region.
      2. Clinical: May present with Parinaud's syndrome (paralysis of upgaze, convergence—retraction nystagmus, light—near dissociation of the pupils) secondary to compression of the tectum of the midbrain. May also cause hydrocephalus.
      3. Location: Pineal region
      4. Radiology: 100% calcified (as opposed to only 40% of normal pineal glands); isointense-to-normal brain on MRI
      5. Pathology: Composed of two cell lines—large malignant germ cells and small reactive lymphocytes
      6. Treatment: XRT ± chemotherapy
      7. Prognosis: 75% 5-year survival rate after XRT
   B. Pineocytoma
      1. Epidemiology: Primarily middle to late adulthood
      2. Location/radiology: Contrast-enhancing solid mass in the pineal region
      3. Pathology

        a. Gross: Slow-growing; displace, do not invade.

        b. Micro: Sheets of small cells resembling normal pineal gland with pineocytomatous rosettes

    4. Treatment: Surgical resection

    5. Prognosis: Favorable following resection

  C. Pineoblastoma (see section on PNET tumors)

IX. Choroid Plexus Tumors

  A. Choroid Plexus Papilloma

    1. Epidemiology: First decade of life

    2. Clinical features: Present with symptoms secondary to CSF obstruction or CSF overproduction

    3. Location

        a. Adults: Fourth ventricle > lateral ventricle > third ventricle

        b. Children: Most common in the lateral ventricles (usually on the left)

    4. Radiology: Homogeneous mass with prominent flow voids (richly vascularized), frequent calcification

    5. Pathology: Large choroid plexus with redundant plexus epithelium

    6. Treatment: Surgical resection, ± XRT

    7. Prognosis: Good with complete resection

  B. Anaplastic Choroid Plexus Papilloma—Choroid plexus carcinoma

    1. Always consider metastatic disease. Very vascular.

        a. In children less than 8 years of age: Think of primary choroid plexus papilloma.

        b. In adults: Think metastatic disease.

X. Other Primary CNS Tumors

  A. Craniopharyngioma (Adamantinomatous)

    1. Epidemiology: First two decades of life; is the most common supratentorial childhood tumor.

    2. Clinical features: Hypopituitarism and visual abnormalities secondary to compression of pituitary and optic chiasm

    3. Radiology: Strongly enhancing, calcified cystic mass in the suprasellar region with frequent intrasellar component

    4. Pathology: Thought to arise from Rathke's pouch

        Rule of 6 Cs: *childhood* tumors that are *calcified* and *cystic*. The cysts contain *cholesterol* crystals and *"crank-case oil"* that, upon rupture, can cause a *chemical* meningitis.

    5. Treatment: Surgical resection (if possible) followed by XRT for residual tumor

    6. Prognosis: 76% 10-year survival rate with surgery and XRT; only 17% with resection alone

  B. Epidermoid Cyst

    1. Epidemiology: Rare

    2. Clinical features: Seizures are the most frequent presentation, but cranial nerve abnormalities and hydrocephalus may also occur.

    3. Location: Most commonly cerebellopontine angle but may occur in the intrasellar and suprasellar regions. Intraspinal lesions are less common.

    4. Radiology: Low-density cyst with irregularly enhancing rim on CT; variable signal on MRI, depending on lipid content

    5. Pathology: Squamous epithelium surrounding a keratin-filled cyst (epidermal structures)

    6. Treatment: Surgical excision preferred. XRT is of no proven benefit.

    7. Prognosis: Recurrence can occur with subtotal excision.

C. Dermoid Cyst

    1. Epidemiology: Most present in childhood

    2. Clinical features: Hydrocephalus common

    3. Location: Midline, related to fontanelle, fourth ventricle or spinal cord

    4. Radiology: Hair and sebaceous content result in heterogeneous MRI signal.

    5. Pathology: Contains both epidermal and dermal structures (hair follicles, sweat glands, sebaceous glands).

    6. Treatment: Surgical resection

    7. Prognosis: Recurrence can occur with subtotal excision.

D. Teratoma

    1. Epidemiology: Rare; comprise only 0.1% of primary intracranial tumors; occur in first decade of life.

    2. Clinical features: Associated with spina bifida if located in the sacrococcygeal area

    3. Location: Favor the midline (pineal region, sellar and suprasellar regions, posterior fossa) and sacrococcygeal area.

    4. Pathology: Composed of cells of all three germ-cell layers—epidermal, dermal, vascular, glandular, muscular, neural, and cartilaginous

    5. Treatment: Resection

    6. Prognosis: Favorable with resection

E. Colloid Cyst

    1. Epidemiology: Young to middle-aged adults

    2. Clinical features: May present with obstruction of the foramen of Monroe with headaches, drop attacks, or sudden death; produces "ball-valve" obstruction of the ventricle, with headache ("thunderclap headache") upon sitting.

    3. Location: Third ventricle (at foramen of Monroe)

    4. Radiology: Thin-walled cyst that is hyperintense on T1-weighted MRI

    5. Pathology: Goblet and ciliated columnar epithelium surrounding a cystic cavity

    6. Treatment: Surgical resection

    7. Prognosis: Cured with complete resection

F. Lipoma

    1. Epidemiology: Rare, benign

    2. Clinical features: Frequently associated with other congenital anomalies, such as agenesis of the corpus callosum

    3. Location: Favors midline sites, such as the corpus callosum.

    4. Radiology: Cat density on all imaging modalities

    5. Pathology: Mature adipose tissue

    6. Treatment: Excision is usually not necessary or possible.

    7. Prognosis: Good; usually an incidental finding

G. Hypothalamic Hamartoma

1. Epidemiology: Rare
2. Clinical features: Associated with gelastic seizures and endocrine abnormalities
3. Location: Hypothalamus
4. Radiology: Small discrete mass near floor of third ventricle
5. Pathology: Well-differentiated but disorganized neuroglial tissue
6. Treatment: Surgical resection or ablation if possible
7. Prognosis: Cured if surgery possible (difficult to resect)

H. Hemangioblastoma
1. Epidemiology: Most frequent between ages 30 and 65 years
2. Clinical features: Frequently associated with von Hippel-Lindau's disease (retinal and cerebellar hemangioblastomas, renal and pancreatic cysts/tumors, polycythemia). This is the most common intraaxial primary neoplasm of the posterior fossa in adults.
3. Location: Cerebellum most common, followed by brain stem and spinal cord
4. Radiology: Cyst with mural nodule that enhances
5. Pathology
   a. Gross: Well-circumscribed cyst that contains yellowish fluid (due to abundant lipid content) and a nodule on the cyst wall
   b. Micro: Richly vascularized; cyst wall may contain Rosenthal fibers, making distinction from pilocytic astrocytoma difficult on biopsy. Clusters of foamy cells (on oil-red-O stain) separated by blood-filled channels.
6. Treatment: Surgical resection
7. Prognosis: Cured after complete resection

I. Primary CNS Lymphoma
1. Epidemiology: Preferentially occurs in immunosuppressed patients (iatrogenically or those with AIDS). Highly malignant. Increasing in incidence, even in the immunocompetent population.
2. Clinical features: Headaches, seizures, and mental status changes are common symptoms.
3. CSF: Lymphocytic pleocytosis (LP) in 50% of cases, increased protein in 85%, monoclonal B cells. Chance of positive cytology—50% with first LP, 90% with third LP.
4. Location: Most frequent site is deep periventricular region; may be multifocal.
5. Radiology: Hypodense on T1, isodense or hypodense on T2 (due to hypercellularity). Usually dense uniform enhancement, but may be only slightly enhancing or nonenhancing.
6. Pathology: Usually of B-cell origin. Cells arranged in an angiocentric pattern.
7. Treatment: Responds to corticosteroids and XRT, but recurs.
8. Prognosis: Overall survival less than 3 months in HIV patients, 19 months in non-HIV patients

CNS TUMORS—QUICK REFERENCE TABLES AND LISTS

I. Metastatic Tumors
  A. General Statements
    1. Metastatic tumors are the most common posterior fossa tumors in adults.
    2. 80% are supratentorial; they tend to occur at the gray/white junction and produce surrounding vasogenic edema.
    3. The most common tumors to metastasize to brain are lung (males) and breast (females).
    4. Melanoma has a strong propensity for the CNS; 40% of patients with systemic disease have CNS metastases. This can produce black CSF on LP.

Tumors that Metastasize to Brain	Tumors that Metastasize to Skull and Dura/Meninges
1. Lung	1. Breast
2. Breast	2. Prostate
3. Melanoma	3. Multiple myeloma
4. GI (especially colon and rectum)	4. Lymphoma
5. Renal cell	5. Leukemia (to pia)
6. Reproductive (especially testicular)	6. Lung
7. Thyroid	
8. Others: liver, gallbladder, pancreas	

Metastatic Tumors that Commonly Bleed
1. Melanoma
2. Choriocarcinoma
3. Renal cell carcinoma
4. Lung

II. Most Common Tumors by Location

Temporal Lobes	Corpus Callosum
1. Ganglioglioma	1. GBM
2. Oligodendroglioma	2. Oligodendroglioma
3. Pleomorphic xanthoastrocytoma	3. Lipoma

Lateral Ventricle	Cerebello-pontine Angle
1. Ependymoma	1. Acoustic neuroma
2. Meningioma	2. Meningioma
3. Subependymoma	
4. Choroid plexus papilloma/carcinoma	
5. Central neurocytoma	

Midline—Sellar Region	Midline—Pineal Region
1. Pituitary adenoma	1. Germ-cell tumor (especially males)
2. Craniopharyngioma	2. Teratoma
3. Meningioma	3. Pineocytoma/pineoblastoma
4. Germ-cell tumor	4. Epidermoid/dermoid cyst
5. Epidermoid/dermoid cyst	
6. Esthesioneuroblastoma	
7. Optic nerve glioma	
8. Hypothalamic glioma/hamartoma	

Conus/Filum Terminale
1. Ependymoma
2. Lipoma
3. Paraganglioma
4. Meningioma
5. Drop metastases

Two Most Common Locations for a Chordoma
1. Clivus
2. Sacrum

Suprasellar Neoplasms (mnemonic: SATCHMOE)
Suprasellar extension of a pituitary adenoma
Aneurysm
Tuberculum sellae meningioma
Craniopharyngioma—Rathke's cysts
Hypothalamic glioma/hamartoma
Metastases
Optic nerve glioma
Epidermoid/dermoid/teratoma

III. Tumors that commonly present radiographically/grossly as a cyst containing a mural nodule
   A. Pilocytic Astrocytoma
   B. Hemangioblastoma
   C. Ganglioglioma
   D. Pleomorphic Xanthoastrocytoma
   E. GBM

IV. Rosenthal Fibers
   A. Intracytoplasmic, eosinophilic, irregular enlargement of astrocytic processes
   B. Most commonly associated with pilocytic astrocytoma and Alexander's disease
   C. May also be seen with other tumors (pleomorphic xanthoastrocytoma, craniopharyngioma, hemangioblastoma) and can be found surrounding other chronic, more benign conditions (around a syrinx, around MS plaques). May also be found in the normal pineal gland.

When You Hear . . .	Think of . . . (most commonly associated with)
Rosenthal fibers	Pilocytic astrocytoma, Alexander's disease
Pseudopallisading/necrosis	Glioblastoma multiforme
"Fried-egg cells"	Oligodendroglioma
Perivascular pseudorosettes	Ependymoma
Homer-Wright rosettes	Medulloblastoma, PNET tumors
Flexner-Wintersteiner rosettes	Retinoblastoma
Verocay bodies	Schwannoma
Antoni A and B tissue	Schwannoma
Psammoma bodies	Meningioma
Whorled pattern of cells	Meningioma
B cells in an angiocentric pattern	Primary CNS lymphoma

V. Miscellaneous cellular alterations of note (not neoplastic)
  A. Alzheimer's Type II Astrocytes—large vesicular, watery nucleus; associated with increased ammonia and hepatic encephalopathy
  B. Alzheimer's Type I Astrocytes—abundant cytoplasm; associated with increased ammonia, but especially Wilson's disease
  C. Opalski Cells—found in basal ganglia; associated with Wilson's disease
  D. Globoid Cells—associated with Krabbe's disease
VI. Nervous System Complications of Chemotherapy
    1. 5-FU—acute cerebellar syndrome, cranial neuropathy, disorientation/confusion, seizures
    2. Altretamine—peripheral neuropathy, ataxia, tremor, visual hallucinations
    3. Amsacrine—seizures
    4. Azacitidine—muscle pain and weakness
    5. Bleomycin—Raynaud's phenomenon
    6. Busulfan—seizures, venous thrombosis, encephalopathy
    7. Carboplatin—peripheral neuropathy, hearing loss, transient cortical blindness
    8. Cisplatin—peripheral neuropathy, autonomic neuropathy, ototoxicity (high-frequency hearing loss, tinnitus), encephalopathy
    9. Cladribine—peripheral neuropathy
   10. Cytarabine (Ara-C)—cerebellar dysfunction, somnolence/confusion, personality change, peripheral neuropathy, rhabdomyolysis, myelopathy
   11. Dacarbazine—paresthesia
   12. Etoposide—peripheral neuropathy
   13. Fludarabine—visual disturbances, peripheral neuropathy, encephalopathy
   14. Interleukin 2—parkinsonism, brachial plexopathy
   15. Isotretinoin—pseudotumor cerebri
   16. L-asparaginase—central vein thrombosis, headache, encephalopathy
   17. Leamisole—peripheral neuropathy
   18. Methotrexate—leukoencephalopathy, myelopathy, chemical arachnoiditis if given intrathecally.
   19. Nitroureas (BCNU)—encephalopathy
   20. Paclitaxel (taxol)—peripheral neuropathy, autonomic neuropathy
   21. Procarbazine—peripheral neuropathy, autonomic neuropathy, encephalopathy, ataxia
   22. Suramin—peripheral neuropathy
   23. Tamoxifen—decreased visual acuity
   24. Teiposide—peripheral neuropathy
   25. Thiotepa—myelopathy
   26. Trimexetrate—peripheral neuropathy
   27. Vinblastine—peripheral neuropathy, muscle pain, cranial neuropathy, autonomic neuropathy
   28. Vincristine—peripheral neuropathy, cranial neuropathy, autonomic neuropathy, decreased ADH secretion
   29. Vincristine—peripheral neuropathy, cranial neuropathy, autonomic neuropathy
   30. Vinorelbine—peripheral neuropathy, autonomic neuropathy

Pathologic Inclusions

Inclusion Body	Disease	Pathology	Location
Intracytoplasmic			
Bunina bodies	ALS	Eosinophilic	Anterior horn cells
Lafora bodies	Myoclonic epilepsy	Basophilic	Dentate nucleus and cortex
Pick bodies	Pick's disease	Argyrophilic	Neurons of frontal and temporal poles
Hirano bodies	Alzheimer's disease	Eosinophilic	In or adjacent to hippocampal pyramidal cells
Lewy bodies	Parkinson's disease	Eosinophilic	Pigmented brainstem neurons
	Diffuse Lewy body disease	Eosinophilic	Diffuse in cortex
Granulovacuolar degeneration (GVD)	Alzheimer's disease	Small vacuoles with central dark granule	Cytoplasm of hippocampal pyramidal cells
Neurofibrillary (NF) tangles	Alzheimer's disease (see footnote for others)	Paired helical filaments Stains with silver	Diffuse, in cortical and subcortical neurons
Corpora amylacea (Polyglucosan bodies)	Nonspecific, aging	Basophilic PAS +	Astrocytes, especially perivacular subpial areas
Negri bodies	Rabies	Eosinophilic	Purkinje cells of cerebellum and pyramidal cells of the hippocampus
Intranuclear			
Cowdry A	Viral infection (HSV, VZV, CMV, measles, rare JC virus)	Large, single, surrounding halo	Diffuse neurons
Marinesco bodies	Nonspecific, aging	Small, multiple, no halo	Pigmented neuron of brainstem (especially substantia nigra and locus ceruleus)
Cowdry B	Acute polio	Small, multiple, no halo	Anterior horn cells
"Ground glass" inclusions	PML-JC virus	Papovavirions in nucleus	Oligodendrocytes

Inclusions found in Alzheimer's disease include NF tangles, Hirano bodies, and GVD.

Note that NF tangles can also be found in PSP, Down's syndrome, postencephalitic parkinsonism, dementia pugilistica, and ALS/parkinsonism/dementia complex of Guam.

ALS, amyotrophic lateral sclerosis; CMV, cytomegalovirus; HSV, herpes simplex virus; PML, progressive multifocal leukoencephalopathy; VZV, varicella zoster virus.

BRAIN EDEMA AND HERNIATION SYNDROMES

I. Three Types of Brain Edema
   A. Vasogenic
      1. Associated with increased permeability of brain capillaries
      2. White matter chiefly affected
      3. Most commonly seen with brain tumors. Can also be associated with abscesses, meningitis, lead encephalopathy, infarction, hemorrhage, and trauma.
      4. In patients with brain tumor, clinical signs/symptoms are often caused more by this edema than by the tumor mass itself.
      5. Treatment: Steroids (Decadron 10 mg IV bolus, then 4 mg po/IV every 6 hours). Also give GI prophylaxis with H2 blockers and antacids.

B. Cytotoxic (Cellular)
   1. Swelling of all cellular elements (neurons, glia, endothelial cells)
   2. Gray and white matter affected
   3. Most commonly associated with hypoxia/ischemia. Also seen in meningitis, Reye's syndrome, water intoxication, and acute hyponatremia.
   4. Edema following stroke is usually maximal 72 to 96 hours after the event. Must monitor patients closely during this period. Decreased level of arousal is often first sign.
   5. Treatment: Steroids are of no proven benefit.
      a. Preventive: Albumin 5% solution, 250 to 500 mL plus Lasix 20 mg; repeat this every 6 to 8 hours.
      b. Acute
         (1) Mannitol 20% solution, 0.5 to 1 g/kg IV load over 10 min, then 0.25 to 0.5 g/kg every 4 to 6 hours. Keep serum OSM = 310 to 320.
         (2) Glycerol 10% solution, 1 g/kg via NGT every 6 h
         (3) Hyperventilation—lower PCO_2 to 25 to 30 mm Hg. Effect of hyperventilation is very short-lived.
         (4) Hypertonic saline
C. Interstitial (Hydrocephalic)
   1. Caused by obstruction of CSF circulation that results in transependymal flow of CSF
   2. Chiefly periventricular white matter involved
   3. Occurs with hydrocephalus, pseudotumor cerebri, and normal pressure hydrocephalus.
   4. Dementia and gait disorder are main symptoms.
   5. Treatment: CSF shunting if needed
II. Herniation Syndromes
   A. Cingulate Herniation
      1. One hemisphere expands and causes lateral/midline shift and forces the cingulate gyrus under the falx cerebri.
      2. Compression of the vessels (especially the ACA) may result in leg weakness.
   B. Lateral/Uncal Herniation
      1. Space-occupying lesion in the middle fossa pushes the uncus and midbrain toward the midline.
      2. Pressure on the ipsilateral CN III → Ipsilateral CN III palsy ipsilateral
         Pressure on the PCA → Occipital infarction/swelling, Contralateral homonymous hemianopia
         Pressure on the ipsilateral cerebral peduncle → Contralateral hemiparesis
      Note: Further lateral displacement of the midbrain can result in denting of the opposite cerebral peduncle on the edge of the tent (Kernohan's notch) resulting in ipsilateral hemiparesis. This is often referred to as a "false localizing sign."
   C. Central/Transtentorial Herniation
      1. May be due to space-occupying lesion or diffuse increase in intracranial pressure.
      2. Downward displacement of the diencephalon through the tentorial notch.

3. First sign is usually decreased level of alertness. May progress to involve the lower midbrain, pons, and medulla, producing further neurologic deterioration.

D. Cerebellar Herniation

   1. May be due to a posterior lesion that causes *upward* herniation through the tentorial notch. This obliterates the aqueduct and cisterns resulting in hydrocephalus with obtundation and/or coma.

   2. May also be due to hemispheric lesions that cause herniation of the cerebellar tonsils *downward* through the foramen magnum (tonsillar herniation). Compression of the medulla associated with this can cause respiratory arrest and death.

9

Neuromuscular Diseases

GENERAL APPROACH TO PERIPHERAL NEUROPATHIES

I. Evaluation and Classification
  A. Thorough History
    1. Nature of chief complaint: Weakness vs. sensory disturbance vs. pain vs. autonomic disturbance vs. atrophy vs. ataxia vs. combination thereof
    2. Time course of symptoms: Acute vs. subacute vs. chronic (relapsing, recurrent, progressive, etc.)
    3. Anatomic pattern of symptoms: Symmetric vs. asymmetric, focal vs. diffuse; with additional help from physical examination, determine if clinically a mononeuropathy, mononeuropathy multiplex, polyneuropathy, radiculopathy, polyradiculopathy, or plexopathy.
    4. Ask specifically about the following:
      a. Trauma
      b. Toxic exposures (including recreationals such as alcohol [ETOH])
      c. Infections or vaccinations
      d. Dietary deficiencies
      e. Medications used
      f. Presence of other medical conditions (diabetes, thyroid disease, vascular disease, liver disease, GI disease, sarcoidosis, renal disease, connective-tissue disease, cancer, etc.)
      g. Constitutional symptoms (weight loss, fever, etc.)
      h. Family history
  B. Thorough Physical Examination
    1. Cranial nerves most commonly involved in Guillain-Barré syndrome (GBS), sarcoid, carcinomatosis, diphtheria
    2. Motor examination
      a. Look for atrophy and distribution thereof.
      b. Distribution of weakness:
        (1) Most polyneuropathies affect distal muscles of lower extremities first.
        (2) Most demyelinating and certain acute motor and toxic neuropathies affect all muscles of limbs, trunk, neck, and some facial muscles.
        (3) With help of history, try to narrow weakness into pattern of mononeuropathy, mononeuropathy multiplex, polyneuropathy, radiculopathy, polyradiculopathy, or plexopathy.

3. Sensory examination
   a. Most neuropathies have distal, symmetric, sensory loss in lower extremities first (stocking-glove distribution).
   b. Sensory loss exceeds weakness in most toxic neuropathies.
4. Reflex examination
   a. Diminution or loss is an invariable sign of peripheral nerve disease (except in small fiber sensory neuropathies, where reflexes may be retained).
   b. May be diminished out of proportion to weakness.
5. Coordination and gait
   a. Proprioceptive loss may result in ataxia of limb movement and gait with positive Romberg test.
   b. Fast frequency action tremor occasionally seen
6. Skin and musculoskeletal examination
   a. Pes cavus: Often seen in hereditary neuropathies secondary to weakness of peroneal and pretibial muscles greater than calf muscles
   b. "Claw" hand: Same principle as lower extremities
   c. Kyphoscoliosis: Secondary to weakness of paravertebral muscles
   d. Skin ulcers, pressure sores, burns, etc., secondary to analgesia
   e. Tight, shiny skin with sparse hair
   f. Analgesic joints become traumatized and deformed (Charcot arthropathy).
   g. Discoloration (erythema and hyperpigmentation)
   h. Hypertrophied nerves (e.g., chronic inflammatory demyelinating polyneuropathy [CIDP], Refsum's disease, leprosy, hereditary sensorimotor neuropathy [HMSN] III > II > I, acromegaly, neurofibromatosis, amyloidosis, etc.)
   i. Check for herpes zoster lesions.
7. General examination
   a. Cardiovascular: Check pulses, listen for murmurs, check orthostatics, etc.
   b. GI: Hepatomegaly (hepatitis, mononucleosis, etc.) or hepatic cirrhosis
   c. Nodes: Lymphadenopathy (HIV, lymphoma, mono, etc.)
C. Laboratory Evaluation
1. Serum for general screening labs—Liver function tests (LFTs), electrolytes, erythrocyte sedimentation rate (ESR), antinuclear antibodies (ANA), rheumatoid factor (RF), thyroid stimulating hormone (TSH), free T4, B12, folate, serum immunofixation electrophoresis (SIFE), hemoglobin A1C. (Also consider the following based on clinical suspicions: anti-MAG, anti-GM-1, and antisulfatide antibodies, ACE level, lead level, RBC protoporphyrins, cryoglobulins, HIV, anti-Hu, etc.)
2. Consider 24-hour urine for heavy metals, porphyrins; urine IEP.
3. Consider chest X-ray (CXR) as work-up for brachial neuropathy, suspected carcinomatous neuropathy, etc.
4. Electrophysiologic studies—can further categorize neuropathies as primarily demyelinating or axonal, sensory or motor, or both; mononeuropathy vs. polyneuropathy vs. mononeuropathy multiplex vs. plexopathy vs. radiculopathy.
   a. *Axonal*—encompasses most neuropathies.

         (1) Clinical correlation: Usually with symmetric distal sensory loss with weakness, atrophy, and lost ankle jerks

         (2) Nerve conduction velocity (NCV) shows mild slowing *without* conduction block or temporal dispersion, plus significantly decreased amplitudes of compound motor action potential (CMAP) and sensory nerve action potential (SNAP) (often no obtainable potential).

         (3) EMG shows evidence of distal denervation.

         (4) Many toxic and metabolic neuropathies are in this category.

    b. *Demyelinating*

         (1) Clinical correlation: Early generalized reflex loss, mild atrophy, proximal and distal muscle weakness, sensory loss of large-fiber > small-fiber modalities, motor usually > sensory involvement, tremor, and hypertrophied nerves common.

         (2) NCV shows marked slowing, conduction block, temporal dispersion, prolonged F-wave, and distal latencies.

         (3) EMG may show denervation, based on chronicity.

         (4) Examples: GBS, CIDP, some hereditary neuropathies, paraproteinemias, anti-MAG- and anti-GM-1-related neuropathies, etc.

    c. Many neuropathies are mixed axonal and demyelinating.

  5. Consider lumbar puncture if suspect GBS, CIDP, etc.

  6. Consider nerve biopsy (sural) if suspect a treatable disease (vasculitic neuropathy, CIDP, sarcoid, leprosy, etc.) or need to make diagnosis of hereditary neuropathy.

  7. If paraprotein is found on SIFE or urine immunofixation electrophoresis (UIFE), consider skeletal survey, bone marrow biopsy, etc.

II. Treatment

  A. Specific treatment modalities aimed at the underlying etiology are not possible in most neuropathies (especially chronic sensorimotor polyneuropathies); nevertheless, the search for a specific, treatable cause should be undertaken.

    1. In approximately 25% of all chronic polyneuropathies, an etiology cannot be determined.

    2. Treatments for specific neuropathies are discussed in a later section of this chapter.

  B. General Treatment Modalities

    1. Management of neuropathic pain

      a. Sympathetically independent pain—seen in most generalized neuropathies; paroxysmal pain, paresthesias, spontaneous burning pain, tactile hyperalgesia, and occasional cold hyperalgesia; *allodynia*—perversion of sensation (touch-induced burning pain); usually worse in feet and hands.

         (1) Treat underlying etiology, if present (e.g., glucose control in diabetes).

         (2) Tricyclic antidepressants (TCAs) (e.g., amitriptyline, nortriptyline, imipramine, desipramine)

           (a) Start at 10 to 25 mg of amitriptyline or nortriptyline qhs and increase q 2 weeks to 75 to 150 mg qhs (may go higher if no side effects).

           (b) Six weeks may be required for proper trial.

(c) Amitriptyline—most studied; highest incidence of side effects (e.g., orthostatics, urinary retention, dry mouth, early-morning "hangover," constipation, somnolence, nightmares)

(d) Side effects usually decrease after first few weeks.

(e) If patient has cardiac conduction defects or orthostatic hypotension, TCAs should be used with caution, *if at all.*

(f) Desipramine may be tried if anticholinergic side effects or somnolence are bothersome (also nortriptyline).

(g) If no response or intolerable side effects after 6 weeks, try another drug.

(3) Antiepileptic drugs (AEDs) (e.g., carbamazepine, clonazepam, phenytoin, valproic acid, gabapentin, tiagabine, levetiracetam)

(a) Start with low doses and increase to effect or clinical toxicity (much like epilepsy treatment).

(b) Always taper (never stop) AEDs if ineffective.

(c) Work well for sharp, lancinating pain.

(4) Local anesthetics (mexiletine)

(a) Start with prognostic IV lidocaine test (if no cardiac conduction defects)—5 mg/kg over 1 hour; perform in blinded fashion using saline infusion as placebo.

(b) If greater than 50% pain relief, try oral mexiletine, 150 mg/d, increased by 150 mg q 3 to 4 days to total dose of 10 mg/kg/d, divided tid.

(c) Side effects: Nausea/vomiting, altered taste, dizziness, uncoordination, tremor, tinnitus

(5) Opiates (e.g., oxycodone, hydromorphone, morphine sulfate sustained-release, codeine/acetaminophen, hydrocodone, fentanyl)

(a) Use with *extreme caution,* if at all.

(b) Use longer-acting preparations.

(c) Maintain control over the number prescribed.

(d) Warn patient of possible side effects: addiction and physical dependence, respiratory depression, nausea/vomiting, constipation, sedation, euphoria, confusion, urinary retention, myoclonus, allergy, headaches, "histamine" reaction.

(6) Topical agents (e.g., capsaicin, lidocaine)

(a) More effective if used with oral agents

(b) Capsaicin—deactivates heat sensitive nociceptors; 0.075% cream bid to qid × 4 weeks; initial intolerable burning sensation common

(c) Lidocaine: 3 to 5 cc ointment applied q day, covered with plastic film

(7) Neurostimulation techniques

(a) TENS unit (transcutaneous electrical nerve stimulation)—more useful in mononeuropathies

        (b) SCS (spinal cord stimulation)—mainly for lower-extremity pain; epidural percutaneous multielectrode device implanted over lower thoracic segments; more effective if radicular component

    (8) Surgery—dorsal root entry zone lesions for selected cases (e.g., postherpetic neuralgia)

  b. Sympathetically maintained pain (causalgia)—distal, severe, burning pain in single extremity associated with hyperalgesia to touch and cold; usually associated with trauma to a major nerve in the affected extremity; associated with vasomotor, sympathetic and trophic changes; relieved with sympathetic block

    (1) Document response to IV phentolamine

    (2) If more than 50% relief of pain with phentolamine, try alpha-adrenergic blockade with phenoxybenzamine (10 mg bid; increase by 10 mg q week to a maximum of 120 mg q day), clonidine (0.1 mg bid to tid), or prazocin (2 mg bid).

    (3) Watch for impotence and postural hypotension.

    (4) Guanethidine regional sympathetic block or surgical sympathectomy, if pharmacologic therapy fails.

2. Other considerations
  a. Hereditary neuropathies
    (1) Proper shoes with sole cushioning
    (2) Ankle foot orthoses (over entire calf) for foot drop
    (3) Physical (PT) or occupational therapy (OT)—stretching and mild strengthening, provide assist devices, encouragement of self-reliance, writing assistance
    (4) Early orthopedics consultation for pes cavus, kyphoscoliosis, etc.
    (5) Counseling
  b. Ataxic neuropathies—PT for gait training and gait prosthetics, home improvement
  c. Many physicians prescribe B vitamins for chronic sensorimotor polyneuropathies, especially if felt to be partially related to nutritional insufficiency (e.g., alcoholic neuropathy)

PERIPHERAL NEUROPATHY SYNDROMES

I. Acute Ascending Motor Neuropathy with Variable Sensory Disturbance

Etiology	Onset	Type	CSF prot	CSF wbc	Special Features
Mononucleosis	Infection midphase	D	I	I	—
Viral hepatitis	Follows jaundice	D	I	N	Hep screen often negative
Uremia	Rapid	D	I	N	Transplant curative
Diphtheria	5–8 wk postinfection	D	I	N	No inflammation, loss of pupil accommodation
Porphyria	Rapid	A	N	N	Retained ankle jerk, bibrachial weakness, whisper
Tick paralysis	Rapid	A	N	N	Rapid recovery with tick removal
Tetanus	Rapid	A	N	N	Asymmetric sensory and motor responses
Hypophosphatemia	Rapid	D	I	N	Resolves with PO$_4$ correction
Organophosphates	Rapid				Acute paralysis, alopecia
Thallium	Rapid	A	I	N	Sensory and autonomic > motor responses
Arsenic	Subacute				
Tetrodotoxin	Rapid	D			Sodium blocker, motor tongue numb
Saxitoxin	Rapid	D			Sodium blocker, motor
Ciguaratoxin	Rapid				Prolongs sodium channel sensory > motor response
Lupus	Rapid	D/V	±	±	—
Polyarteritis nodosa	Chronic	A/V			Occurs in 70% of these patients
Lymphomatous HIV	Acute at conversion	D	I	I	HIV often negative, p24 PCR +

A, axonal; D, demyelinating; I, increased; N, normal; PCR, polymerase chain reaction; V, variable.

II. Subacute Sensorimotor Paralysis
 A. Symmetric Polyneuropathies—usually *axonal* in type
  1. Deficiency states

Vitamin	Neuropathy	Type	CSF Protein	Special Features
Thiamine (beriberi)	Axonal	S>M	Increased	Postural hypotension, burning pain
Niacin (pellagra)	Axonal	S>M	Increased	Delirium, dementia
Vitamin B$_{12}$	Axonal	S>M	Normal	Subacute combined degeneration
Vitamin B$_6$ (pyridoxine)	Neuronopathy	S>M	Normal	Occurs with INH/hydralazine
Pantothenic acid	Axonal	S>M	Normal	
Folate	Axonal	S>M	Normal	
Vitamin E	Axonal	S	Normal	Increased CK, ataxia, ophthalmoplegia

2. Metals/solvents

Substance	Course	Neuropathy	Type	Special Features
Arsenic	Acute	Axonal	S	Mees lines
Lead	Chronic	Axonal	M	Radial (wrist drop)
Mercury	Chronic	Axonal	S	Encephalopathy, acrodynia
Thallium	Chronic	Axonal	S/M	Imitates GBS
Gold	Chronic	Axonal	S	Myokymia
N-Hexane	Chronic	Axonal	S	Giant axonal neuropathy (slowing)

3. Medications

Medication	Course	Neuropathy	Type	Special Features
Isoniazid	Chronic	Axonal	S>M	Treat with vitamin B_6
Hydralazine	Chronic	Axonal	S>M	Treat with vitamin B_6
Pyridoxine	Chronic	Axonal	S	Sensory neuronopathy
Nitrofurantoin	Chronic	Axonal	S/M	Uremic patients
Vincristine	Chronic	Axonal	M	Dose related
Cisplatin	Chronic	Axonal	S	Dose related
Phenytoin	Chronic	Axonal	S	
Chloramphenicol	Chronic	Axonal	S	
Amitriptyline	Chronic	Axonal	S/M	
Colchicine	Chronic	Axonal	S/M	Vacuolar degeneration
Dapsone	Chronic	Axonal	M	
Ethambutol	Chronic	Axonal	S	Optic neuropathy
Lithium	Chronic	Axonal	S/M	
Metronidazole	Chronic	Axonal	S	
Disulfiram	Chronic	Axonal	S/M	Giant axons
Nitrous oxide	Chronic	Axonal	S	Giant axons, myelopathy
Amiodarone	Chronic	Demyel	S/M	
Perhexiline	Chronic	Demyel	S/M	

Demyel, demyelinating; M, motor; S, sensory.

B. Asymmetric Polyneuropathies (Mononeuropathy Multiplex)
   1. Major players: Diabetes, vasculitides
   2. Definition: Simultaneous or sequential involvement of three individual noncontiguous nerves in a random fashion (two or more nerves in more than one extremity)
   3. Diabetic neuropathy
      a. Most common cause of neuropathy in United States
      b. 15% to 25% of diabetics have both symptoms and signs of neuropathy, and 50% have either neuropathic symptoms or slowing of NCV. (Some say 75% to 85% of diabetics have NCV evidence of peripheral nerve dysfunction.)
      c. Most common over 50 years of age, uncommon under 30 years
      d. Pathology: Loss of myelinated fibers most prominent finding; segmental demyelination/remyelination; axonal degeneration; location in posterior roots, posterior columns, sympathetic ganglia.

e. Pathogenesis: Ischemic vs. Metabolic—Ischemic etiology favored in painful, asymmetric neuropathy of sudden onset, mononeuropathy, and cranial neuropathy; metabolic etiology favored in other forms (although this is debated).

f. NCV/EMG: "Gray zone"—both axonal and demyelinating features; NCVs mildly reduced with diminished amplitudes; focal slowing at sites of infarct or compression/trauma; sensory NCVs more sensitive; peroneal NCV best predictor of severity; NCV worse in poorly controlled and long-standing diabetics

g. CSF protein may be elevated (50 to 200 mg/dL).

h. Neuropathy can be initial manifestation of diabetes.

i. Types (Remember, traumatic neuropathies are more common in diabetics.)

   (1) Symmetric, distal, sensory greater than motor, chronic polyneuropathy (most common)

       (a) Nighttime paresthesias (painful) in feet

       (b) Lost ankle jerks; skin ulcers and neuropathic joints present

       (c) Occasionally combined with proximal weakness and wasting and sensory loss on lower abdomen

       (d) May have severe sensory loss (dorsal column) with ataxia, bladder atony, unreactive pupils, limb weakness, neuropathic joints (diabetic pseudotabes).

   (2) Ophthalmoplegia

       (a) Usually pupil-sparing third-nerve lesion; may affect sixth and seventh nerves.

       (b) Usual spontaneous recovery in 6 to 12 weeks

   (3) Mononeuropathy or mononeuropathy multiplex

       (a) Mononeuropathies most commonly involve femoral and sciatic nerves, and, less commonly, median and ulnar nerves and lumbosacral plexus.

       (b) Compression neuropathies more common in diabetics

       (c) Acute onset, painful, motor > sensory, usually remits, ischemic in nature

   (4) Diabetic amyotrophy

       (a) Painful, asymmetric, unilateral or bilateral—lumbosacral plexopathy/mononeuropathy multiplex

       (b) Begins with pain in low back or hip, spreads to thigh/knee (aching with lancination), worse at night.

       (c) Pelvofemoral muscle weakness and atrophy with lost knee jerks

       (d) Sphincters may be involved; sensation may be spared.

       (e) Subacute onset in elderly diabetics with poorly controlled or unrecognized diabetes and severe weight loss

       (f) Tendency for recurrence on opposite side

       (g) Improvement or recovery in 6 to 18 months

       (h) Femoral NCV abnormal in two-thirds of cases, and EMG invariably shows denervation.

(5) Diabetic polyradiculopathy
- (a) Syndrome of severe thoracoabdominal pain and dysesthesia, usually in elderly male type II diabetics who have experienced weight loss
- (b) Subacute onset with maximal intensity in weeks
- (c) Initial symptoms are sensory, but motor weakness develops in most patients, unilaterally in one-third of them.
- (d) Increased CSF protein almost universal
- (e) Thoracic roots most commonly involved, especially T8 to T12
- (f) Usually asymmetric and involves two or more contiguous roots.
- (g) May occur in association with severe diffuse polyneuropathy, producing diabetic neuropathic cachexia.
- (h) EMG is essentially sole means of confirming diagnosis—shows fibrillations and positive sharp waves in involved thoracic paraspinous muscles.
- (i) Commonly associated with sensorimotor polyneuropathy
- (j) Good prognosis for recovery

(6) Autonomic neuropathy
- (a) Often superimposed on sensorimotor polyneuropathy
- (b) Pupillary and lacrimal dysfunction, impairment of sweating and vascular reflexes, nocturnal diarrhea, atonicity of GI and GU tracts, impotence, postural hypotension
- (c) Pathology shows degeneration of neurons in sympathetic ganglia, loss of myelinated fibers in vagus and splanchnic nerves, and loss of neurons in intermediolateral cell column.
- (d) Therapy
  - (i) Postural hypotension—elevate head of bed 5° to 20°, avoid certain drugs, liberal salt diet, elastic stockings; fludrocortisone (0.1 mg/d, increase to 0.5 mg bid), indomethacin (25 to 50 mg tid), DHE and caffeine (30 minutes before breakfast).
  - (ii) Delayed gastric emptying—metoclopramide (10 mg q AC and qhs)
  - (iii) Diarrhea—tetracycline (250 to 500 mg po at onset)
  - (iv) Facial sweating after meals—propantheline bromide (15 mg 30 minutes q AC and at social occasions)

(7) Proximal symmetric polyneuropathy
- (a) Symmetric, proximal weakness and wasting usually without pain; insidious onset and chronic progression
- (b) Lower extremities more commonly involved
- (c) Sensory changes usually mild, if present
- (d) Possible association with distal, sensory polyneuropathy

(8) Treatment
- (a) Control glucose (NCV improves with normalization of glucose.)

      (b) Meticulous foot care

      (c) Pain control (glucose control, tricyclics for burning pain, anticonvulsants for stabbing pain, fluphenazine for deep aching pain, mexiletine or capsaicin cream for painful mononeuropathies)

      (d) Avoid trauma.

      (e) Myoinositol, aldose reductase inhibitors, gangliosides may improve NCV.

      (f) May be subcategories of patients who would respond to immune-modulating therapy, including those who have demyelinating neuropathy similar to CIDP and those who have mononeuropathy multiplex picture with inflammatory vasculopathy on biopsy pathology.

4. Vasculitic neuropathies—Most commonly mononeuropathy multiplex, but also see symmetric or asymmetric distal sensorimotor polyneuropathy; associated with systemic symptoms (weight loss, fever, malaise, anorexia) and evidence of multiple end-organ involvement and high erythrocyte sedimentation rate. Pathologically, see axonal degeneration, usually secondary to systemic necrotizing vasculitis; NCV shows sensory conduction more often affected. Diagnosis made by sural nerve biopsy; treatment with steroids and other immune-modulating therapies is often beneficial.

    a. Polyarteritis nodosa

    b. Rheumatoid arthritis

    c. Systemic lupus erythematosus

    d. Wegener granulomatosis

    e. Progressive systemic sclerosis

    f. Sjögren's syndrome

    g. Churg-Strauss syndrome

    h. Temporal arteritis

    i. Lymphomatoid granulomatosis

    j. Hypersensitivity vasculitis

    k. Amphetamine-induced vasculitis

    l. Hypereosinophilic syndrome

    m. Nonsystemic vasculitic neuropathy

5. Multifocal motor neuropathy (multifocal demyelinating neuropathy)

    a. Subacute progression of mononeuropathy multiplex usually in arms, with pure motor weakness in 50% of cases

    b. More common in males; two-thirds of patients are younger than 45 years.

    c. Asymmetric, distal weakness, beginning in hands in more than 80% of cases

    d. Slow progression up to 20 years

    e. Pain prominent with tender nerves

    f. Possibly associated with optic neuropathy

    g. Possible mimicking of motor neuron disease (fasciculations in 25%, normal reflexes in 15%)

    h. CSF protein increased in one-third of cases

     i. High anti-GM-l titer (350 or more) in 60% to 80% of cases, most common neuropathy associated with anti-GM-l antibodies (primarily polyclonal IgM)

     j. NCV shows nonuniform demyelinating pattern with focal conduction block in multiple motor nerves, usually in short segments and *not* confined to usual sites of compression.

     k. Pathology shows demyelination—remyelination in 60% of cases and inflammatory cells in a third.

     l. Majority respond to immunomodulating therapy in a few weeks (cyclophosphamide greater than prednisone; also plasma exchange and intravenous immunoglobulin [IVIg]).

6. Sarcoidosis
   a. Nervous system involvement in 5% of patients; 15% of this number have neuropathy.
   b. Mononeuropathy multiplex most common, but also see cranial neuropathy (CN VII most common), symmetric or asymmetric polyneuropathy, or mononeuropathy.
   c. Neuropathy may be associated with myopathy or CNS involvement (basilar meningitis—pituitary stalk and hypothalamus).
   d. Large, irregular zones of sensory loss over the trunk sometimes seen; said to distinguish sarcoidosis from other causes of mononeuropathy multiplex
   e. Pathology shows axonal degeneration, sometimes combined with segmental demyelination.
   f. NCVs most consistent with axonal degeneration
   g. Clinically improves with steroids.

7. Lyme disease
   a. Neuropathy occurs in 36% to 40% of patients with symptomatic late disease.
   b. Acute and chronic forms of neuropathy
      (1) Acute—more severe; cranial nerve palsy and CSF pleocytosis are present.
      (2) Chronic—less severe; most common CSF finding is increased protein.
      (3) Features in common:
         (a) Frequent radicular involvement
         (b) Features of mononeuropathy multiplex
         (c) Nerve biopsy findings of perivascular inflammation and axonal degeneration
         (d) Good response to antibiotics
   c. Three patterns of Lyme neuropathy
      (1) Cranial neuropathy
      (2) Painful radiculopathy
      (3) Peripheral neuropathy
   d. Sensory peripheral neuropathy most common, followed by painful radiculopathy and CN VII palsy
   e. Barnwarth syndrome—Triad of lymphocytic meningitis with increased protein, cranial neuritis, and radiculoneuritis following days to weeks after erythema chronicum migrans appears.

  f. Cranial neuropathy occurs early (often facial diplegia).
  g. Peripheral neuropathy characterized by painful intermittent asymmetric paresthesias, with rare motor weakness and hyporeflexia
  h. Carpal tunnel syndrome incidence increased in patients with Lyme disease
  i. NCV compatible with axonal degeneration
  8. Leprosy—mononeuropathy multiplex occurs in the tuberculoid form of this disease secondary to local granuloma formation (see later section).
  9. Ischemic neuropathy
  10. Bacterial endocarditis
  11. HIV disease
III. Syndrome of Chronic Sensorimotor Polyneuropathy (less chronic acquired forms)
  A. CIDP (see later section)
  B. Diabetes (most common diabetic neuropathic syndrome—see previous section)
  C. Alcoholic Neuropathy and Neuropathic Beriberi (see previous section)
  D. Neuropathy Associated with Connective-Tissue Diseases (see previous section)
  E. Paraneoplastic Polyneuropathy—neuropathy in 2% to 5% of patients with malignancy
    1. Sensorimotor polyneuropathy—not truly paraneoplastic, distal, symmetric, and axonal, CSF protein usually normal
    2. Subacute sensory neuronopathy—small-cell lung cancer, breast cancer, proprioceptive loss, paraneoplastic encephalomyelitis, anti-Hu antibodies found in 86% of cases in one series, CSF protein usually high, sensory neuronopathy inflammation and degeneration of dorsal root ganglion (DRG) cells, degeneration of posterior roots and columns
    3. Subacute to acute, primarily motor polyradiculoneuropathy—similar to GBS; lymphoma
    4. Chronic, primarily motor polyradiculoneuropathy—similar to CIDP; demyelinating, CSF protein high
    5. Paraneoplastic vasculitis—rare; lymphoma and lung cancer; high ESR and CSF protein; axonal mixed pattern
    6. Autonomic neuropathy—small-cell lung cancer, pulmonary carcinoid, and Hodgkin's disease
    7. Paraneoplastic motor neuron syndrome—very rare; lymphoma (primarily), lung cancer, and renal cell carcinoma; mimics ALS
  F. Paraproteinemic or Dysproteinemic Polyneuropathies
    1. Osteolytic multiple myeloma
      a. Neuropathy present clinically in 13% of patients and electrophysiologically in another 26%.
      b. Two types
        (1) With amyloidosis (two-thirds)
        (2) Without amyloidosis (one-third)
      c. Neuropathy without amyloidosis is heterogeneous and resembles axonal carcinomatous neuropathy.
      d. Neuropathy with amyloidosis resembles that of nonhereditary systemic amyloidosis (see later section).
      e. Treatment of myeloma usually *does not* affect neuropathy.

2. Osteosclerotic multiple myeloma
   a. Associated with neuropathy 50% of time
   b. Demyelinating, primarily motor neuropathy, with high CSF protein (similar to CIDP)
   c. Usually with IgG or IgA lambda light chain in serum
   d. Treatment of tumor may result in remission of neuropathy.
3. Monoclonal gammopathy of undetermined significance (MGUS)
   a. Of neuropathies associated with M-protein, 50% have MGUS.
   b. Usually affects males older than 50 years.
   c. Insidious onset, distal (feet more so than hands) symmetric sensory (mainly large fiber) and motor dysfunction.
   d. Associated with Raynaud's phenomenon, ataxia, and action tremor
   e. Demyelinating
   f. CSF protein high
   g. Anti-MAG antibodies seen in 50% of cases
   h. Biopsy shows loss of myelinated fibers with monoclonal antibodies on myelin sheaths, hypertrophic changes.
   i. Treatment with immune modulating therapy
      (1) Therapeutic plasma exchange (TPE)
      (2) Prednisone
      (3) IVIg
      (4) Azathioprine
4. Waldenström's macroglobulinemia
   a. Neuropathy rare; usually chronic, sensorimotor, and symmetric, but may be chiefly sensory, chiefly motor, subacute, and asymmetric
   b. Demyelinating and increased CSF protein
   c. Treatment: May respond to chemotherapy and/or TPE but less predictable and not immediate (should continue treatment at least 3 months)
5. Cryoglobulinemia
   a. Neuropathy occurs in 7% of patients and is axonal and usually vasculitic (secondary to intravascular immune complex deposition and associated vasculitis).
   b. Usually symmetric or asymmetric sensory neuropathy, associated with Raynaud's, purpuric lesions of ulcers of legs
   c. Neuropathy precipitated by cold
   d. Occasionally see mononeuropathy multiplex and may be acute
   e. Treatment: Prednisone, chlorambucil, cyclophosphamide, or TPE
6. Nonhereditary amyloid neuropathy
   a. Neuropathy primarily sensory with prominent early loss of small-fiber function, followed by progressive weakness and large-fiber involvement
   b. Dysautonomia often severe and debilitating, as is pain associated with small-fiber damage
   c. Sural nerve biopsy shows axonal degeneration with amyloid identifiable.
   d. Carpal tunnel syndrome seen in 20% of patients
   e. Secondary amyloidosis associated with malignant dysproteinemias; familial amyloid neuropathy also seen (see later section)

       f. Poor response to therapy

G. Uremic Polyneuropathy

    1. Most common complication of chronic renal failure

    2. 66% to 70% of patients on dialysis affected

    3. Does not occur in acute renal failure.

    4. Duration and severity of renal failure and symptomatic uremia are the important factors in development of neuropathy.

    5. Clinically, painless distal sensory loss followed by motor weakness of leg more so than arm

    6. May begin with burning dysesthesias of feet and restless legs syndrome (creeping, crawling, itching of legs at night).

    7. Pathology shows primary axonal degeneration and secondary segmental demyelination.

    8. Hemodialysis stabilizes or arrests the clinical and electrophysiologic signs.

    9. Renal transplantation usually results in complete recovery after 6 to 12 months.

   10. Uremia associated with two focal neuropathies:

       a. Carpal tunnel syndrome

       b. Ischemic monomelic neuropathy

H. Leprous Polyneuritis

    1. Most common neuropathy in the world

    2. Neuropathy due to direct invasion by *Mycobacterium leprae*

    3. Initial lesion is anesthetic, hypopigmented skin macule or papule caused by invasion of cutaneous nerves (indeterminate leprosy); after this stage, disease may take one of two forms—tuberculoid leprosy or lepromatous leprosy.

    4. Tuberculoid leprosy—causes mononeuropathy multiplex by inclusion of larger nerves in region of granuloma formation (most frequently involved are ulnar, median, peroneal, posterior auricular, and facial); these nerves, as well as involved superficial sensory nerves, may be palpably enlarged.

    5. Lepromatous leprosy—lack of resistance permits hematogenous spread to skin, ciliary bodies, testes, nodes, nerves; causes symmetric or asymmetric polyneuropathy with pain and temperature loss involving cooler body areas (pinnae of ears, dorsal hands and feet, anterolateral leg); motor dysfunction follows from invasion of nerves close to skin (ulnar at elbow, deep peroneal at ankle, superficial facial, median at wrist).

    6. DTRs usually spared in face of widespread sensory loss (relatively sparing vibration/proprioception—syringomyelic pattern)

    7. Trophic ulcers, Charcot's joints, and mutilated digits common secondary to anesthesia

    8. Pathology shows segmental demyelination (organisms proliferate in Schwann cells).

    9. Treatment: Sulfone (Dapsone), rifampin, and clofazimine; thalidomide for skin lesions

I. Hypothyroid Polyneuropathy

    1. Infrequent complication

    2. Two types seen:
       a. Carpal and tarsal tunnel syndromes
       b. Diffuse sensory more so than motor polyneuropathy
    3. Axonal degeneration with segmental demyelination
    4. CSF protein often increased
    5. Reversible with thyroid hormone replacement

J. Chronic Benign Polyneuropathy of the Elderly

K. Acromegalic Neuropathy
    1. Carpal and tarsal tunnel syndromes
    2. Pathology shows segmental demyelination with onion-bulb formation

L. Critical Illness Polyneuropathy (CIP)
    1. Sepsis and critical illness occur in approximately 5% of ICU patients, and CIP occurs in 50% of these; incidence is 70% in patients with sepsis and multiorgan system failure.
    2. Usually patients in ICU at least 1 week when earliest signs develop (e.g., difficulty weaning from the ventilator)
    3. Later signs—distal weakness, decreased DTRs; if severe, complete quadriplegia and respiratory paralysis (signs occur in 50% of patients; the other 50% are diagnosed by NCV/EMG)
    4. NCVs are compatible with primary axonal degeneration, and EMG shows signs of denervation. (Decreased diaphragmatic CMAPs and signs of chest wall denervation establish CIP as the cause of difficulty of weaning; may be the most common cause of difficulty of weaning.)
    5. Pathology shows primary axonal degeneration distally, motor > sensory fibers, without inflammation; CSF protein usually normal.
    6. CIP may occur outside the ICU in patients who develop sepsis in the course of severe renal failure.
    7. Mild polyneuropathies may improve; severe ones may not.
    8. Pathophysiology—sepsis itself is the likely cause (disturbs the microcirculation of nerves, increases capillary permeability, causing endoneural edema with resultant hypoxia and axonal damage)

M. Neuropathy Associated with Antisulfatide Antibodies
    1. Sensory > motor involvement
    2. Numbness or pain in feet and spreads proximal within 1 year
    3. Loss of ankle jerks; other DTRs preserved
    4. Axonal degeneration with little, if any, demyelination
    5. Antisulfatide antibodies > 1,000 in 20% to 30% of cases
    6. IVIg may be helpful.

N. Neuropathy Associated with Liver Disease
    1. Clinical peripheral neuropathy reported in 9% of patients with chronic liver disease, and NCVs abnormal in 14% to 68% of patients
    2. Segmental demyelination
    3. Neuropathy associated with primary biliary cirrhosis is painful; xanthoma formation in and around nerves

O. AIDS Neuropathy
   1. Types
      a. Chronic predominantly sensory polyneuropathy (most common)
      b. AIDP or CIDP
      c. Mononeuritis multiplex (see earlier section)
      d. Sensory ataxic neuropathy
      e. Lumbosacral polyradiculopathy
P. Chronic Ataxic Neuropathy
   1. Characterized by slow progression, distal paresthesias, sensory ataxia with profound loss of proprioceptive and kinesthetic sense, with normal strength
   2. Clinically not different from paraneoplastic sensory neuropathy except that carcinoma is not found in these patients
   3. Monoclonal or polyclonal gammopathy may be found.
   4. EMG/NCV shows sensory neuronopathy pattern (absent sensory CNAP with normal motor NCV and EMG).
   5. Sural nerve biopsy shows loss of myelinated fibers (large > small); regeneration of myelinated fibers may be seen; these findings are secondary to selective destruction of the DRG neuron.
Q. Neuropathy Associated with HTLV-1 Myelopathy—subclinical inflammatory demyelinating neuropathy has been described in this disorder (motor > sensory).
R. GALOP Antibody Syndrome
   1. Gait disorder, autoantibody, late age onset, polyneuropathy
   2. Age at onset approximately 70 years
   3. Weakness and sensory loss primarily distal
   4. IgM to sulfatides and central myelin antigen
S. POEMS Syndrome
   1. Polyneuropathy, organomegaly, endocrinopathy, M protein and skin changes
   2. Age at onset approximately 40 to 50 years
   3. Weakness common
   4. CSF protein elevated

IV. Syndrome of Hereditary Chronic Polyneuropathy (tends to be more chronic than acquired, progressive, symmetric, and degenerative neuropathies)
   A. Hereditary Neuropathy with Autonomic Features

Type	Inheritance	Onset	Lesion
HSAN I	AD	Second decade	Degeneration of small DRG neurons
HSAN II	AR	Infancy	Absence of myelinated fibers
HSAN III	AR	Birth	Absence of myelinated fibers
HSAN IV	AR	Birth	Absence of small DRG neurons and Lissauer's tracts
Friedreich's ataxia	AR	Before age 20 years	Loss of large myelinated fibers
Ataxia telangiectasia	AR	Before age 5 years	Loss of large unmyelinated fibers
Olivo-pontocerebellar degeneration	AD	Adult	Loss of large unmyelinated fibers

HSAN, hereditary sensory autonomic neuropathy.

B. Hereditary Motor and Sensory Neuropathy

Type	Inheritance	Onset	Neuropathy	Lesion
HMSN I (CMT I)[a]	AD 17	Childhood	D	Onion bulb
HMSN II (CMT II)[a]	AD 1p	Second decade	A	Degeneration of large myelinated fibers
HMSN III (Dejerine-Sottas syndrome)	AR 1q or 17p	Infancy	D	Interstitial hypertrophy onion bulbs
Rousy-Levy syndrome	AD	Infancy	D	Onion bulbs
HMSNIV (Refsum's syndrome)	AR	Childhood	D	Hypertrophic nerves onion bulb

A, axonal; D, demyelinating; HMSN, hereditary motor sensory neuropathy.

[a]Charcot-Marie-Tooth (CMT) disease is characterized by distal muscle atrophy beginning in the lower extremities, equinovarus deformity, champagne bottle legs, clawed hands, lost deep tendon reflexes, paresthesias, and sensory loss.

ACUTE AND CHRONIC INFLAMMATORY DEMYELINATING POLYNEUROPATHIES

I. Acute Inflammatory Demyelinating Polyneuropathy (AIDP) (Guillain-Barré Syndrome)
  A. Epidemiology
    1. Most frequent cause of acute generalized weakness
    2. Incidence: 1 or 2/100,000 each year
    3. Nonseasonal, nonepidemic; occurs in all ages, all parts of the world, both sexes
    4. Incidence increases with increasing age (highest in ages 50 to 74 years)
    5. Two-thirds have preceding event 1 week to 1 month prior to onset (URI, 60%; GI syndrome, 20%; surgery, 5%; vaccinations, 5%)
       a. Antecedent infections associated with GBS:
          (1) Cytomegalovirus (CMV)
          (2) Epstein-Barr virus (EBV)
          (3) HIV
          (4) Hepatitis B
          (5) Herpes simplex virus (HSV)
          (6) *Mycoplasma pneumoniae*
          (7) *Campylobacter jejuni*—associated with poor outcome and Miller-Fisher variant
          (8) *Borrelia burgdorferi*—Lyme disease
          (9) Influenza and others
       b. Lymphoma (particularly Hodgkin's disease) has been associated with GBS
       c. Spinal/epidural anesthesia
  B. Etiology/Pathology and Pathogenesis
    1. Immune-mediated segmental demyelination initiated by an undetermined antigenic reaction (may be viral)
       a. Cell-mediated component: T-cell lines are sensitized to P2, a basic protein found in peripheral nerve myelin. A clinically and pathologically indistinguishable disease called *experimental allergic neuritis (EAN)* develops in ani-

mals 2 weeks after immunization with a peripheral nerve homogenate containing P2; EAN can be transferred via these cells.

    b. Antibody-mediated component: IGs and complement are found on myelinated fibers, and antiperipheral nerve myelin antibodies found in some patients' serum (titers correlate with clinical course). An antibody to the GD1a ganglioside has been associated with a worsened clinical course. GBS serum demyelinates rat nerve.

  2. Pathology specimens show endoneural perivascular mononuclear cell infiltrates early, associated with perivenular demyelination. (Changes are initially present in ventral roots and proximal spinal nerves.) Later segmental demyelination and secondary Wallerian degeneration occur, affecting entire peripheral nerve, cranial nerves, dorsal and ventral roots, and dorsal root ganglia. Lymphocytic infiltrates also seen in lymph nodes, liver, spleen, and heart. Some cases show intense axonal damage with paucity of inflammation (axonal variant).

C. Clinical Features

  1. Rapidly progressive symmetric weakness with areflexia; may be associated with cranial nerve palsies, autonomic instability, and respiratory failure

    a. Weakness usually ascending (distal to proximal): lower extremities first, then trunk, arms, and cranial muscles

      (1) Proximal muscles can be affected first.

      (2) Cranial nerves rarely affected first; more than 50% have cranial nerve involvement, with facial diplegia most common (some sources say occurs in half of all cases).

      (3) Maximum deficit occurs within days to maximum of 4 weeks and then plateaus (90% have maximum deficit at 14 days, with mean of 12 days).

        (a) Total motor paralysis with respiratory failure and death may occur in a few days.

        (b) Weakness is so rapid that atrophy is not seen.

    b. Hypotonia and decreased, then absent, reflexes

    c. Pain and paresthesias/sensory symptoms

      (1) Low back pain and myalgias in greater than 50% (hips, thighs)

        (a) Consider acute cord lesion in patients with LBP, areflexia, leg paralysis.

        (b) Severe myalgia with increased CPK is rarely seen.

      (2) Paresthesias are frequent and early symptom.

        (a) Resolve rapidly (usually).

        (b) Objective sensory loss usually mild and usually affects large fiber modalities (vibration and position sense).

    d. Autonomic instability not uncommon and highly variable in expression

      (1) Sinus tachycardia and bradycardia, other tachyarrhythmias, orthostatic hypotension, hypertension, anhidrosis, diaphoresis, sphincter dysfunction, pupil changes, gut atony, flushing

      (2) Usual duration of less than 1 to 2 weeks

      (3) Urinary retention in 15% of cases

      e. Rare variations of signs
        (1) Babinski sign
        (2) Pseudotumor cerebri with papilledema—possibly due to increased CSF protein with CSF block
2. Associated clinical findings
    a. Minor ECG changes—T-wave changes
    b. Hyponatremia—usually secondary to syndrome of inappropriate anti-diuretic hormone secretion (SIADH)
    c. Transient diabetes insipidus
3. Clinical variants
    a. Miller-Fisher syndrome (MFS)
      (1) Gait ataxia, ophthalmoparesis, and areflexia, with normal limbs (some patients have mild proximal limb weakness)
      (2) May have pharyngeal weakness, diminished position sense, and paresthesias
      (3) Associated with IgG antibody to ganglioside GQ_1b.
      (4) Associated with prior *Campylobacter jejuni* infection
      (5) Differentiation from brain stem encephalitis often difficult (lesion in MFS is peripheral, most likely)
    b. Pharyngeal—cervical—brachial
      (1) Blurred vision or diplopia; ptosis; marked oropharyngeal, neck, and shoulder weakness; respiratory failure; areflexia in arms only; normal sensation (occasionally leg areflexia present)
      (2) Simulates botulism and diphtheria clinically
        (a) No dry mouth, dizziness, or GI symptoms that are seen in botulism
        (b) Differentiation by electrophysiologic studies
    c. Paraparesis
      (1) Areflexia in legs *only*; normal to near-normal power and reflexes in arms, face, and respiratory muscles
      (2) Differentiation from acute cord lesion difficult
    d. Severe ptosis without ophthalmoplegia
      (1) Mild facial weakness present
      (2) These may later develop into typical GBS or pharyngeal-cervical—brachial variant.
      (3) Clinically similar to myasthenia gravis
    e. Polyneuritis Cranialis
      (1) Rapid onset of multiple symmetric cranial neuropathies
      (2) Rule out sarcoid, carcinomatosis, diphtheria.
    f. Acute pandysautonomia
      (1) Minimal weakness
      (2) Rule out thallium poisoning (additional sensory findings and alopecia usually present)
    g. Acute axonal form
      (1) Quadriplegia, bulbar dysfunction, respiratory impairment
      (2) Axonal degeneration in nerve roots and distal nerves

(3) Muscle atrophy present early

(4) Minimal inflammation and demyelination on biopsy

(5) More common in China—associated with IV ganglioside treatment and *C. jejuni*—both with increased anti-GM-1 antibody titers

(6) Poor prognosis

    h. Sensory GBS (rare)

D. Laboratory Features

    1. Electrophysiologic studies: NCV shows focal slowing, motor conduction block, temporal dispersion, and prolongation of F-wave and terminal latencies.

        a. All parameters may be normal for first few days.

        b. First noted abnormality is prolonged (or absent) F-waves.

        c. Persistent normal NCVs in 10% of cases.

    2. CSF studies: Elevated protein with normal cell count (albuminocytologic dissociation)

        a. 10% of patients have 10 to 50 cells/mm^3 (mostly lymphs).

        b. Protein may be normal in first few days, rising to peak in 4 to 6 weeks.

        c. CSF protein remains normal in 10% of patients.

        d. Transient oligoclonal bands and elevated myelin basic protein may be present.

        e. Pressure and glucose usually normal

E. Differential Diagnoses

    1. Diphtheria—impaired visual accommodation, EOM, and oropharyngeal paresis

    2. Poliomyelitis—epidemic, meningismus, fever

    3. Porphyria—abdominal crisis and psychologic symptoms

    4. Acute myelopathy—sensory level, sphincter dysfunction

    5. Basilar artery thrombosis—positive Babinski sign, brisk reflexes

    6. Acute myasthenia gravis—no sensory symptoms, reflexes usually obtainable, weak mandibular muscles (usually spared in GBS)

    7. Botulism—pupillary reflexes lost, bradycardia present

    8. Tick paralysis—can exactly mimic GBS, except no sensory loss and CSF protein normal

    9. Hypophosphatemia and hypokalemia

   10. Hexane inhalation

   11. Thallium, arsenic, or lead poisoning

   12. Lyme disease

   13. HIV seroconversion

   14. Complication of IV methylprednisolone

   15. Saxitoxin from contaminated shellfish, tetrodotoxin from puffer fish, and ciguatera toxin, which accumulates in various fish

   16. Hysteria

   17. Rare cases that were misdiagnosed as GBS: Polyarteritis nodosa, vasculitis, children with severe musculoskeletal pain, polymyositis, critically ill polyneuropathy, encephalomyeloneuritis, alcoholic neuropathy, sarcoid, *Mycoplasma pneumoniae*

F. Work-up

    1. Good H and P (preceding illness, time course, thorough physical examination)

2. Lumbar puncture (albuminocytologic dissociation)
3. Electrophysiologic studies (may need to be repeated as chronology progresses)
4. Serum for CBC, FBP with Ca, Mg, Phos, LFTs, HIV ESR. (Consider ANA, rheumatoid factor [RF], RBC protoporphyrins, urine porphobilinogen, 24-hour urine for heavy metals, Lyme titer.)
5. EKG and CXR

G. Treatment
  1. Supportive therapy—essence of therapy is respiratory assistance and careful nursing
    a. Frequent forced vital capacity (FVC) measurements
      (1) Intubate if FVC < 12 to 15 mL/kg, regardless of ABG.
      (2) If significant bulbar weakness and good FVC, may need intubation for airway protection.
      (3) Aggressive pulmonary toilet
      (4) Consider tracheostomy if intubated for more than 10 days.
    b. Cardiac monitoring and frequent vitals; pressors and IVF prn.
    c. Deep vein thrombosis prophylaxis
    d. Ulcer prophylaxis
    e. Early PT for range of motion
    f. Decubitus prevention
    g. Careful monitoring for infection (UTI and pneumonia)
    h. Artificial tears and eye patch if facial weakness (qhs)
    i. Emotional support and communication devices for patient and family
    j. Pain control
  2. Immune modulating therapy
    a. Mild cases: Careful observation and supportive care may be all that is needed. Patients who are progressing, are ambulatory only with assistance or recently have become nonambulatory, or those with respiratory compromise or autonomic instability should be considered for immune modulating therapy.
    b. Therapeutic plasma exchange (TPE)
      (1) Mainstay of therapy
      (2) Most effective if given within 7 days of disease onset and for patients who require intubation
      (3) Should be instituted before 3 weeks after onset
      (4) Predictions of response (most important)—younger age and preserved CMAP amplitudes on NCV
      (5) 200 to 250 mL/kg removed during four to six treatments on alternate days with saline and 5% albumin as replacement fluid
      (6) Results in decreased hospitalization time, mechanical ventilation time, and time until patient walks again; results in more patients returning to full muscle strength at 1 year.
      (7) Side effects—hypotension, bleeding, arrhythmias, infection
      (8) Avoid in patients with significant dysautonomia.
      (9) Possible increased relapse rate if started early

       c. IVIg
         (1) Proven effective in one multicenter trial at dosage of 400 mg/kg/d × 5 days
         (2) Increased strength over TPE and improved median time to improvement
         (3) Reduced complication rate over TPE, and less need for mechanical ventilation
         (4) Superiority or equivalence of IVIg to TPE in doubt; questionable biased selection of worse cases in TPE arm of study; also concern about increased relapse rate with IVIg
         (5) Alternative to TPE in children, in cases where TPE is not available, in patients with severe autonomic dysfunction or with cardiac disease
         (6) Side effects—allergic reactions, renal failure, aseptic meningitis, increased serum viscosity with vasoocclusive phenomena, headache
         (7) Always check IgA level before beginning IVIg; increased anaphylaxis in IgA-deficient patients
       d. Glucocorticoids are ineffective.
   H. Prognosis
     1. Mortality rate of 3%
       a. Early deaths—cardiac arrest (secondary to dysautonomia, ARDS, mechanical failures, etc.)
       b. Later deaths—pulmonary embolism, bacterial infections
     2. 35% have permanent residual deficits.
       a. Of these, 10% have severe disability—patients with rapid progression (bedridden first week), early mechanical ventilation, elderly, and early decreased amplitude of CMAP on NCV.
       b. 10% to 25% have minor signs/symptoms.
     3. 10% to 20% develop respiratory failure.
     4. 3% to 10% have biphasic course with partial recovery, then relapse.
     5. 65% to 75% make full neurologic recovery.
     6. Children have a better prognosis.
     7. Speed of recovery varies from a few weeks to months in less severe cases, 6 to 18 months or longer in severe cases. Little or no improvement is expected after 2 years.
 II. Chronic Inflammatory Demyelinating Polyneuropathy (CIDP)
   A. Synonyms: Chronic inflammatory demyelinating polyradiculoneuropathy, chronic relapsing GBS, chronic relapsing polyneuritis, relapsing corticosteroid-dependent polyneuritis
   B. Epidemiology
     1. Represents one-third of all initially undiagnosed acquired neuropathies.
     2. Peak incidence: 40 to 60 years of age, but can occur from infancy to late adulthood.
     3. Less than 10% have preceding viral infection.
     4. Age of onset can influence disease course. Younger patients tend to have relapsing course; older patients, a more chronic, progressive course.
     5. Pregnancy is associated with relapse.
     6. Males outnumbered females in one large series by 5:3.

      7. CIDP may be associated with MS.
- C. Etiology/Pathology and Pathogenesis
  1. Immune-mediated segmental demyelination
     a. Evidence for cell-mediated component based on mononuclear cell infiltration of spinal roots, ganglia, and proximal nerve trunks
     b. Evidence for humoral component based on detection of IgM (less often IgG) and complement fragment C3d on myelin sheaths of sural nerve biopsies and also the fact that CIDP patients respond to plasmapheresis
  2. Possible association with certain HLA haplotypes (A1, B8, DRw3, Dw3)
  3. Pathology specimens (usually sural nerve biopsy) show interstitial and perivascular inflammatory cell infiltrates, loss of many myelinated fibers, and degeneration of others with segmental demyelination/remyelination (onion-bulb formations). Large fibers are more severely involved.

  Note: In predominantly motor disease, changes in sensory nerves may not be fully representative of the pathologic process (i.e., in one series, demyelination seen in 50%, axonal in 20%, mixed in 13%).

- D. Clinical Features
  1. Insidious onset and steady or step-wise progression of symmetric (occasionally asymmetric) proximal and distal muscle weakness of both upper and lower extremities
     a. Weakness must be present for at least 2 months.
     b. Weakness varies from mild to severe, requiring assisted ambulation, but rarely assisted ventilation.
     c. Proximal muscle weakness may be equal to or greater than distal. (This sets CIDP apart from most other neuropathies.)
     d. Arms and legs affected, but legs are usually more severely involved.
     e. Neck flexor weakness is also a distinguishing feature of CIDP.
     f. Facial muscles may be involved, but cranial nerves are usually spared.
  2. Diffuse areflexia or hyporeflexia
  3. Sensory findings are usually mild; sensory involvement more prominent than in GBS.
     a. Touch, vibration, and proprioception are more commonly involved than pain/temperature.
     b. Numbness, paresthesias, and dysesthesias of hands may be initial symptoms. (Painful paresthesia is uncommon.)
     c. Some patients may have severe proprioceptive loss, with ataxia, wide-based gait, and positive Romberg sign. Rule out paraproteinemia in this group.
     d. CIDP may present as a pure sensory neuropathy, but first think of paraneoplastic syndrome, Sjögren's syndrome, etc.
     e. Patients may describe loss of balance, even if position sense remains intact.
  4. Papilledema and optic neuritis may be seen.
  5. Hypertrophic, firm nerves may be palpated.
  6. Four types of clinical courses usually described.
     a. Monophasic (may mimic GBS in rapidity of evolution)

      b. Step-wise progressive—earlier onset (accounts for one-third of cases)

      c. Relapsing/remitting—earlier onset (one-third of cases)

      d. Chronic progressive—later onset (along with monophasic, accounts for one-third of cases)

   7. Usually attains maximum severity after several months to 1 year or longer

E. Laboratory Features

   1. Electrophysiologic studies: Nerve conduction velocity findings:

      a. Nonuniform reduction in NCV in the demyelinating range in at least two motor nerves

      b. Conduction block or abnormal temporal dispersion in at least one motor nerve

      c. Prolonged distal latencies in at least two nerves

      d. Absent F-waves or prolonged F-wave latencies in at least two motor nerves

   2. CSF studies: Albuminocytologic disassociation

      a. CSF protein > 55 mg/dL (found in 95% of patients)

      b. Cell count < 10/mm^3

   3. Nerve biopsy: see the immediately preceding section C.3.

F. Diagnostic Criteria

   1. Definite CIDP—all mandatory clinical features and major laboratory features must be present (50% of patients). Mandatory clinical features include

      a. Progression of proximal and distal upper- and lower-extremity weakness for at least 2 months

      b. Areflexia or hyporeflexia

   2. Probable CIDP—all mandatory clinical features and two of three major laboratory features

   3. Possible CIDP—all mandatory clinical features and one of three major laboratory features

   4. Mandatory exclusion criteria must be met in all groups. (For an extensive list refer to Mendell JR. Chronic inflammatory demyelinating polyradiculoneuropathy. *Ann Rev Med* 1993;44:211–219.)

G. CIDP with Concurrent Illness: These patients have underlying illness associated with a neuropathy identical to CIDP.

   1. Inflammatory bowel disease

   2. Hodgkin's disease

   3. Chronic active hepatitis

   4. Connective tissue disorders

   5. HIV infection

   6. Monoclonal gammopathy of undetermined significance (MGUS)

      a. Onset is slightly older than in idiopathic CIDP.

      b. More likely to affect males

   7. Demyelinating neuropathy associated with multiple sclerosis

H. Other Neuropathies in Differential Diagnoses of CIDP

   1. Diabetes mellitus

   2. Hereditary leukodystrophies

   3. Hereditary motor/sensory neuropathies

Note: Family history should settle these issues.

I. Work-up
  1. Good history and physical (including family history)
  2. Electrophysiologic studies
  3. Serum for ESR, ANA, RF, B_{12}, folate, TFTs, SIFE, hemoglobin A1C, LFTs, HIV. (Consider RBC protoporphyrin, urine porphobilinogen, serum lead level, 24-hour urine for heavy metals, anti-GM-1, and anti-MAG antibodies.)
  4. Lumbar puncture with MS profile (if demyelinating features on NCV)
  5. Nerve biopsy (if demyelinating features on NCV)
  6. Consider CXR (further neoplastic work-up if paraprotein found—e.g., skeletal survey, bone marrow biopsy, etc.)

J. Treatment
  1. Mainstays of treatment are prednisone and therapeutic plasma exchange (TPE).
    a. Prednisone is initial treatment, 60 to 100 mg/d po for adults (1.5 mg/kg/d in children); continue until significant improvement in weakness is apparent.
      (1) Mean time to initial response is 2 months.
      (2) Following improvement, change to alternate-day, single-dose regimen at 100 mg; continue until patients reach maximum therapeutic response (50% do so by 6 months, 95% by 12 months).
      (3) Taper by 5 mg q 2 weeks after maximum response seen. Taper may result in relapse; if so, reinitiate high-dose prednisone and a course of plasmapheresis. Taper should be *slow* with frequent reevaluation.
      (4) Begin calcium therapy with steroids and watch for side effects (e.g., increased BP, hyperglycemia, cataracts, weight gain).
    b. Plasma exchange added to initial prednisone treatment for nonambulatory patients; usually do five exchanges of one plasma volume (40 to 50 mL/kg) each, over 7 to 14 days (total of 200 to 250 mL/kg).
  2. Other modalities
    a. IVIg—usually used when prednisone or TPE is contraindicated or unsuccessful
      (1) Side effects—see preceding section.
      (2) Guidelines are not yet established, but many use 400 mg/kg/d for 5 days with follow-up treatments q 1 to 3 weeks × 3 months or more.
    b. Azathioprine (Imuran)—often used as steroid-sparing agent or if steroids not tolerated or ineffective
      (1) Start with 1 mg/kg/d × 2 weeks and increase to 2 to 3 mg/kg/d.
      (2) Check CBC with SGOT q 2 weeks × 3 months, then q month.
    c. Cyclosporine A and cyclophosphamide—used infrequently
    d. Physical and occupational therapy

K. Prognosis
  1. 95% of patients initially improve with immunosuppression, but most relapse. In one series, 50% of patients relapsed after 49 months mean follow-up, and 50% made complete recovery.
  2. Inform patients of the chronicity of their disease.

MYASTHENIC SYNDROMES

I. Myasthenia Gravis (MG)
  A. Etiology/Pathogenesis
    1. Abnormal production of autoantibodies to nicotinic acetylcholine receptors (AChR)
    2. Overall, 80% to 90% of patients with MG are positive for AChR antibodies.
    3. It is thought that the 10% to 20% of patients who have "antibody-negative" MG do have autoantibodies that may be directed at epitopes not present in the AChR extract used in testing or they may have too low an affinity for detection in the assay system.
    4. AChR antibodies are synthesized by B cells in the thymus gland.
    5. The thymus gland of MG patients is almost always abnormal.
      a. Most (>75%) have lymphoid hyperplasia.
      b. 15% have thymomas (slightly more common in older patients).
    6. AChR antibodies directly interfere with ACh binding, and there is a decrease in the number of ACh receptors with "simplification" of the postsynaptic folds and a widened synaptic cleft.
    7. The amplitude of the MEPPs are not sufficient to trigger an action potential in some fibers. When transmission fails at many junctions, the power of the whole muscle is reduced (weakness). When contractions are repeated, muscle power progressively declines as a result of the failure of transmission at more and more NMJs (fatigue, decremental response on EMG).
  B. Epidemiology
    1. Relatively common disorder. Approximately 2 to 10/100,000 people in the United States are affected.
    2. Before age 40 years, MG is three times times more common in women than men.
    3. May begin at any age but is rare before age 10 years or after age 60 years.
    4. Bimodal age-related peaks:
      a. Ages 10 to 40 years: Mostly women
      b. Ages 50 to 70 years: Slightly more men; patients more often have thymomas.
    5. Patients and their first-degree relatives have an increased incidence of other autoimmune disorders (e.g., SLE, rheumatoid arthritis [RA], thyroiditis, Grave's disease); 3% to 8% of patients have hyperthyroidism. Must screen for these disorders on initial work-up.
  C. Symptoms—three cardinal features
    1. Fluctuating weakness
      a. Weakness varies from day to day or during the course of a single day.
      b. Excessive fatigability with exercise
    2. Characteristic distribution of weakness
      a. Ocular muscle weakness—ocular muscles affected at presentation in 40% of patients and are eventually affected in 85%. This produces the characteristic symptoms of diplopia and ptosis.
      Note: Purely ocular myasthenia differs from generalized myasthenia. Only 50% of these patients have AChR antibodies (as opposed to 80% to 90% with generalized

MG). If myasthenia remains restricted to the eye muscles for more than 3 years, it is likely to remain restricted.

    b. Bulbar muscle weakness—common; produces dysphagia, dysarthria, facial weakness.

    c. Limb/neck weakness—proximal > distal. Limbs almost never affected alone.

3. Response to cholinergic drugs

    a. Acetylcholinesterase Inhibitors—see later section on treatment.

D. Diagnosis

1. History compatible, supported by physical examinations findings:

    a. General exam: Normal, vital signs stable (unless in crisis)

    b. Speech: May be "mushy" or nasal

    c. Cranial nerves: Facial weakness, ptosis, EOM weakness, fatigability on prolonged upgaze

    d. Motor: Proximal muscle weakness, fatigability with repeated contractions, improves with rest. Wasting only in patients with malnutrition secondary to severe dysphagia

    e. Sensory/cerebellar/DTRs: Normal

2. Tensilon test (Edrophonium)

    a. Short-acting acetylcholinesterase inhibitor; onset of action 30 seconds, duration about 5 minutes

    b. How to do the test:

        (1) Decide on a readily observable sign of weakness that you can measure (e.g., ptosis, FVC).

        (2) Make sure that the patient has a functioning IV line.

        (3) Keep 10 mg tensilon and 1 mg atropine at bedside.

        (4) Inject 2 mg tensilon and watch for side effects (bradycardia, hypotension, arrhythmias).

        (5) If patient tolerates the test dose well, inject the remaining 8 mg tensilon.

        (6) Observe the patient for improvement (and keep watching for side effects).

        (7) If at any point during the test the patient has serious side effects or becomes unstable, abort the test and give atropine 0.5 to 1 mg IV.

Note: Placebo injections with NS are sometimes used in evaluation of limb weakness but are not usually necessary when evaluating cranial muscle weakness as this is difficult for most patients to simulate.

Alternate test: This is the ice-pack test. Cooling the eyelids can improve ptosis.

3. Repetitive nerve stimulation (Jolly test)

    a. Decremental response to low rates of stimulation (2 to 5 Hz)

4. Acetylcholine receptor antibody assay

    a. Positive in 80% to 90% of patients with generalized MG and in 50% with pure ocular MG

    b. Antibody titers do *not* correlate with severity of disease.

5. Single-fiber EMG (SFEMG)

    a. May be helpful in difficult cases

    b. Increased "jitter" and blocking are seen.

      c. Positive in about 90% of patients but very nonspecific

E. Further work-up in newly diagnosed myasthenia
  1. Labs
     a. ANA, RF, ESR ± anti-double-stranded DNA (screen for lupus [SLE], rheumatoid arthritis [RA], etc.)
     b. T4, TSH (R/O hyperthyroidism and R/O hypothyroidism, which can exacerbate MG)
     c. CBC with differentials, U/A with culture (R/O infection, which can exacerbate MG)
     d. Blood sugar, electrolytes. (Screen for diabetes mellitus [DM], renal disease, or anything that may interfere with future immunosuppressive treatment.)
     e. ± Antistriated muscle antibody (positive in 85% of patients with thymoma)
  2. Chest X-ray and chest CT scan: R/O infection, R/O thymoma
  3. PPD skin test: Should be dome prior to beginning any immunosuppressive treatment.
  4. Pulmonary function tests/FVC: Assess extent of respiratory comprise, if any.
  5. Review medication list; eliminate/avoid drugs that may exacerbate MG.
     a. D-Penicillamine
     b. Aminoglycoside and polymyxin antibiotics (e.g., gentamicin)
     c. Antiarrhythmics (quinidine, procainamide)
     d. Beta blockers (propranolol)
     e. Thyroid hormones
     f. Lithium, chlorpromazine

F. Myasthenic Crisis
  1. If respiratory weakness becomes severe enough to require mechanical ventilation, the patient is in crisis. This can also result from severe dysphagia with airway compromise secondary to inability to clear secretions.
  2. May be provoked by infection (particularly respiratory), surgical procedures, drugs, IV contrast dye, emotional stress, or systemic illness.
  3. Two types of crisis:
     a. Myasthenic crisis: due to underlying disease
     b. Cholinergic crisis: due to overmedication. Symptoms include miosis, increased salivation and secretions, diarrhea, cramps, fasciculations. Treat by withdrawal of medications.
     c. If unsure which type the patient has, you can challenge with tensilon. If the patient improves, this is myasthenic crisis and the patient needs more drug. If the patient worsens, this is cholinergic crisis and the patient needs less drug. (Be prepared for marked worsening!)
  4. For myasthenic exacerbation, not yet crisis:
     a. Check FVC every 4 to 6 hours. Intubate if <1 L (or <12 to 15 mL/kg). (Must follow FVC, not arterial blood gas!)
     b. Monitor bulbar function closely. Intubate if needed to prevent aspiration.
     c. Aggressively treat underlying infections/precipitating factors.
     d. Avoid drugs known to worsen myasthenia (such as aminoglycoside antibiotics).

   e. Patients can decompensate quickly. Must monitor very closely.
   f. Plasma exchange should be used for those in crisis.
   g. Avoid incentive spirometry, which can cause fatigue of respiratory muscles.
G. Treatment
   1. Acetylcholinesterase inhibitors (anticholinesterases)
      a. Pyridostigmine (Mestinon)
         (1) Onset is 30 minutes. Peak 2 hours. Lasts 3 to 6 hours.
         (2) Dosage—30 to 90 mg every 3 to 4 hours. Maximum of 120 mg every 3 hours.
         (3) IV dose = 1/30 of the po dose
         (4) Timespan: 180 mg hs for morning weakness. Lasts 6 to 8 hours.
         (5) Side effects: Diarrhea, nausea/vomiting, sweating, increased salivation, miosis, bradycardia, hypotension
            (a) Glycopyrrolate (Robinul)—anticholinergic, can be used for the GI side effects caused by Mestinon. Dosage: 1 to 2 mg po tid.
   2. Immunosuppressive agents: Used when symptoms not adequately controlled by anticholinesterases alone.
      a. Prednisone
         (1) Patients should be hospitalized when high-dose steroids are initiated because they can precipitate weakness.
         (2) Dosage: 1 to 1.5 mg/kg (60 to 100 mg) qd until remission, then change to qod dosing. Taper to lowest dose needed to maintain patient.
         (3) May try slow, low-dose outpatient upward titration.
            (a) Ten to 20 mg qd to begin, then increase by 5 mg every 2 to 3 days until patient has satisfactory response or reaches a dose of 60 mg/d.
            (b) If weakness worsens, drop the dosage and go up more slowly.
            (c) After the patient is better (usually takes 2 to 6 months), change to a qod schedule. Increase "on" day by 5 mg and decrease "off" day by 5 mg every week or so. Usual dosage is 10 to 100 mg qod.
            (d) Monitor for side effects: hyperglycemia, sodium and water retention (HTN, edema, CHF), psychosis, PUD, osteoporosis, aseptic necrosis, etc.
      b. Azathioprine (Imuran)
         (1) For use when steroids are contraindicated or there is insufficient response to steroids alone, or to permit a decrease in steroid dose ("steroid sparing").
         (2) Dosage: Start at 50 mg/d for 1 week. Check CBC. If CBC is okay, begin maintenance dose of 100 to 300 mg/d (2 to 3 mg/kg/d).
         (3) Side effects: Leukopenia/bone marrow suppression (dose limiting), macrocytic anemia, elevated LFTs, pancreatitis.
         (4) Monitor: CBC with differentials and platelets (expect slight increase in MCV), LFTs.
         (5) Works slowly, may take longer than 1 year to see maximal benefit.
      c. Cyclosporine (Sandimmune)

             (1) Works more quickly than Imuran (1 to 2 months); expensive

             (2) Dosage: 5 mg/kg/d in two divided doses with meals (125 to 200 mg bid)

             (3) Side effects: Nephrotoxicity, hepatotoxicity, HTN, tremor, hirsutism, gum hyperplasia

             (4) Monitor: CBC, electrolytes, BUN/Cr, LFTs, blood pressure, and CsA levels

      3. Total plasma exchange (TPE)/plasmapheresis

        a. Used to stabilize patients in crisis or prior to thymectomy to optimize the patient's condition

        b. One exchange qod × 5 to 6 treatments (total of 200 to 250 mL of plasma/kg)

        c. Improvement correlates roughly with a reduction in antibody titers.

        d. Complications: BP fluctuations, arrhythmias, bleeding (due to depletion of coagulation factors), hypocalcemia, complications from large-bore intravenous catheter insertion

      4. Intravenous immunoglobulin (IVIg)

        a. Indications basically the same as TPE (to produce rapid improvement to help a patient through a difficult period of weakness)

        b. Dosage: 400 mg/kg/d × 5 days

        c. Improvement usually begins within 4 to 5 days and may last weeks to months.

        d. Advantages over TPE: No need for large-bore IV access, patients with autonomic or cardiovascular instability tolerate IVIg better. Disadvantage—possibly less effective.

        e. Adverse reactions: Headache (most common), aseptic meningitis, acute renal failure, hyperviscosity (stroke, especially in elderly), anaphylaxis (mainly in IgA deficiency), nausea/vomiting, fever/chills, abdominal pain, low back pain

      5. Thymectomy

        a. Recommended for virtually all patients with thymoma (except those with poor surgical risk, elderly, and those with limited life expectancy because it may take years before a benefit is noted)

        b. Also advocated for patients (usually less than 65 years of age) with severe generalized myasthenia without thymoma and for selected patients with severe, disabling ocular myasthenia requiring immunosuppressants

II. Special Forms of Myasthenia

  A. Neonatal Myasthenia

    1. Occurs in approximately 15% of infants born to mothers with MG

    2. Due to placental transfer of AChR antibody

    3. Begins 1 to 3 days after birth with weak suck and cry, limp limbs, and sometimes respiratory weakness. Resolves within about 3 weeks.

    4. Treatment: Respiratory and nutritional supportive care. Mestinon

  B. Congenital Myasthenia

    1. Rare, often familial

    2. No AChR antibodies but does have a decremental response to RNS (Jolly test)

    3. Heterogeneous disorder due to various pre- and postsynaptic anomalies of the NMJ

    4. Present with ophthalmoplegia in infancy

C. Drug-Induced Myasthenia
   1. D-penicillamine best example
   2. Clinical manifestations and AChR antibody titers similar to MG, but both disappear after the drug is stopped.

III. Lambert-Eaton Myasthenic Syndrome
   A. Etiology/Pathogenesis
      1. Abnormal production of antibodies to voltage-gated calcium channels on presynaptic cholinergic nerve terminals
      2. This causes decreased release of ACh-containing vesicles from the nerve terminal.
   B. Epidemiology
      1. Two types: (1) Paraneoplastic form and (2) primary autoimmune form
      2. Approximately two-thirds of cases are associated with small (oat) cell carcinoma of the lung (and rarely other tumors).
      3. Onset of LEMS usually precedes the diagnosis of cancer by about 10 months.
      4. The paraneoplastic form usually has a more rapid onset and progression than the autoimmune form.
      5. The nonparaneoplastic form is often associated with other autoimmune disorders.
   C. Symptoms
      1. Proximal leg and arm weakness ± myalgias (seen in one-third of patients)
      2. May complain of dry mouth (and less commonly other autonomic symptoms of decreased ACh, such as decreased sweating, impotence, constipation, blurred vision).
      3. Cranial nerve/bulbar involvement is rare initially. (May develop in later stages.)
   D. Diagnosis
      1. Physical examination
         a. General: May have systemic symptoms/signs to suggest underlying malignancy.
         b. CN: Usually normal
         c. Motor: Proximal weakness, legs > arms. May get stronger with sustained contraction but then later fatigues. Muscle wasting is mild if present.
         d. Sensory/cerebellar: Normal
         e. DTRs: Absent (or significantly diminished) in more than 90%. May see facilitation after the muscle is exercised for 10 to 15 seconds, a reflex may appear (or increase).
      2. Repetitive nerve stimulation (Jolly test)
         a. An incremental response seen at high rates of stimulation (>10 Hz).
         b. This results from increased calcium in the nerve terminal and increased release of ACh.
      3. Voltage-gated calcium channel antibodies
         a. Positive in 50% of patients overall (in 75% of those with paraneoplastic form and in 30% of those with the primary autoimmune form).
   E. Treatment
      1. Search for and treat the underlying tumor if present. Removal or treatment of the tumor may induce remission of LEMS. The diagnosis of LEMS may precede the

tumor by several months to 3 or 4 years. If the first chest CT is negative, follow the patient with serial scans.

    a. For smokers: CT every 3 months for 1 year, then every 6 months for 3 years

    b. For nonsmokers: CT every year for 4 years

2. 3,4 DAP (Diaminopyridine)

    a. Acts as a depolarizing agent at the motor terminal by blocking K efflux

    b. Dosage: 15 mg po qid (about 1 mg/kg/d)

    c. Side effects: Increased salivation, lightheadedness, rare seizures

    d. 4 AP was tried in the past but cannot be used due to frequent seizures.

3. Guanidine

    a. Facilitates release of ACh

    b. Dosage: 10 to 30 mg/kg/d

    c. Side effects: Bone marrow suppression, severe tremor, cerebellar syndrome

    d. Monitor: CBC

4. Acetylcholinesterase inhibitors (Mestinon)

    a. Limited benefit but improves some patients

5. TPE/IVIG/steroids and immunosuppressive agents

    a. Helpful in some patients, particularly those with autoimmune LEMS (i.e., those not associated with underlying malignancy)

Myasthenia Gravis and Lambert-Eaton Myasthenic Syndrome Quick Reference Table

	Myasthenia Gravis	Lambert-Eaton Syndrome
Antibodies to	Ach receptors	Voltage-gated calcium channels
Associated tumor	Thymoma (15%)	Oat-cell carcinoma of the lung (>60%)
Clinical features		
Ocular/bulbar Sx	Very common	Rare (until late in the disease)
Limb weakness	Proximal>distal	Proximal>distal
Sustained contraction	Fatigability (weaker)	Facilitation (get stronger)
Autonomic Sx	Rare complaint	Very common (dry mouth)
Myalgias	Rare complaint	Common (33%)
Physical examination		
CN involvement	Common (40%–85%)	Rare (until late in the disease)
DTRs	Normal	Absent (or significantly decreased)
Diagnosis		
Tensilon test	+Response	±Response
RNS (Jolly) test	Decremental response to low rates of stimulation	Incremental response to high rates of stimulation
SFEMG	Increased jitter/blocking	Increased jitter/blocking
Treatment	Mestinon	Mestinon
	±Prednisone	3, 4 DAP
	±Azathioprine	±Guanidine
	±TPE/IVIG	±TPE/IVIG/steroids
	Thymectomy if appropriate	Rx/removal of tumor if found

DAP, di-amino pyradine; DTR, deep tendon reflex; IVIG, intravenous immunoglobulin; RNS, repetitive nerve stimulation test; SFEMG, single-fiber EMG; TPE, therapeutic plasma exchange.

IV. Botulism
   A. Etiology/Pathogenesis
      1. Caused by the exotoxin of *Clostridium botulinum*
      2. The toxin interferes with the presynaptic release of ACh from the nerve terminal.
   B. Epidemiology: Three types of botulism
      1. Food—most often due to ingestion of *C. botulinum* in home-preserved foods. Less commonly due to improperly canned commercial products. Must notify public health authorities.
      2. Wound—secondary to penetrating injury or IV drug abuse. Due to colonization of the wound by *C. botulinum* from the soil. Can see gas production in the wound on X-ray.
      3. Infant—peak incidence 2 to 7 months of age. May be a cause of SIDS. Due to colonization of the GI tract by *C. botulinum* after ingestion of spores or during periods of constipation.
   C. Symptoms
      1. Usually appear within 12 to 36 hours after ingestion of contaminated food
      2. Symptoms evolve rapidly over 2 to 4 days.
      3. Characteristic progression of symptoms: Begins with ophthalmoparesis → loss of pupillary reactions → bulbar weakness (dysphagia, dysarthria) → generalized weakness and respiratory compromise
      4. Severe constipation and paralytic ileus frequently occur.
      5. Infantile form also has similar progression of symptoms: 24 to 48 hours of constipation → ophthalmoparesis → bulbar weakness → generalized hypotonia
   D. Diagnosis
      1. Symptoms compatible, clustering of cases, supported by physical examination findings:
         a. General examination: Patient alert, consciousness usually retained
         b. Pupils: often unreactive
         c. CN: Ptosis, ophthalmoparesis, facial/oropharyngeal weakness, dry mouth, decreased secretions
         d. Motor: Progressive weakness
         e. DTRs: Decreased or absent due to severe weakness
         f. Sensation: Normal
      2. Labs: Send stool and serum for toxin assay, send stool for *C. botulinum* culture.
      3. Repetitive nerve stimulation: Incremental response to high rates of stimulation
      4. SFEMG: Increased jitter and blocking
   E. Treatment
      1. Trivalent antiserum (Antitoxin)—obtain from Centers for Disease Control and Prevention
         a. Dosage: 10,000 units IV, then 50,000 units IM qd until improvement begins
      Note: This is a horse serum product and can cause serum sickness or anaphylaxis.
      2. Guanidine

   3. Penicillin—may help in wound and infant forms
   4. Surgical debridement—for wound form
   5. Supportive care (respiratory, fluid/electrolytes, etc.)
F. Prognosis
   1. Improvement, in those who recover, begins within a few weeks, but complete recovery may take many months.
   2. Approximate order of recovery: Ocular movement → other cranial nerves → limb/trunk and respiratory muscles. (Mirrors order of symptom onset.)
   3. Recovery in large part depends on aggressive supportive care, especially ventilatory support, care of the GI tract, and prevention of complications (such as infection).
G. Differential Diagnosis
   1. Miller-Fisher variant of Guillain-Barré syndrome
   2. Diphtheria
   3. Tick paralysis
   4. Sepsis, acute polio (in infants)
   5. Initial phase of brain stem ischemic event
   6. MG/LEMS (Pupillary involvement + Loss of DTRs should help distinguish)

MYASTHENIC SYNDROMES IN CHILDHOOD

Three forms of myasthenia affect children:
1. Juvenile (autoimmune)
2. Neonatal (transient)
3. Congenital (genetic)
   I. Juvenile Myasthenia
      A. Sporadic, Autoimmune
      B. Due to antibodies to acetylcholine receptors (AChR) and subsequent changes in the NMJ
      C. Similar to adult-onset myasthenia gravis
      D. Special Characteristics of Juvenile Myasthenia:
         1. Children less often have detectable AChR antibodies.
            a. Only 40% of children with ocular myasthenia are Ab+ (50% in adults).
            b. Only 58% of children with generalized MG are Ab+ (80% to 90% in adults).
            c. As with adults, titers do not correlate with severity of disease.
         2. Children, like adults, have other associated autoimmune disorders.
            a. Most commonly: DM, rheumatoid arthritis, asthma, thyroid disease
         3. Children also commonly have other nonimmune disorders associated with their MG.
            a. Seizure disorder (in 3% to 12% of patients)
            b. Rarely neoplasm, such as breast, uterine, pineal, colon tumors
         4. Sex ratio depends on age and race. The likelihood of being Ab+ depends on age.
            a. Whites, prepuberty: Males = Females. There is less severe disease in general in this group with more spontaneous remissions and shorter disease duration. More patients in this group are seronegative (50%).

      b. Whites, peripuberty and postpuberty: More females than males (4.5:1). Females in this group tend to have more severe disease than males. 32% of peripubertal children are seronegative, and 9% of postpubertal children are antibody negative.

      c. Blacks, all ages: More females than males (2:1). The percentage of black children negative for AChR antibodies is the same as that for whites.

  5. Thymectomy is recommended for those with moderate to severe generalized MG and disabling ocular MG not responsive to medical management. The following features favor better response to thymectomy:

      a. Surgery performed early (<1 year after onset of symptoms). This is the most important indication.

      b. Bulbar symptoms

      c. White race (58% of whites, 15% of blacks remit after surgery)

      d. Presence of other autoimmune disorders

      e. Onset of symptoms between 12 and 16 years of age

  6. There has been little or no correlation with thymus pathology and response to the surgery. (Approximately 77% have hyperplasia, 16% normal, 3% thymoma.)

II. Neonatal Myasthenia

  A. Transient Disorder seen in 15% of infants born to mothers with MG

  B. Due to placental transfer of AChR antibodies

  C. Symptomatic babies are thought to synthesize the Ab *de novo* as well (this explains why only 15% of babies are affected instead of the expected 100%)

  D. Symptoms

    1. May appear prenatally with intrauterine hypotonia and can be born with arthrogryposis.

    2. Usually become evident within the first 24 hours of life. (Always by day 3 of life.)

    3. Mean duration of symptoms is 18 days. (Range is 5 days to 2 months.)

    4. Most common symptoms: Paresis of bulbar muscles with weak cry, weak suck, and difficulty feeding. Half have generalized hypotonia. Respiratory insufficiency is uncommon.

  E. Diagnosis

    1. AChR antibody positive. Positive tensilon test. Mother with MG.

  F. Treatment

    1. For those with severe generalized weakness and respiratory distress, may need exchange transfusion.

    2. For others, neostigmine 0.1 mg IM (or 1 mg prior to feeds; supportive care nasogastric tube.

III. Congenital Myasthenia

  A. Heterogeneous disorder due to genetic defects in the presynaptic or postsynaptic neuromuscular junction

  B. *Not associated* with antibodies to the AChR

  C. Classification

    1. Presynaptic defects (most AR)

      a. Defect in ACh resynthesis/packaging (Familial Infantile Myasthenia)

b. Decreased number of synaptic vesicles and reduced quantal release
2. Postsynaptic defects (most AR)
    a. Endplate acetylcholinesterase deficiency
    b. Defect in AchR ligand-binding affinity
    c. AchR deficiency with paucity of secondary synaptic clefts
    d. Abnormal kinetic properties of the AchR channel with or without AchR deficiency:
       (1) Slow-channel syndrome—(AD)
       (2) High-conductance fast-channel syndrome
D. Symptoms
    1. Usually begin in the neonatal period
    2. Ocular, bulbar, respiratory weakness, worse with crying or activity
    3. Ptosis, ophthalmoplegia, or ophthalmoparesis
    4. Heterogeneous disorder, however, and some disorders may not cause symptoms until the second or third decade of life (i.e., slow-channel syndrome)
E. Diagnosis
    1. Positive family history in some (but not required)
    2. Tensilon test negative in most forms (± in the Slow- and Fast-Channel Syndromes)
    3. AchR antibodies must be negative.
    4. RNS: Decremental response; SFEMG: Increased jitter
F. Course usually protracted with mild to moderate symptoms refractory to both medical and surgical treatments.

MYOPATHY

I. Duchenne's Muscular Dystrophy
    A. Epidemiology
        1. Incidence: 1:3,500
        2. 30% spontaneous mutation rate
    B. Inheritance: X-linked recessive
    C. Defect: Absence of dystrophin
    D. Clinical Features
        1. Onset in childhood
        2. Calf hypertrophy (pseudohypertrophy)
        3. Delayed walking
        4. Toe walking
        5. Waddling
        6. Gower's maneuver
        7. Lordosis
        8. Limb weakness (proximal > distal)
        9. Wheelchair bound by age 12 years
        10. Contractures common
        11. Bulbar weakness late
        12. Cardiac conduction defects late

      13. Death in second or third decade
- E. Lab
  1. CK and aldolase high (20 to 50 times normal) early in course
  2. Genetic test
- F. EMG: Myopathic changes
- G. Path (Muscle)
  1. Type I fiber predominance
  2. Rounded, split fibers
  3. Fiber size variation
  4. Central migration of nuclei
  5. Fibrosis and fatty infiltration of muscle
  6. No staining with dystrophin stain
  7. Quantitative dystrophin analysis: Absent
- H. Treatment
  1. Prednisone until wheelchair bound
  2. Muscular Dystrophy Association referral

II. Becker's Muscular Dystrophy
- A. Inheritance: X-linked recessive
- B. Defect: Dystrophin decreased or defective
- C. Clinical Features
  1. Onset later than Duchenne's
  2. Weakness less severe than Duchenne's
  3. Patient ambulates beyond 12 years of age
  4. Death in fifth decade
- D. Lab
  1. CK and aldolase high (20 to 50 times normal)
  2. Genetic testing
- E. EMG: Myopathic changes
- F. Path
  1. Similar to Duchenne's
  2. Partial dystrophin staining
  3. Quantitative dystrophin analysis: Low

III. Limb Girdle Dystrophy
- A. Inheritance
  1. AR, chromosome 15
  2. AD, chromosome 5
  3. SCARMD, chromosome 13
- B. Clinical Features
  1. Slowly progressive weakness
  2. Able to ambulate into the fifth or sixth decade
  3. Proximal weakness
     a. Iliopsoas
     b. Quadriceps
     c. Hamstrings

   d. Deltoids

   e. Biceps

   f. Triceps

  4. Facial and extraocular muscles are spared.

  5. Patellar reflexes lost before achilles reflexes

 C. Lab: Slightly elevated CK

 D. EMG: Myopathic changes

 E. Path

  1. Fiber size variation

  2. Fiber splitting

  3. Degeneration/regeneration

IV. Facioscapulohumeral Muscular Dystrophy

 A. Inheritance: AD, chromosome 4

 B. Clinical Features

  1. Onset at end of first decade

  2. Slowly progressive weakness

  3. Weakness

   a. Facial (Bell's phenomenon)

   b. Serratus anterior (scapular winging)

   c. Biceps

  4. Deltoids preserved usually

  5. Forearm muscles preserved (Popeye appearance)

  6. Scapuloperoneal form

   a. Face spared

   b. Anterior tibialis and peroneals affected

   c. AD, chromosome 5

 C. Lab: CK slightly elevated

 D. EMG: Myopathic changes

 E. Path: Early and minimal myopathic changes

V. Emery-Dreifuss Muscular Dystrophy (Humeroperoneal)

 A. Inheritance: X-linked recessive

 B. Clinical Features

  1. Biceps weakness

  2. Triceps weakness

  3. Distal leg muscle weakness

  4. Contractures early in course

  5. Rigid spine

  6. Cardiac conduction block

 C. Treatment

  1. Pacemaker

VI. Oculopharyngeal Dystrophy

 A. Epidemiology

  1. Most common in French-Canadian or Spanish-American people

 B. Inheritance: AD

    C. Clinical Features
        1. Onset in fifth decade
        2. Slowly progressive
        3. Ptosis first
        4. Pharyngeal weakness later (difficulty swallowing)
        5. Extraocular muscle weakness
    D. Lab: CK slightly elevated
    E. EMG: Myopathic features
    F. Path
        1. Myopathic changes
        2. Rimmed vacuoles
        3. Intranuclear tubulofilamentous inclusions
VII. Myotonic Dystrophy
    A. Epidemiology
        1. Incidence: 13.5:100,000
        2. Prevalence: 5:100,000
    B. Inheritance: AD, chromosome 19. Trinucleotide repeat disease.
    C. Clinical Features
        1. Onset in early adulthood
        2. Myotonia early (delayed relaxation)
           a. Active
           b. Percussion
           c. Grasp
        3. Weakness
           a. Neck
           b. Prominent finger flexor weakness
           c. Foot drop
        4. Cold causes flaccidity.
        5. Premature frontal balding
        6. Protuberant lips
        7. Temporalis and masseter atrophy
        8. Nasal voice
        9. Hypersomnia
        10. Cardiac conduction abnormalities
        11. Testicular or ovarian atrophy
        12. Cataracts
        13. Retinal degeneration
    D. Lab: CK normal
    E. EMG: Myotonia
        1. Spontaneous bursts of high-frequency and high-amplitude discharges
    F. Path
        1. Type I fiber hypertrophy
        2. Ring fibers
    G. Treatment

       1. Dilantin or mexiletine
       2. Diamox
       3. Pacemaker
       4. Testosterone replacement
       5. Cataract extraction

VIII. Congenital Myotonic Dystrophy
    A. Inheritance: Children of mothers with myotonic dystrophy
    B. Clinical Features
       1. Present at birth
       2. No myotonia at birth
       3. Severe hypotonia
       4. Dysphagia
       5. Facial diplegia
       6. Floppiness transforms into myotonia
       7. Mental retardation
       8. High neonatal mortality

  IX. Myotonia Congenita (Thomsen's Disease)
    A. Inheritance: AD, chromosome 7
    B. Defect: Chloride channel decreased conductance
    C. Clinical Features
       1. Seen at birth
       2. Muscle hypertrophy (mini-Hercules)
       3. No weakness
    D. EMG
       1. Myotonic discharges
       2. No myopathic features

   X. Central Core Disease
    A. Inheritance: AR, chromosome 19
    B. Clinical Features
       1. Floppy baby
       2. Motor delay (begin walking at 4 to 5 years)
       3. Weakness (proximal > distal)
       4. Slowly progressive
       5. Spine abnormalities
       6. Associated with malignant hyperthermia
    C. Lab: CK normal
    D. EMG: Normal or mild myopathic features
    E. Path
       1. Central core in fibers devoid of mitochondrial activity
       2. PAS-positive core

  XI. Centronuclear (Myotubular) Myopathy
    A. Inheritance: X-linked recessive
    B. Clinical Features
       1. Bilateral ptosis

    2. No ophthalmoplegia
    3. Facial weakness
    4. Diffuse extremity weakness
  C. Lab: CK normal
  D. EMG: Myopathic features or normal
  E. Path
    1. Central nuclei in 85% of fibers
XII. Nemaline Rod Myopathy
  A. Inheritance
    1. AR, chromosome 1
    2. Occasionally AD
  B. Clinical Features
    1. Weakness
      a. Proximal > distal
      b. Facial
      c. Lingual
      d. Pharyngeal
    2. Decreased reflexes
    3. Marfanoid features
    4. Narrow face
    5. Scoliosis
    6. Cardiomyopathy
  C. Lab: CK normal
  D. EMG: Myopathic features or normal
  E. Path
    1. Subsarcolemmal rods
XIII. Neuromyotonia (Isaac's Disease)
  A. Clinical Features
    1. Childhood onset
    2. Myokymia
    3. Abnormal limb posture
    4. Cramps
    5. Hyperhidrosis
    6. Stiffness and myokymia persist in sleep
  B. EMG
    1. Myokymia
    2. Persists after nerve block
  C. Treatment
    1. Phenytoin
    2. Carbamazepine
    3. Plasmapheresis
XIV. Stiff-Person Syndrome (Moersch-Woltman Syndrome)
  A. Epidemiology: Males = Females
  B. Clinical Features

      1. Progressive muscular rigidity
      2. Aching discomfort
      3. Axial muscles predominantly affected
      4. Facial muscles may be affected
      5. Lordosis
      6. Spasms

   C. Lab: Associated with anti-GAD antibodies (glutamic acid decarboxylase)

   D. EMG
      1. Continuous MUPs
      2. Abolished by:
         a. Nerve block
         b. Spinal anesthesia

   E. Treatment: Benzodiazepines

XV. Polymyositis

   A. Epidemiology
      1. Females > Males
      2. Most patients are between 30 and 60 years old.
      3. Most common acquired myopathy

   B. Clinical Features
      1. Progressive over weeks or months
      2. Symmetric proximal muscle weakness
      3. Occasionally begins asymmetrically
      4. Dysphagia
      5. Dysphonia
      6. Painless (<30% complain of pain)
      7. Extraocular muscles are spared
      8. Atrophy
      9. Contractures
     10. Cardiomyopathy
     11. Carcinoma in 9%

   C. Lab
      1. CK high in 90%
      2. Aldolase high
      3. IgG and IgA levels may be elevated.
      4. ANA positive in <50%
      5. Myoglobinuria
      6. Antimyosin antibodies in 90%

   D. EMG
      1. Myopathic features (small, short MUPs)
      2. Fibrillations
      3. Positive sharp waves

   E. Path
      1. Inflammatory cell infiltrate in the muscle fiber membrane and endomysium

      2. Increased numbers of subsarcolemmal nuclei
      3. Small residual fibers
      4. Phagocytosis
  F. Treatment
      1. Prednisone
      2. Methotrexate
      3. Azathioprine
      4. Plasmapheresis
      5. IVIG
XVI. Dermatomyositis
  A. Epidemiology: Females > Males
  B. Clinical Features
      1. Progressive over weeks
      2. Skin lesions usually precede muscle involvement.
      3. Skin lesion types:
         a. Diffuse erythema
         b. Maculopapular eruption
         c. Heliotrope rash of the face
         d. Eczematoid dermatitis of extensor surface of joints
      4. Raynaud's phenomenon
      5. Esophageal weakness in 30%
      6. Proximal muscle weakness
      7. Usually painless
      8. Cardiomyopathy
      9. Carcinoma in 15% (affects many more adults than children)
  C. Lab
      1. CK high
      2. Aldolase high
      3. IgG and IgA levels may be elevated.
      4. ANA positive in < 50%
      5. Myoglobinuria
  D. EMG
      1. Myopathic features (small, short MUPs)
      2. Fibrillations
      3. Positive sharp waves
  E. Path
      1. Perifascicular muscle fiber degeneration and atrophy
      2. Tubular aggregates present in endothelial cells
      3. Inflammatory infiltrate predominantly in the perimysial connective tissue
  F. Treatment
      1. Prednisone
      2. Methotrexate/Azathioprine
      3. Plasmapheresis/IVIg

XVII. Inclusion Body Myositis
    A. Epidemiology: Males:Females = 3:1
    B. Clinical Features
      1. Most common after age 50 years
      2. Proximal weakness (legs > arms)
      3. Distal weakness occurs in 50%.
      4. Early loss of patellar reflexes secondary to predilection for quadriceps
      5. Painless
      6. Autoimmune disorders in 15%
    C. Lab: CK normal or slightly elevated
    D. EMG
      1. Myopathic features
      2. Fibrillations
      3. Positive sharp waves
    E. Path
      1. Filamentous inclusions
      2. Rimmed vacuoles
      3. Inflammatory infiltrate (T-cell mediated)
    F. Treatment: Rarely responsive to treatment
XVIII. Laboratory Evaluation for Muscle Diseases
    A. CK, Aldolase, Lactic Acid
    B. Calcium, Phosphate, Magnesium
    C. ANA, RA
    D. ESR
    E. TSH, Free T4
    F. Urinalysis
    G. Fluid Balance Profile
    H. EKG
    I. EMG/NCS
    J. Muscle Biopsy
    K. Forearm Ischemic Exercise Test
      1. Explain procedure. Get informed consent.
      2. Patient should rest for 30 minutes.
      3. Obtain urine for myoglobin.
      4. Place blood pressure cuff around arm.
      5. Insert IV.
      6. Obtain baseline ammonia, lactic acid, and CK.
      7. Inflate cuff to 20 mm Hg above systolic BP.
      8. Patient should squeeze dynomometer 40 times in the first minute.
      9. Patient should squeeze the dynomometer 120 times in the second minute.
      10. Release the blood pressure cuff after exercise.
      11. Collect blood for ammonia, lactic acid, and CK at 1, 3, 5, 10, and 20 minutes.
      12. Collect urine for myoglobin after completion of the test.

I. Periodic Paralysis Quick Reference Table

	Hypo K	Hyper K	Paramyotonia
Age	10–20	10–20	Birth
Frequency	Infrequent	Frequent	Rare
Severity	Severe	Moderate	Variable
Duration	Hours to days	Minutes to hours	Hours
Trigger	Rest	Rest	Exercise
	Cold	Cold	Cold
	Stress	Hunger	
Serum K	Low	High	Normal
Myotonia	None	Occasional	Prominent
Inheritance	AD	AD	AD
Channel	Calcium	Sodium	? Sodium
Treatment	Diamox	Diamox	Mexiletine
	Potassium	Low potassium	

II. Other Periodic Paralysis Subtypes
   A. Thyrotoxic Periodic Paralysis
      1. Males to Females = 70:1
      2. Hypo-K periodic paralysis secondary to hyperthyroidism
      3. Treat with beta blockers, PTU
   B. Barium Periodic Paralysis
      1. Barium blocks K channels
   C. Myotonia Congenita—chloride channels
   D. Malignant Hyperthermia—calcium channels
   E. Central Core Disease—calcium channels
   F. Episodic Ataxia and Myokymia—potassium channels

DYSTONIA

I. Dystonia
   A. Definition—Dystonia is a clinical syndrome characterized by sustained or spasmodic repetitive muscle contractions that produces twitching, flexing, rotating, extending or squeezing movements, or abnormal postures. The disorder may be generalized, hemibody, segmental, multifocal, or focal. It is either idiopathic (including genetic forms) or secondary. It often starts insidiously and slowly progresses.
II. Treatment
   A. Lioresal (Baclofen)
   B. Tizanidine (Zanaflex)
   C. Clonazapam
   D. BOTOX
      1. Type A—100 units per bottle
      2. One unit is the LD50 for a 20 g mouse. US botox is four times stronger than UK version.
      3. Diffuses through muscle and fascia for approximately 30 mm

4. Causes chemical denervation-prevents ACh release
5. Onset: 24 to 72 hours
6. Maximal effect: 5 to 14 days
7. Duration of action: 12 to 16 weeks
8. Results
    a. Atrophy
    b. Decreased involuntary discharges
    c. Decreased CMAPs
    d. EMG: Fibrillations and sharp waves
    e. SFEMG: Increased jitter in muscles remote from injection
9. Good candidates
    a. One abnormal movement
    b. Easily identified muscle
    c. No essential movement of muscle
    d. No vital muscles nearby
10. Contraindications
    a. Pregnancy
    b. Preexisting neuromuscular disease
    c. Aminoglycosides
11. EMG guidance
    a. EMG guidance can increase efficacy and decrease required dose.
    b. EMG guidance is especially helpful with:
        (1) Deep muscles (dysphonia)
        (2) Small muscles (blepharospasm)
        (3) Specific muscle required (toe)
12. Dosing
    a. Multipoint injections (more than one injection per muscle) are especially helpful for treating pain, posture deformity, range of motion, and activity endurance.
    b. Blepharospasm: 5 to 20 mouse units (MU)
    c. Hand (writer's cramp): 10 to 300 MU
    d. Cervical dystonia
        (1) Sternocleidomastoid   25 to 200 MU (initial dose 80 MU)
        (2) Splenius capitis   25 to 200 MU (initial dose 80 MU)
        (3) Splenius cervicis   25 to 200 MU (initial dose 80 MU)
        (4) Levator scapulae   20 to 100 MU (initial dose 20 MU)
        (5) Trapezius   25 to 200 MU (initial dose 80 MU)
        (6) Scalene   25 to 100 MU (initial dose 40 MU)
        (7) Deep retrocollis   25 to 200 MU (initial dose 80 MU)
13. Side effects
    a. Paralysis of injected muscle
    b. Paralysis of distant muscles by diffusion
    c. SFEMG change in distant muscles
    d. Brachial plexus neuropathy (rare)

      e. Development of resistance (anti-botox antibodies)
      f. Pain and local bruising
      g. Blurred vision
      h. Nausea
      i. Hypotension
      j. Biliary stasis
      k. Pruritis
      l. Flulike symptoms
    m. Psoriatic rash
      n. Myasthenic syndrome
      o. Hypotension
      p. Long-term effect and safety is unknown.
14. No response
      a. Wrong injection site
      b. Inadequate dose
      c. Anti-botox antibodies

10

Epilepsy

SEIZURES

I. Definitions
   A. Seizure—a sudden temporary change in brain function caused by an abnormal rhythmic excessive electrical discharge
   B. Epilepsy—a state of recurrent seizures
   C. Generalized status epilepticus—two or more generalized seizures without full recovery of consciousness or a single seizure lasting longer than 10 minutes
   D. Aura—simple partial seizure producing sensory, autonomic, or psychic manifestations
   E. Prodrome—the sensation or feeling that a seizure is about to occur
II. Classification
   A. Generalized
      1. Generalized tonic-clonic seizures
         a. Prodrome: apathy, fatigue, irritability
         b. Aura: None
         c. Tonic Phase: 10 to 15 seconds; jaw snaps shut, tonic spasm, cyanosis
         d. Clonic Phase: 1 to 2 minutes; rhythmic, generalized muscle contractions; apnea; increased blood pressure
         e. Terminal Phase: 5 minutes; coma, pupils react, breathing resumes
         f. Postictal Phase: Minutes to hours; confusion, somnolence, agitation
         g. Ictal EEG: Generalized spike wave or polyspike
         h. Drug of Choice: Valproate, phenytoin, phenobarbital
         i. Epidemiology
            (1) Newborns—rare
            (2) Children—febrile, metabolic
            (3) Age under 30 years—idiopathic epilepsy, metabolic
            (4) Age 30 to 60 years—idiopathic epilepsy, tumor, metabolic
            (5) Age more than 60 years—tumor or ischemia with secondary generalization, metabolic
      2. Absence seizures
         a. Prodrome: None
         b. Aura: None
         c. Seizure: Seconds to minutes; sudden interruption of consciousness, staring, 3-Hz blinking, automatisms
         d. Postictal Phase: None

  e. Ictal EEG: 3-Hz spike and wave

  f. Drug of choice: Ethosuximide, valproate

  g. Epidemiology: Onset at age 4 to 10 years; usually resolves by age 20 years

 3. Atypical absence seizures

  a. Similar to absence seizures but often associated with other seizure types

  b. Ictal EEG: Spike and wave usually less than 3 Hz

  c. Drug of Choice: Valproate

  d. Epidemiology: Usually occurs in patients who are neurologically or developmentally abnormal

 4. Febrile seizures

  a. Prodrome: Fever

  b. Seizure:

   (1) Simple—brief generalized tonic-clonic seizure occurring after the onset of fever

   (2) Complicated—prolonged seizure activity or focal seizure activity

  c. Drug of choice: No therapy indicated for isolated seizure; phenobarbital if frequent or severe

  d. Epidemiology: 6 months to 5 years old with no other identifiable etiology; seizures occur in 2% to 5% of all children; only 10% have more than three febrile seizures.

 5. Juvenile myoclonic epilepsy

  a. Prodrome: Morning myoclonus

  b. Aura: None

  c. Seizure: Generalized tonic-clonic ± absence

  d. Drug of choice: Valproate, lamotrigine

  e. Epidemiology: Age of onset is 10 to 20 years. Patients are usually developmentally and neurologically normal.

 6. Progressive myoclonic epilepsy

  a. Unverricht-Lundborg disease (Baltic myoclonus)

   (1) Onset: Age 6 to 16 years; mean age, 11 years

   (2) Genetics: AR, chromosome 21q

   (3) Clinical features

    (a) Myoclonus > ataxia, dementia

    (b) IQ drops 10 points each decade.

    (c) Some develop absence or atonic seizures.

   (4) Pathology: Neuronal loss and gliosis of cerebellum medial thalamus and spinal cord

   (5) Epidemiology: Most common in Finland

  b. Myoclonic epilepsy and ragged red fibers (MERRF)

   (1) Onset: Variable

   (2) Genetics: Familial or sporadic; maternal inheritance in mitochondrial disorders

   (3) Clinical: Myopathy, neuropathy, deafness, lipomas, optic atrophy, myoclonus

   (4) Pathology: Ragged red fibers on muscle biopsy; degenerative changes in dentate nucleus and inferior olive

c. Lafora's disease
  (1) Onset: 10 to 18 years
  (2) Genetics: AR, chromosome 6
  (3) Clinical: Dementia, ataxia > myoclonus; death by age 20 in most cases
  (4) EEG: Shows occipital spikes in 50% of patients.
  (5) Pathology: Lafora bodies (intracytoplasmic basophilic) in eccrine sweat glands or brain
  (6) Epidemiology: Most common in southern Europe
d. Neuronal ceroid lipofuscinosis (NCL) (also known as Batten's disease)
  (1) Infantile (Santavori's disease)
    (a) Onset: Age 1 to 2 years
    (b) Genetics: AR, chromosome 1
    (c) Clinical features: Massive myoclonus, vanishing EEG, common in Finland
  (2) Late infantile (Bielschowsky-Jansky disease)
    (a) Onset: Age 2.5 to 4 years
    (b) Genetics: AR
    (c) Clinical features: Seizures (myoclonic, generalized tonic—clonic, absence) followed by dementia, ataxia, and blindness; death usually occurs by age 5 years; is the most common NCL outside of Finland.
  (3) Juvenile (Spielmeyer-Vogt disease)
    (a) Onset: Age 4 to 10 years
    (b) Genetics: AR, chromosome 16
    (c) Clinical features: Starts with visual failure followed by ataxia, dementia, and seizures; the most common neurodegenerative disorder of childhood
  (4) Adult (Kuf's disease)
    (a) Onset: Age 30 years
    (b) Genetics: AR or AD
    (c) Clinical features: Seizures, dementia, ataxia; no visual failure
  (5) Pathology: Diagnose with skin or brain biopsy. Accumulation of lipopigments in lysosomes. Electromicroscopy shows curvilinear or fingerprint inclusions.
e. Sialidosis
  (1) Type I
    (a) Onset: Adolescence
    (b) Genetics: AR, chromosome 20
    (c) Clinical features: Severe myoclonus, gradual visual failure, ataxia and cherry-red spots. No dementia.
    (d) Pathology: Decrease in neuraminidase
  (2) Type II
    (a) Onset: Adolescence
    (b) Genetics: AR, chromosome 10
    (c) Clinical features: Type I plus coarse facies and corneal clouding
    (d) Pathology: Decrease in neuraminidase and beta-galactosidase

f. Noninfantile Gaucher's disease
  (1) Genetics: AR, chromosome 1
  (2) Clinical features: Supranuclear gaze palsy, splenomegaly, pancytopenia, myoclonus. No dementia.
  (3) Pathology: Increased acid phosphatase. Decreased glucocerebrosidase.
g. Late infantile and juvenile GM2 gangliosidosis
  (1) Genetics: AR, chromosome 15
  (2) Clinical features: Myoclonus, dementia. No cherry-red spots.
  (3) Pathology: Decreased hexosaminidase
h. Juvenile neuroaxonal atrophy
  (1) Clinical features: Myoclonus, dementia, ataxia, neuropathy, choreoathetosis. Choreoathetosis appears when the myoclonus is suppressed, and myoclonus appears when the choreoathetosis is suppressed.
  (2) Pathology: Axonal spheroids in autonomic terminals
i. Dentorubral—pallidoluysian atrophy
  (1) Genetics: AD

Genetics

Autosomal Dominant	Maternal Inheritance
Dentatorubral-pallidoluysian atrophy Kuf's disease	MERRF

Geography

Japan Sialidosis type II Dentatorubral pallidoluysian atrophy	Finland Unverricht-Lundborg disease Santavori's disease
Sweden Gaucher's disease	Canada Myoclonus—renal failure

Clinical Features

Severe Dementia Lafora's disease Late infantile NCL GM2 gangliosidosis Juvenile neuroaxonal dystrophy	Little or No Dementia Unverricht-Lundborg disease Sialidosis type I Noninfantile Gaucher's disease Myoclonus-renal failure Biotin-responsive encephalopathy
Severe Myoclonus Lafora's disease MERRF Sialidosis	Focal Occipital Spikes Unverricht-Lundborg disease MERRF
Deafness MERRF Sialidosis type II Biotin-response encephalopathy	Chorea Juvenile neuroaxonal dystrophy Dentorubral-pallidoluysian atrophy Juvenile Gaucher's disease

(2) Clinical features: Chorea, ataxia, dementia, myoclonus

(3) Epidemiology: Most common in Japan

7. Infantile spasms

  a. West's syndrome

    (1) Onset: 3 months to 3 years

    (2) Seizure: Jack-knifing, myoclonus

    (3) EEG: Hypsarrhythmia

    (4) Clinical features: Infantile spasms, mental retardation; varies according to etiology of spasms.

    (5) Drug of choice: Adrenocorticotropic hormone (ACTH) start at $150/m^2$ and taper.

  b. Aicardi syndrome

    (1) Onset: Birth

    (2) Genetics: X-linked dominant

    (3) Seizure: Infantile spasms, alternating hemiconvulsions

    (4) EEG: Bursts of asynchronous slow waves, spikes, and sharp waves alternating with suppressed EEG

    (5) Clinical features: Coloboma, chorioretinal lacunae, agenesis of the corpus callosum, vertebral anomalies, and seizures

    (6) Drug of choice: ACTH

8. Lennox-Gastaut syndrome

  a. Onset: Age 1 to 10 years

  b. Seizure: Multiple seizure types

  c. EEG: Slow spike wave complex 1 to 2.5 Hz, multifocal spikes, generalized paroxysmal fast activity (GPFA)

  d. Clinical features: Multiple seizure types, retardation

  e. Drug of choice: Felbamate (use restricted because of side effects), lamotrigine

B. Partial Seizures

1. Simple partial seizures

  a. Definition: Partial seizures with no alteration in consciousness

  b. Origin: Any part of the cortex

  c. Jacksonian motor seizures

    (1) Clinical features: Begins with tonic contractions of the face, fingers, or feet and transforms into clonic movements that march to other muscle groups on the ipsilateral hemibody. There is no alteration in consciousness, but postictal aphasia if the seizure occurs in the dominant hemisphere.

  d. Autonomic

  e. Sensory

  f. Motor

  g. Psychic

2. Complex partial seizures

  a. Definition: Partial seizure with alteration of consciousness

  b. Benign rolandic epilepsy

    (1) Epidemiology: Incidence is 21/100,000 children less than 15 years old, usually 5 to 10 years old

        (2) Clinical features: Single nocturnal seizure with clonic movement of the mouth and gurgling. Secondary generalization is common. Alteration in consciousness, aura, and postictal confusion are rare. Resolves by age 16 years.

        (3) Interictal EEG: Central- and mid-temporal high-amplitude spike and wave

        (4) Genetics: Autosomal dominant with low penetrance

        (5) Drug of Choice: Carbamazepine, phenobarbital

3. Temporal lobe epilepsy

    a. Epidemiology: Accounts for approximately 70% of partial seizures. Many patients have a history of febrile seizures or head trauma.

    b. Prodrome: Lethargy

    c. Aura: Common

    d. Seizure: Oral or motor automatisms. Alteration of consciousness. Head and eye deviation. Contralateral twitching or tonic-clonic movements. Some seizures are brief episodes of staring and behavior arrest. Posturing. Right temporal lobe seizures are often hypermobile. Left temporal lobe seizures often result in behavior arrest.

    e. Postictal phase: Typically minutes to hours of confusion and somnolence

4. Frontal lobe epilepsy

    a. Epidemiology: Accounts for approximately 20% of partial seizures

    b. Prodrome: Rare

    c. Aura: Unusual

    d. Seizure: Typically consists of combinations of behavior alteration and automatisms and very brief duration. Frontal seizures often have atypical presentations.

        (1) Orbitofrontal

            (a) Characteristics include brief duration, blink or stare, complex automatisms, and sometimes aura.

        (2) Dorsolateral (Brodman's area 4, 6, 8, 9, and 46)

            (a) Characteristics include tonic eye and head contraversion, very brief duration, all simple partial.

        (3) Anteromedial (Brodman's area 6, 8, and 32)

            (a) Characteristics include somatosensory aura, tonic posture, very brief duration, contralateral eye and head version, frequent generalization.

        (4) Frontopolar (Brodman's area 10)

            (a) Characteristics include no aura, loss of tone, rapid generalization.

        (5) Cingular (Brodman's area 24)

            (a) Characteristics include "psychotic" appearance, facial expressions of fear and anger, amnesia.

        (6) Opercular/insular (Brodman's area 4, 6, 43, and 44)

            (a) Characteristics of simple seizures include gustatory sensation, salivation, gagging.

            (b) Characteristics of complex seizures include gagging, swallowing, chewing, amnesia, genital manipulation.

(7) Supplementary motor area (Brodman's area 6)
    (a) Characteristics include simple motor seizure, vocalizes, somatosensory aura, contralateral tonic posture, tonic eye and head contraversion.
  e. Postictal phase: Rare
5. Occipital lobe epilepsy
  a. Epidemiology: Accounts for less than 10% of partial seizures
  b. Prodrome: Rare
  c. Aura: Unusual
  d. Seizure
    (1) Striate cortex—elemental visual hallucination
    (2) Lateral occipital—twinkling, pulsing lights
    (3) Temporooccipital-formed visual hallucination
6. Reflex epilepsy
  a. Seizure occurs secondary to a stereotypical sensory stimulus. There are various types:
    (1) Visual—flashing lights (most common), colors
    (2) Auditory—music, clapping
    (3) Somatosensory
    (4) Reading
    (5) Eating

III. Etiology of Seizures
  A. Idiopathic
  B. Fever
  C. Trauma
  D. Congenital Malformations
  E. Genetic Diseases
    1. Phakomatoses—tuberous sclerosis, von Hippel-Lindau disease
    2. Sturge-Weber syndrome
    3. Amino acidurias
    4. Phenylketonuria (PKU)
    5. Storage diseases
  F. Infection
    1. Bacterial—meningitis, encephalitis, abscess
    2. Fungal—abscess
    3. Toxoplasmosis
    4. Viral—herpes simplex virus (HSV), cytomegalovirus (CMV), viral encephalitis
  G. Toxic/Metabolic
    1. Electrolyte—hypo/hypernatremia, hypo/hyperglycemia, hypocalcemia, hypomagnesemia
    2. Uremia (3 days of anuria)
    3. Thyroid storm
    4. Porphyria
    5. Pyridoxine deficiency

     6. Heavy metals—lead, mercury

     7. Liver failure

     8. Hyperosmolarity

     9. Hypoxia

  H. Drug Withdrawal

     1. Ethanol

     2. Barbiturates

     3. Benzodiazepines

     4. Antiepileptic drugs (AEDs)

  I. Drug Intoxication

     1. Tricyclic antidepressants

     2. Theophylline

     3. Lidocaine

     4. Cocaine

     5. Amphetamines

  J. Cerebral Ischemia

  K. Eclampsia

  L. Tumors

IV. Evaluation

  A. History is the most important diagnostic tool and should include information on the following:

     1. Aura

     2. Seizure description by an eyewitness

     3. Postictal state

     4. Exacerbating factors (sleep, emotion, stress, menstrual cycle, substance abuse)

     5. Birth and developmental history

     6. Head trauma

     7. CNS infections

     8. Family history of epilepsy

  B. Evaluation

     1. MRI head with temporal lobe protocol (thin coronal slices through hippocampi)

     2. EEG

     3. Laboratory tests as indicated by history

     4. Emergency room

       a. CT head

       b. Arterial blood gas (ABG)

       c. Fluid balance profile (FBP), Ca, Mg, PO_4, liver function tests (LFTs)

       d. Urine drug screen

       e. EKG

V. Treatment

  A. See Antiepileptic Drug Selection and Summary Tables

  B. Special Situations

     1. Catamenial Seizures—Tegretol and Diamox

     2. Eclampsia—Magnesium

     3. Alcohol Withdrawal—No long-term therapy

VI. Prognostic Factors for Stopping AEDs

Favorable	Unfavorable
Primary generalized epilepsy	Partial epilepsy
Idiopathic epilepsy	Identifiable lesions
Childhood onset	Adult onset
Easy to control	Difficult to control
Normal neurologic examination	Abnormal neurologic examination
Normal intelligence	Mental retardation
More than 3 years seizure-free	Less than 3 years seizure-free
Normal EEG	Epileptiform EEG

VII. Drug-Drug Interactions

Effects on Serum Concentration of Adding a Second Antiepileptic Drug to First Antiepileptic Drug

Original Drug	Added Drug	Effects of Added Drug on Serum Concentration of Original Drug
Carbamazepine	Clonazepam	No change
	Phenobarbital	Decrease
	Phenytoin	Decrease
	Primidone	Decrease
Clonazepam	Phenobarbital	Decrease
	Phenytoin	Decrease
	Valproate	No change
Ethosuximide	Carbamazepine	Decrease
	Methylphenobarbital	Increase
	Phenobarbital	No change
	Phenytoin	No change
	Primidone	No change
	Valproate	Increase or no change
Phenobarbital	Carbamazepine	No change
	Clonazepam	Data conflicting
	Methsuximide	Increase
	Phenytoin	Increase
	Valproate	Increase
Phenytoin	Carbamazepine	Increase or decrease
	Clonazepam	Data conflicting
	Ethosuximide	No change
	Methsuximide	Increase
	Phenobarbital	Decrease, increase, or no change
	Primidone	No change
	Valproate	Decrease
Primidone	Carbamazepine	Increased concentration of derived phenobarbital
	Clonazepam	No change
	Ethosuximide	No change
	Phenytoin	Increased concentration of derived phenobarbital
	Valproate	Increase
Valproate	Carbamazepine	Decrease, increase, or no change
	Clonazepam	No change
	Ethosuximide	No change
	Phenobarbital	Decrease
	Phenytoin	Decrease
	Primidone	Decrease

Anti-Epileptic Drug Summary Table

Drug	T1/2 (hr)	Protein Binding	Metabolism	Levels (µgm/mL)	Mechanism	Loading Dose	Maintenance	Side Effects
Phenytoin (PHT)	22	90%	Hepatic	10–20	Na channel blocker	20 mg/kg IV 50 mg/min max	5 mg/kg/d titrate	Ataxia, rash, sedation, neuropathy, gingival hyperplasia, hirsuitism
Fosphenytoin is available for faster IV loading as well as IM loading.								
Carbamazepine (CBZ)	11–24	75%	Hepatic toxic-epoxide	4–12	Na channel blocker	10 mg/kg	15–40 mg/kg/d titrate	Diplopia, ataxia, hyponatremia, rash, liver dysfunction, dyscrasias
Valproate (VPA)	8–16	90%	Hepatic	50–150	Na channel blocker	15 mg/kg	20–40 mg/kg/d titrate	Nausea, tremor, weight gain, hair loss, hepatic toxicity
Phenobarbital (PHB)	96	40%	Hepatic	15–40	GABA-receptor agonist 15 mg/kg child	10 mg/kg adult 3–8 mg/kg/d child	2–4 mg/kg/d adult	Sedation, irritability, rash
Primidone	6–8	70%	Hepatic to PEMA & Phb	6–12	GABA-receptor agonist	250 mg/kg	250–1,000 mg/d titrate	Sedation, irritability, rash, impotence
Ethosuximide (ETX)	18–40	0%	Hepatic	40–100	T-type Ca channel blocker		750–1,500 mg/d divided bid	Nausea, lethargy, headache, rash
Methsuximide	38	0%	Hepatic	10–40	T-type Ca channel blocker		300–900 mg/d	Dizziness, somnolence, fatigue, irritability

Drug								
Felbamate (FBM)	20	25%	50% Hepatic 50% Renal	50–110	Glutamate-receptor glycine blocker	15 mg/kg	Titrate	Bone marrow failure (1/3,000), liver failure, weight loss, GI complaints
Gabapentin (GBP)	5	0%	Renal	NA	Unknown	300 mg/d titrated to 900 mg/d over 3d	Titrate to 3,600 mg/d	Dizziness, fatigue, ataxia
Lamotrigine (LTG)	24	50%	Hepatic	2–12	Voltage-gated Na channel blocker	25 mg qd	200–500 mg/d slowly titrated	Elevated epoxide, dizziness, ataxia, rash, headache, Stevens-Johnson syndrome
Tiagabine (TGB)	7	25%	Hepatic	NA	Blocks glial GABA uptake		Up to 56 mg/d	Dizziness, headache, somnolence, tremor
Topiramate (TPM)	22	20%	75% Renal 25% Hepatic	NA	Na channel blocker	25 mg qd	100–600 mg/d slowly titrated	Somnolence, confusion, paresthesias, psychosis
Levetiracetam (LEV)	8	66%	Primarily renal	NA	Unknown	500 mg bid	Titrate to 3,000 mg/d	Dizziness, sleepiness, headache
Oxcarbazepine (OXC)	2		73% Hepatic, 23% Renal		Na channel blocker	600 mg bid	Titrate to 2,400 mg/d	Sleepiness, dizziness, ataxia, rash
Zonisamide (ZNS)	50–70	35%	Renal	NA		100 mg qd	Titrate to 600 mg/d	

Frequency of Aura Types by Location

Aura Type	Temporal	Frontal	Occipital
Somatosensory	5%	15%	0%
Epigastric	50%	15%	5%
Cephalic	5%	15%	5%
General	10%	15%	5%
Psychical	15%	5%	15%
Visual	10%	5%	50%
Auditory	10%	0%	0%
Olfactory	10%	0%	10%
Gustatory	10%	0%	10%
Vertiginous	10%	2%	0%
None	15%	40%	5%

Aura Types

Psychical auras	Illusion	Hallucination
Memory	Déjà vu, jamais vu, strangeness	Flashbacks
Vision	Macropsia, micropsia, near, far, blurred	Objects, faces, scenes
Sound	Advancing, receding, louder, softer, clearer	Voices, music
Self-image	Depersonalization, remoteness	Autoscopy
Time	Stand-still, rushing, slowing	

Antiepileptic Drug Selection

Seizure Type	VPA	LTG	ETX	ACTH	GBP	CBZ	PHT	PHB
Infantile spasms				1				2
Absence	2		1					
Tonic—Clonic	1	2				3	2	4, 1 (infants)
Myoclonic	1	2						
Atypical absence	1	2						
Simple partial	3				2	1	2	1 (infants)
Complex partial	3	2			2	1	2	1 (infants)

Numbers refer to order of preference for use in specific seizure types.

VIII. Neonatal Seizures
- A. Seizure Types
  1. Subtle—more common in premature, ± EEG changes, tonic horizontal eye movements, sustained eye opening, chewing, apnea, "boxing" movements
  2. Clonic—rhythmic and slow (1 to 3 Hz)
     a. *Focal*—usually involve one side of the body, not clearly unconscious
     b. *Multifocal*—involve several body parts, often in migrating pattern
     c. *Generalized*—rarely observed in newborn
  3. Tonic
     a. *Focal*—sustained posturing of a limb or trunk/neck; usually show EEG changes.
     b. *Generalized*—tonic extension of all limbs (mimicking decorticate posturing) or tonic flexion of upper limbs and tonic extension of lower limbs (mimicking decerebrate posturing). No EEG changes in 85% of cases.

4. Myoclonic
  a. *Focal*—usually involve flexor muscles of an upper extremity, often without EEG changes.
  b. *Generalized*—bilateral jerks of both upper and lower limbs, resemble infantile spasms, more likely to have EEG changes
B. Etiology
  1. Hypoxic-ischemic encephalopathy (60%)—most common cause of seizures in both premature and term infants, usually occur within first 24 hours of life (or earlier), status epilepticus not uncommon
  2. Intracranial hemorrhage (10%)
    a. Subarachnoid—the well baby with seizures, usually on second day of life
    b. Germinal matrix—premature, onset of seizures after 3 days of age
    c. Intraventricular—term infant usually with associated hemorrhagic infarction
    d. Subdural—seizures in first 48 hours of life, usually focal
  3. Metabolic
    a. Hypoglycemia (3%)—most common in infants who are small for gestational age and in the setting of diabetes; onset usually on second day of life
    b. Hypocalcemia (3%)—two peaks of incidence
      (1) First 48 to 72 hours; mostly in low birth weight and in infants of diabetic mothers
      (2) Later neonate; large full-term infants drinking cow's milk or improper formula. Increased DTRs, clonus, jitteriness. Seizures often focal.
    c. Hypomagnesemia—onset of seizures at 2 to 4 weeks of age
    d. Local anesthetic intoxication—usually into scalp following pudendal block characteristic features:
      (1) Decreased APGAR scores, bradycardia, pupils fixed and often dilated, doll's eyes absent
    e. Other—hyponatremia, amino acids, ammonia, pyridoxine deficient
  4. Infection (10%)—usually in first 3 days of life; beta streptococcus and *E. coli* most common bacterial causes, toxoplasmosis, HSV, coxsackie B, rubella, CMV
  5. Development—most secondary to migration disorder (lissencephaly, pachygyria, and polymicrogyria)
  6. Drug withdrawal—narcotics, sedatives, TCA, cocaine, ETOH; usually in first 3 days after discontinued use
  7. Unknown (5%)
C. Syndromes
  1. Benign familial neonatal seizures—Usually on day 2 or 3 of life; may have 10 to 20 per day; self-limiting benign; 10% progress to AED, requiring seizure d/o; neurologic development normal; AD inheritance with high penetrance, chromosome 20q
  2. Fifth-day fits
    a. Onset at age 4 to 6 days; usually multifocal clonic; often with apnea; usually last less than 24 hours; status epilepticus in 80% of cases
  3. Benign neonatal sleep myoclonus
    a. Onset in first week of life; bilateral myoclonic jerks that last for several minutes and occur only during NREM sleep; EEG normal or slow; worsened with benzodiazepines; resolve within 2 months; neurologic outcome normal

4. Benign myoclonus of early infancy
   a. Usual onset at age 3 to 9 months, can be much earlier; resemble infantile spasms but EEG normal; usually while awake; may continue for 1 to 2 years; neurologic outcome normal

D. Diagnosis
   1. Lab: Must quickly rule out hypoglycemia and bacterial meningitis, check electrolytes.
   2. EEG: Must use caution since many neonatal seizures are not associated with changes detectable by normal scalp electrodes. Also, the reverse is sometimes true—electrical seizures are often not accompanied by clinical seizure phenomena.
   3. Imaging: Particularly in the setting of focal seizures

E. Prognosis
   1. Relation to background EEG
      a. Normal EEG—less than 10% have neurologic sequelae.
      b. Moderate abnormalities—about 50% have neurologic sequelae.
      c. Severe abnormalities—more than 90% have neurologic sequelae.
   2. Relation to etiology

Etiology	Normal Development
Hypoxic-Ischemic encephalopathy	50%
Intraventricular hemorrhage	10%
Subarachnoid hemorrhage	90%
Hypocalcemia, early onset	50%
Hypocalcemia, late onset	100%
Hypoglycemia	50%
Bacterial meningitis	50%
Developmental defect	0%

F. Treatment
   1. Acute cases
      a. Hypoglycemia—glucose 10% solution 2 mL/kg IV
      b. No hypoglycemia
         (1) Phenobarbital—20 mg/kg load over 10 to 15 min. If necessary add:
            (a) More phenobarbital in 5 mg/kg boluses
            (b) Dilantin—20 mg/kg at 1 mg/kg/min
            (c) Ativan—0.1 mg/kg
         (2) Other (as indicated)
            (a) Calcium gluconate, 5% solution, 4 mL/kg IV
            (b) Magnesium sulfate, 50% solution
            (c) Pyridoxine, 50 to 100 mg IV
   2. Chronic cases
      Duration of therapy has not been fully studied.

11

Neurophysiology

ELECTROENCEPHALOGRAPHY (EEG)

I. Origin of the EEG
   A. Sum of excitatory postsynaptic potentials (EPSPs) and inhibitory postsynaptic potential (IPSPs)
   B. EEG rhythm depends on thalamic pacemaker cells and the reticular activating formation.
   C. One-third of the cortex can be seen by scalp electrodes.
   D. At least 6 cm^2 of cortex must be involved to be detected by surface electrodes.
II. EEG Recording
   A. Electrical Resistance: 1,000 to 5,000 ohms
      1. R > 5,000 ohms attenuates signal and causes 60-Hz noise.
      2. R < 100 ohms results in a short circuit.
   B. Filters: Low frequency is 0.5 to 1 Hz; high frequency is 70 Hz. Filters are variable but may alter spike morphology.
   C. Amplifier Sensitivity: Variable; typically set at 7 μV/mm
   D. Paper Speed: Variable; typically 3 cm/sec
   E. Montages
      1. Bipolar
         a. Localizes potential by *direction* of pen deflection (phase reversal).
         b. Distorts wave shape and amplitude.
      2. Referential
         a. Localizes potential by *amplitude* of pen deflection.
         b. Potentials at the reference electrode may appear in all channels.
         c. Interelectrode distance alters the amplitude.
   F. Activation Procedures
      1. Hyperventilation
         a. Normal: Generalized slowing (3 to 5 min)
         b. Abnormal: Prolonged slowing caused by hypoglycemia or anoxia; 75% of absence seizures are elicited.
      2. Photic stimulation
         a. Normal: Occipital driving at stimulus frequency or no response
         b. Abnormal:
            (1) Photomyoclonic (photomyogenic) response
            (2) Photoparoxysmal (photoconvulsive) response
            (3) Asymmetric response

III. Normal Adult EEG
    A. Alpha 8 to 13 Hz
        1. Voltage: 15 to 45 μV; decreases with age; higher on right; maximal at occiput.
        2. Attenuates with eye opening and concentration.
        3. Drops out with drowsiness.
    B. Mu 7 to 11 Hz
        1. Arch-shaped alpha variant. Best seen in bipolar montage in the centroparietal areas.
        2. Attenuates with contralateral hand movement (e.g., fist).
        3. Enhanced by immobility and hyperventilation
    C. Beta > 13 Hz
        1. Voltage < 25 μV
        2. Frontocentral attenuates with movement.
        3. Global does not attenuate with movement.
        4. Posterior is a fast alpha variant.
        5. Increases with benzodiazepines, barbiturates, and anxiety.
        6. Found over skull defects (less filtered by skull)
    D. Lambda
        1. Occipital positive sharp saw-tooth transients
        2. Occur with visual scanning (VEP)
    E. Vertex Waves
        1. Negative sharp transients at the vertex
        2. Normal with sleep
    F. Kappa
        1. Temporal bursts of low-amplitude alpha or theta. Occur with deep thought.
    G. Posterior Slowing of Youth, Ages 8 to 14 Years
        1. Delta range mixed with alpha
        2. Duration of each wave equals 4 to 6 alpha waves (a subharmonic of alpha)
    H. Temporal Slowing of the Elderly
        1. Medium-to-high-amplitude bursts of theta or delta (<1% of the record)
    I. Six per second spike and wave discharges (phantom spike and wave)
        1. Posterior low-amplitude waves increase with Benadryl.
        2. Frontal high-amplitude waves
    J. Small Sharp Spikes of Sleep (SSSS) or (BETS)
        1. Temporal monophasic or biphasic spikes that may have a broad field
IV. Sleep
    A. Components
        1. POSTS—positive occipital sharp transients of sleep
        2. Vertex waves
        3. Sleep spindles 11 to 15 Hz
            a. Duration more than 0.5 sec
            b. Maximal centrally
        4. K complexes
            a. Negative sharp wave followed immediately by a slower positive component
            b. Duration at least 0.5 sec.

   c. Location: maximal at vertex

B. Stages

 1. Stage W (wakefulness)

  a. Alpha rhythm

  b. Blinks occur (vertical deflections)

 2. Stage I

  a. Alpha replaced by slow 2- to 7-Hz activity.

  b. Muscle artifact decreases.

  c. Vertex waves occur.

  d. POSTS appear at the end of Stage I.

 3. Stage II

  a. Vertex waves

  b. Sleep spindles

  c. K complexes

  d. POSTS

  e. Slow waves at 2 to 7 Hz

 4. Stage III

  a. Sleep spindles

  b. POSTS

  c. K complexes

  d. Less than 50% delta activity

 5. Stage IV

  a. More than 50% delta activity

 6. Rapid eye movement (REM)

  a. Eye movements

  b. Low voltage

  c. Decreased muscle activity

  d. Increased heart rate

V. Neonatal EEG

A. EEG depends on conceptual age.

 1. Less than 29 weeks of age

  a. Discontinuous with bursts of moderate to high amplitude on a flat background

  b. Interval between bursts is approximately 6 sec.

  c. Interhemispheric synchrony develops at this age.

  d. Delta brush (0.3 to 1.5 Hz) is central and occipital.

 2. Twenty-nine to 31 weeks of age

  a. Abundant delta brushes over central temporal and occipital regions

 3. Thirty-two to 34 weeks of age

  a. EEG becomes more continuous and reactive. Multifocal sharp transients.

 4. Thirty-four to 37 weeks of age

  a. Decreased multifocal sharp waves. Frontal sharp waves appear.

 5. Thirty-seven to 42 weeks of age

  a. Continuous theta and delta activity

 6. Less than 44 weeks of age

  a. Multifocal spikes normal

       7. Six months of age
         a. Occipital rhythm at 6 Hz
       8. Three years of age
         a. Occipital rhythm at 8 Hz

VI. Abnormal EEG
  A. Amplitude
    1. Decreased generalized activity
      a. Bilateral cortical damage (bilateral infarcts, anoxia)
      b. Widespread cerebral damage (Huntington's disease, Creutzfeldt-Jakob syndrome)
      c. Widespread disturbance of cortical function (hypothermia, hypothyroidism, postictal)
      d. Bilateral subdural hematomas
    2. Decreased alpha rhythm activity
      a. Mild metabolic disturbances (hepatic, hypothyroidism, hypoparathyroidism)
      b. Functional subcortical disturbances (anxiety)
    3. Decreased focal activity (stroke, tumor, subdural hematoma)
    4. Increased beta rhythm activity (benzodiazepines, hyperthyroidism)
  B. Frequency
    1. Generalized asynchronous slow waves
      a. Widespread structural damage of both hemispheres (stroke, anoxia, postictal, degenerative disease)
      b. Medication effect
    2. Persistent Polymorphic Delta Activity (PPDA)—seen in white matter lesions, postictal states, or ipsilateral thalamic lesions
    3. Intermittent Rhythmic Delta Activity (IRDA)—possibly from dysfunction of subcortical centers influencing activation of cortex
    4. Focal slow waves
      a. Local structural damage (stroke, tumor, multiple sclerosis, tuberous sclerosis, porencephaly)
  C. Epileptiform discharges
    1. Spike <70 msec
    2. Sharp wave, 70 to 200 msec

VII. Epilepsy
  A. Thirty-minute EEG in a Patient with Known Epilepsy
    1. 50% abnormal
    2. Absence—95% abnormal
    3. Simple partial—75% abnormal
    4. Complex partial—50% abnormal
    5. Tonic-clonic—30% abnormal
    6. 2% to 4% of nonepileptic people have interictal epileptiform activity.
  B. Three 30-minute EEGs should diagnose 90% of the cases with epilepsy.
  C. Maneuvers to Increase Sensitivity
    1. Sleep—complex partial
    2. Sleep deprivation—complex partial, juvenile myoclonic epilepsy (JME)

      3. Hyperventilation—absence
      4. Extra electrodes
      5. Sphenoidal—mesial temporal sclerosis
      6. FT9/FT10—mesial temporal sclerosis
      7. Longer recording time
D. Spike
      1. Neuronal burst firing
      2. Possible thalamic recruitment
E. Wave
      1. Neuronal inhibitory response to spike
      2. Recruitment
F. Anticonvulsant Effects
      1. Anticonvulsants suppress the change from interictal to ictal.
      2. Most antiepileptic medications do not tend to suppress interictal firing. (Benzodiazepines and barbiturates are exceptions.)
G. Generalized Epileptiform Activity
      1. 3 Hz spike and wave
         a. Absence seizures
         b. 35% of siblings have similar epileptiform abnormalities.
         c. 10% of parents have similar epileptiform abnormalities.
         d. Autosomal dominant with age-dependent penetrance
      2. Polyspike and wave
         a. GTC seizures, atonic seizures, massive myoclonus, akinetic, hypsarrhythmia, infantile spasms
      3. Spike and wave (>10 Hz fast waves with occasional spike and wave)
         a. Clonic seizure
      4. Slow spike and wave (10 Hz with decreasing frequency)
         a. Tonic seizure
      5. Spike and wave
         a. GTC seizure
      6. Generalized paroxysmal fast activity (GPFA)
         a. Lennox-Gastaut syndrome
      7. Three- to 5-Hz spike and wave and polyspike activity with a normal background
         a. Juvenile myoclonic epilepsy
         b. Photoparoxysmal response in 38%
H. Specific Disorders Causing Generalized Epilepsy
      1. Unverricht-Lundborg syndrome
      2. Myoclonic epilepsy
      3. Lafora inclusion body epilepsy
      4. Creutzfeldt-Jakob disease
      5. Ramsay-Hunt's syndrome of dyssynergia cerebellaris myoclonica
      6. Stürge-Weber syndrome
      7. Riley-Day's familial dysautonomia
      8. Micogyria, agyria, holoprosencephaly
      9. Metabolic and toxic encephalopathies

      a. Addison's disease

      b. Hyperglycemia/hypoglycemia, hypocalcemia, hypomagnesemia

      c. Hyponatremia, acute intermittent porphyria, uremia

      d. Pyridoxine deficiency

  10. Toxic agents—alcohol, phenothiazines, tricyclic antidepressants, haloperidol, isoniazid (INH), heavy metals (lead, mercury), barbiturate withdrawal

  11. Hyperthermia

I. Focal Epileptiform Activity

  1. Benign childhood epilepsy with centrotemporal spikes

      a. Centrotemporal with a horizontal dipole

      b. Short runs of spike and wave at 1.5 to 3 Hz

  2. Childhood epilepsy with occipital paroxysms

      a. Interictal spikes at 1 to 3 Hz

      b. Visual seizures during wakefulness and ictal vomiting possible

  3. Landau-Kleffner syndrome

      a. Multifocal, temporal, and parietooccipital spikes

      b. Continuous spike wave of sleep

      c. Moderate- to high-amplitude interictal spikes

  4. Simple/complex partial epilepsy

  5. Developmental disorders

  6. Tuberous sclerosis

  7. Sturge-Weber syndrome

  8. Porencephaly

  9. Polymicrogyria, pachygyria, heterotopias, etc.

  10. Acute metabolic encephalopathies

  11. Inborn errors of metabolism

  12. Acute infarct, ischemia

  13. Trauma

  14. Tumors

      a. Common in slow-growing cortical tumors

  15. Infection

      a. Abscess (bacterial, toxoplasmosis, cysticercosis)

      b. Herpes (temporal lobes with PLEDS)

  16. Venous sinus thrombosis

J. Periodic Complexes

  1. Periodic lateralizing epileptiform discharges

      a. Etiology: Infarction, tumor, encephalitis

      b. Duration: 0.06 to 0.5 sec

      c. Frequency: 1- to 2-sec interval

  2. Periodic generalized sharp waves

      a. Creutzfeldt-Jakob disease

      b. Generalized 0.15- to 0.6-sec duration spikes

      c. Frequency: 0.5- to 2-sec interval

      d. Exaggerated photic response to low flash frequencies in Creutzfeldt-Jakob

  3. Periodic generalized complexes

a. Subacute sclerosing pan encephalitis (PCP overdose may look similar)
b. Generalized symmetric 0.5- to 3-sec sharp wave complexes
c. Frequency: 3- to 20-sec interval
   4. Triphasic waves
a. Metabolic encephalopathy
b. Generalized maximal frontal 0.2- to 0.5-sec major positive wave preceded and followed by minor negative waves
c. Frequency: 0.5- to 2-sec interval
   K. Burst Suppression
1. Anesthesia, anoxia, hypothermia
a. Intermittent sharp complexes interrupting delta or no activity for a 2-sec to many-minutes interval
VIII. Electrocerebral Silence—EEG Settings and Results
   A. Sensitivity: 2 μV
   B. Interelectrode Distance: 10 cm
   C. Impedance: 100 to 10,000 ohms
   D. Minimum of 8 Scalp Electrodes
   E. Low-Frequency Filter: <1 Hz
   F. High-Frequency Filter: >30 Hz
   G. No Cerebral Electrical Activity

ELECTROMYOGRAPHY (EMG)/NERVE CONDUCTION STUDIES (NCS)

I. Neuromuscular Junction
   A. Presynaptic Components
1. Motor neuron
2. Axon
3. Terminal bouton
a. Synaptic vesicles
   (1) Contain 1 quanta of ACh—1 quanta = 5,000 to 10,000 molecules of ACh
b. Active zone: Opposite junctional folds
c. Voltage-gated calcium channels
   B. Synaptic Cleft
1. Two hundred to 500 μm wide
   C. Postsynaptic Components
1. Motor endplate
2. Junctional folds
a. Acetylcholine receptors
b. Voltage-gated sodium channels
II. Miniature Endplate Potential (MEPP)
   A. Depolarization of postsynaptic membrane caused by the release of one vesicle
   B. Amplitude: 1 mV
   C. Occurs every 5 sec
   D. Frequency increases with increasing temperature.
   E. Frequency increases with increasing nerve depolarization.

    F. Frequency decreases with calcium deficiency.
    G. Curare decreases amplitude.
    H. Neostigmine increases amplitude.
    I. Amplitude decreased in myasthenia gravis (normal frequency)
    J. Amplitude normal in Lambert-Eaton myasthenic syndrome (LEMS) and botulism (decreased frequency)

III. End-Plate Potential (EPP)
    A. Nonpropagated Graded Response
    B. Summation of Many MEPPs (approximately 100 quanta)
    C. Always supramaximal in normal subjects
    D. EPPs depolarize the membrane for an action potential.

IV. Motor Unit Potential (MUP)
    A. Action potential recorded from the muscle fibers in one motor unit
    B. Rise time should be less than 500 μsec in an acceptable MUP

V. Compound Motor Action Potential (CMAP)
    A. Obtained by stimulating a motor nerve and recording over the muscle
    B. Terminal Latency: Time from stimulation of nerve to recording over muscle

VI. Compound Nerve Action Potential (CNAP)
    A. Usually refers to sensory nerves or mixed nerves.
    B. Stimulate nerve and record over that nerve at another site.
    C. Orthodromic: Direction nerve normally conducts.
    D. Antidromic: Direction opposite normal conduction (back-firing)
    E. Sural sensory nerve action potentials may be absent in normal older adults.

VII. Nerve Conduction Studies (NCS)
    A. Neuropathy
        1. Axonal
            a. Decreased amplitude
            b. Mild slowing (>70% axonal loss before slowing)
            c. Reduced recruitment
            d. Giant motor unit potentials
            e. Fibrillations
        2. Demyelinating
            a. Slowing to less than 60% of normal
            b. Conduction block
            c. Temporal dispersion
            d. Latency prolonged
            e. Area under curve remains the same.
    B. H-Reflex
        1. Neurophysiologic counterpart of ankle jerk
        2. Seen only in the ankle in adults
        3. Submaximal stimulus
        4. Stimulate IA afferent sensory nerve, and measure reflex arc.
        5. Involves a synapse (monosynaptic).
        6. Represents nerve conduction velocity (NCV) near cord (both afferent and efferent limbs).

7. Faster than F-wave (sensory fibers are faster)
8. Gendrassic maneuvers enhance the H-reflex.
9. H-reflex latency is approximately half the adult value.

C. F-Wave
1. Measure in any motor nerve
2. Supramaximal stimulus
3. Antidromic conduction and measure reflected impulse
4. No synapse
5. Tests entire length of the motor nerve
6. Slower than H-reflex
7. Very early finding in Guillain-Barré syndrome

D. M-wave
1. Muscle compound action potential
2. Requires supramaximal stimulation.
3. Waveform is usually diphasic.
4. Motor latency is measured to the onset of the first phase.

E. NCV Facts
1. Renervation
   a. Begins 1 to 3 weeks after nerve injury.
   b. Progresses at 1 mm/day.
   c. EMG evidence is not seen for weeks or months.
2. Following trauma, neuromuscular transmission fails before NCV change.
3. Sensory NCV preserved more than motor NCV
4. Motor nerves degenerate faster than sensory nerves.
5. Sensory nerve NCV change little as the nerve degenerates.
6. Lesion proximal to the dorsal root ganglion (DRG) causes loss of sensation but normal NCVs.
7. Term infant NCV is half that of adult NCV.

Electrophysiological Findings in Neuropathy

Characteristic	Axonal Degeneration	Demyelination
Motor nerve conduction		
Amplitude	Decreased	N/decreased/block
Duration	N	Dispersion
Shape	N	N or multiphasic
Terminal latency	N or increased (<150%)[a]	Increased (>150%)[a]
Velocity	N or decreased (>60%)[a]	Decreased (<60%)[a]
Sensory nerve conduction		
Amplitude	Decreased/absent	N/decreased/absent
Duration	N	Increased
Shape	N	Rarely multiphasic
Velocity	N or decreased (>60%)[a]	Decreased (<60%)[a]
F-wave	Increased (<150%)[a]/absent	Increased (>150%)[a]
H-reflex	Increased (<150%)[a]/absent	Increased (>150%)[a]

[a]Refers to % of normal mean.
N; normal.

VIII. Electromyography (EMG)
    A. Insertional Activity
        1. Recorded with muscle at rest
        2. Crisp burst of activity as needle enters
        3. Increased (prolonged runs of activity after needle movement ceased) with denervation or irritation (polymyositis)
        4. Decreased when muscle replaced by fat or connective tissue
    B. Motor Unit Potentials
        1. Recorded with minimal muscle contraction
        2. Amplitude: 0.5 to 5 mV
            a. Decreased in myopathy
            b. Increased with renervation and axonal sprouting
        3. Duration: 5 to 14 msec
            a. Increased in renervation
            b. Decreased in myopathy
        4. Polyphasic (greater than five turns) in myopathy and renervation
    C. Interference Pattern
        1. Recorded during maximal muscle contraction
        2. Decreased recruitment seen in neuropathic processes
        3. Increased recruitment seen in myopathic processes
    D. Endplate
        1. Normal spontaneous firing near the endplate
        2. Ocean surf sound
        3. Fibrillations
        4. Positive sharp waves
        5. Nerve potentials
    E. Positive Sharp Waves
        1. Monophasic downward (positive) deflection
        2. Dull thuds, sound like rain on a tin roof
        3. Duration: 4 to 20 msec
        4. Amplitude: 50 to 4,000 mV
        5. Indication of denervation or myopathy
        6. In up to 80% of patients with radiculopathy
        7. Seven to 10 days following an injury
    F. Fibrillation
        1. Spontaneous firing of a single muscle fiber
        2. Diphasic with initial downward (positive) deflection
        3. Sound like crisp tics
        4. Duration: 0.5 to 3 msec
        5. Amplitude: 50 to 200 mV
        6. Indication of hypersensitivity of muscle to ACh or axonal injury or myopathy; 10% of normal muscles have areas of fibrillations.
        7. Possible disappearance relatively quickly with isolated compressive radiculopathies because of collateral sprouting.

8. Typically seen 10 to 14 days following an injury
G. Fasciculation
　1. Spontaneous firing of a single motor unit potential
　2. Large deflections
　3. Usual occurrence with proximal lesions
　　a. Nerve root
　　b. Anterior horn cells
　4. In 15% of normal population
H. Myotonic Potentials
　1. Spontaneous discharges that wax and wane in frequency and amplitude.
　2. "Dive bomber" sound
　3. Indication of myotonic disorders and periodic paralysis
　4. Resolution in true myotonia
I. Giant MUPs
　1. MUP greater than 5 mV during active contraction
　2. Indicate renervation with axonal sprouting and chronic changes.
J. Recruitment
　1. First MUP begins firing at approximately 5 Hz.
　2. At 15 Hz, a second MUP begins firing.
　3. At maximal contraction, MUPs are too numerous to count.
　4. Early recruitment and normal frequency in myopathy
　5. Late recruitment with individual fibers firing faster in neuropathy
K. Myokymic potentials
　1. Rhythmic bursts of normal motor unit potentials
　2. Bursts of potentials occurring at 2 to 60 Hz
　3. Caused by ephaptic firing of anterior horn cells or peripheral nerves
　4. Seen in myokymia-cramp syndrome, radiation-induced plexopathy, demeylinating neuropathy, multiple slerosis, brain stem lesions
L. Neuromyotonic discharges
　1. Bursts of motor unit potentials firing at more than 150 Hz for 0.5 to 2 sec
　2. Amplitude typically wanes during the discharge.
　3. Frequency 100 to 300 Hz
　4. Caused by hyperexcitable peripher nerves
　5. Seen in Isaac's syndrome; irritated, exposed nerves
M. EMG Facts
　1. EMG evidence of denervation
　　a. May not be present for up to 3 weeks after injury.
　　b. Positive sharp waves typically appear at 8 days after injury.
　　c. Fibrillations typically appear at 14 days after injury.
　2. Myopathic pattern
　　a. Active
　　　(1) Small CMAP
　　　(2) Short-duration CMAP
　　　(3) Increased recruitment

            (4) Decreased interference pattern amplitude
            (5) Fibrillations
            (6) Positive sharp waves
        b. Chronic
            (1) Decreased CMAP amplitude
            (2) Decreased insertional activity
            (3) No fibrillations or positive sharp waves
    3. Motor neuron disease
        a. Denervation in three or more limbs
        b. Sensory NCVs spared

Myopathic and Neurogenic MUPs

Motor Unit Potential	Myopathic	Neurogenic
Size	Small (<500 μV)	Large (>5 mV)
Duration	Short (<5 ms)	Prolonged (>14 ms)
Recruitment	Increased	Decreased
Polyphasia	Usually present	Usually absent

IX. Single-Fiber EMG
    A. Recorded during minimal muscle contraction
    B. Electrode positioned between two muscle fibers of the same motor unit
    C. Jitter—fluctuations in conduction time
        1. Sensitive for any defect of muscle or nerve
        2. Poorly specific
    D. Blocking—second motor unit fails entirely.
X. Repetitive Nerve Stimulation Test

Repetitive Stimulation

| | MEPP amplitude | CMAP | | Rest | Exercise | Low Stimulation Rate (2–5 Hz) | High Stimulation Rate (10–50 Hz) |
		Resting frequency	Quantal content				
Normal	1mV	0.2/sec	60	>5mV	>5mV	>5mV	>5mV
MG	Low	Normal	Normal	Normal	Normal	Decremental	N/Decremental
LEMS	Normal	Normal	Low	Low	Incremental	Decremental	Incremental

LEMS, Lambert-Eaton myasthenic syndrome; MG, myasthenia gravis.

EVOKED POTENTIALS

I. Visual Evoked Potentials (VEP)
   A. Produced by either flashing light or shifting checkerboard.
   B. Shifting checkerboard pattern is more sensitive.
   C. Tests visual pathway from optic nerve to occipital cortex.
   D. VEP is a single wave, the P-100.
   E. Normal VEP has a latency from 90 to 110 msec.
   F. Demyelination results in:
      1. Prolonged latency
      2. Normal amplitude
      3. Optic neuritis
         a. Prolonged VEP in >90%
         b. Fewer than 5% normalize after 10 years.
   G. Compression of optic nerve prolongs VEP.
   H. Glaucoma prolongs VEP.
   I. Impaired visual acuity results in:
      1. Normal latency
      2. Decreased amplitude

Full Field Stimulation Interpretations

Best Eye	Worst Eye	Interpretation
Normal	Prolonged p100 latency	Lesion anterior to the chiasm
Normal	Increased interocular p100 difference	Lesion anterior to the chiasm
Normal	Absent VEP	Lesion anterior to the chiasm
Low amplitude	Increased p100 latency	Suspect lesion anterior to the chiasm
		Chiasmal lesion
Absent VEP	Absent VEP	Technical problem
		Cannot be further localized

II. Brain Stem Auditory Evoked Potentials (BAEP)
   A. Auditory stimulus of 1,000 to 2,000 clicks in each ear independently
   B. Normal BAEP duration is approximately 9 msec.
   C. BAEP produces seven waves corresponding with:
      1. N cochlear nerve
      2. C cochlea
      3. S superior olive
      4. L lateral lemniscus
      5. I inferior colliculus
      6. M medial geniculate body
      7. A auditory cortex
   D. Demyelinating Disease—prolonged III to V latency most common
   E. Acoustic Neuromas—prolonged I to III latency

Localization	Waves	Normal limits
Lower brain stem:	I–III	2.6 msec
Upper brain stem:	III–V	2.3 msec
Between acoustic nerve and upper midbrain:	I–V	4.6 msec

BAEP Interpretation

Abnormality	Interpretation
Absent bilaterally	Bilateral acoustic nerve lesions
	Brain death
	Technical problems
Low amplitude or increased latency of entire BAEP	Peripheral hearing loss
	Acoustic nerve lesions
	Low stimulus intensity
Unilateral absent BAEP	Unilateral acoustic nerve or cochlear lesions
Absent waves after normal wave I	Unilateral proximal acoustic nerve lesion
	Pontomedullary junction lesion
	Brain death
Increased latency of all waves and normal III–V IPL	Peripheral hearing loss
	Acoustic nerve lesion
Decreased V/I amplitude ratio	Ipsilateral pontine lesion
Absent wave V	Upper brain stem lesion
	Multiple sclerosis
Increased I–III IPL	Lower brain stem lesion
Increased III–V IPL	Upper brain stem lesion

III. Somatosensory Evoked Potentials (SSEP)
    A. Predominantly evaluates large sensory fibers (proprioception and vibration)
    B. Produced by stimulation at 5 Hz over:
        1. Median nerve
        2. Ulnar nerve
        3. Peroneal nerve
        4. Tibial nerve
    C. Recorded over:
        1. Erb's point
        2. C2-spine
        3. Contralateral parietal cortex
        4. L-spine in lower extremity SSEPs
    D. Peripheral Nerve Disease
        1. Prolongation between stimulus point and Erb's point
    E. Nerve Root Disease
        1. Prolongation from Erb's point to C-spine
    F. Posterior Column Disease
        1. Prolongation from L-spine to C-spine
    G. Central Lesion
        1. Prolongation from C-spine to parietal cortex
    H. For Median SSEP:
        1. EP-Erb's point
        2. N11—cervical cord
        3. N13/P13—lower medulla
        4. N19—thalamus
        5. P22—cortex

Median/Ulnar SSEP Interpretations

Abnormality	Interpretation
Increased N9–N13 interpeak latency	Defect in conduction between the brachial plexus and the lower medulla
Increased N13–N20 interpeak latency	Defect in conduction between the lower medulla and the somatosensory cortex
Absent N13 with absent or delayed N20	Defect in conduction between the brachial plexus and the somatosensory cortex
Absent N20 with normal EP-N13	Defect in conduction between the lower medulla and the somatosensory cortex
Absent N20 with preserved N18	Thalamic lesion

12

Central Nervous System Degenerative Disorders

DELIRIUM/DEMENTIA

I. Definitions
  A. *Confusional State*—characterized by inability to think with proper speed, clarity, and coherence and associated with disorientation, decreased attention and concentration, impaired immediate recall, and diminution of all mental activity.
  B. *Delirium*—an acute confusional state marked by prominent alterations in perception and consciousness and associated with vivid hallucinations, delusions, heightened alertness and agitation, hyperactivity of psychomotor and autonomic functions, insomnia, a tendency to convulse, and intense emotional disturbances.
  C. *Dementia*—syndrome characterized by a deterioration of function in multiple cognitive/ intellectual areas in an individual who had previously possessed a "normal" mind with little or no disturbance of perception or consciousness.
II. Characteristics of Delirium (think delirium tremens)
  A. Symptoms develop over 2 to 3 days.
  B. Initial Signs/Symptoms
    1. Decreased concentration, irritability, tremulousness, insomnia, poor appetite
    2. Convulsions (perhaps a "flurry"—30% of cases)
    3. Dreams (unpleasant and vivid)
    4. Disorientation (transient illusions and hallucinations)
  C. Later Signs/Symptoms
    1. Clouding of sensorium/inattention
    2. Paranoia
    3. Altered perception
    4. Tremor
    5. Insomnia
    6. Autonomic hyperactivity
  D. Duration of 2 days to a few weeks
  E. Recovery is usually complete. Heralded by increased lucid intervals and sound sleep.
  F. Continuum of severity from patient to patient
III. Causes of Delirium
  A. Intoxication
    1. Drugs
      a. Alcohol
      b. Anticholinergics
      c. Sedative hypnotics

      d. Opiates
      e. Digitalis derivatives
      f. Steroids
      g. Salicylates
      h. Antibiotics
      i. Anticonvulsants
      j. Antiarrhythmics
      k. Antihypertensives
      l. H2 blockers
      m. Antineoplastics
      n. Lithium
      o. Antiparkinsonians
      p. Disulfiram
      q. Indomethacin
      r. Cocaine
      s. Glutethimide
      t. Antipsychotics
      u. Meprobamate
      v. Phencyclidine hydrochloride (PCP)
      w. Antidepressants
      x. Others
   2. Inhalants
      a. Gasoline
      b. Glue
      c. Ether
      d. Nitrous oxide
      e. Nitrates
   3. Toxins
      a. Industrial
         (1) Carbon disulfide
         (2) Organic solvents
         (3) Bromide
         (4) Methyl chloride
         (5) Heavy metals
         (6) Organophosphates
         (7) Carbon monoxide
      b. Plants and mushrooms
      c. Venom
B. Withdrawal Syndromes
   1. Alcohol
   2. Sedatives/hypnotics
      a. Barbiturates
      b. Benzodiazepines
      c. Glutethimide
      d. Meprobamate

    e. Others
  3. Amphetamines
C. Metabolic Disorders
  1. Hypoxia
  2. Hypoglycemia
  3. Hepatic, pulmonary, renal, pancreatic insufficiency
  4. Errors of metabolism
    a. Porphyria
    b. Carcinoid
    c. Wilson's disease
D. Nutritional Disorders
  1. Vitamin deficiencies
    a. B_{12}
    b. Nicotinic acid
    c. Thiamine
    d. Folate
    e. Pyridoxine
  2. Hypervitaminosis—vitamin A and D intoxication
  3. Fluid/electrolyte disorders
    a. Dehydration or water intoxication
    b. Alkalosis/acidosis
    c. Excesses or deficiencies of Na, Ca, Mg, etc.
E. Hormonal Disorders
  1. Hyper/hypothyroidism
  2. Hyperinsulinism
  3. Hypopituitarism
  4. Addison's disease
  5. Cushing's syndrome
  6. Hypo/hyperparathyroidism
F. Infection
  1. Systemic—almost anything, especially pneumonia and urinary tract infection (UTI) in elderly; also typhoid, septicemia, rheumatic fever
  2. Intracranial (acute, subacute, chronic)
    a. Viral encephalitis
    b. Aseptic meningitis
    c. Herpes
    d. Rabies
    e. Fungal meningitis
    f. Bacterial meningitis
G. Neoplasms
  1. Metastases or meningeal carcinomatosis
  2. Paraneoplastic (limbic encephalitis)
  3. Primary tumors of temporal lobe, parietal lobe, and brain stem
H. Inflammatory—central nervous system (CNS) vasculitis
 I. Trauma

        1. Subarachnoid hemorrhage
        2. Postconcussive delirium
        3. Cerebral contusions or lacerations
    J. Miscellaneous
        1. Postconvulsive
        2. Postoperative/ICU
        3. Mixed
        4. Poststroke

IV. Evaluation
    A. History and Physical Examination
        1. Query family.
        2. Get good time course.
        3. Look for evidence of systemic disease, intoxication, seizure, etc.
        4. Conduct good mental status examination.
    B. Computed Tomography (CT) Scan (usually without contrast)
    C. Chest x-ray
    D. Electrocardiogram (EKG)
    E. Urinalysis and Urine Drug Screen
    F. Serum ETOH Level
    G. ABG
    H. Serum for the Following: Complete blood count (CBC), Chem 18 [with electrolytes and liver function tests (LFTs)], amylase, B_{12}, folate, thyroid function tests (TFTs), rapid plasma reagin (RPR), ± blood cultures (if febrile), erythrocyte sedimentation rate (ESR), antinuclear antibody (ANA), rheumatoid factor (RF); Consider obtaining HIV antibody titer and cardiac enzymes.
    I. Electroencephalogram (EEG): May show nonfocal slow activity (5 to 7 Hz); may show fast activity or may be normal; Triphasic waves may be present.
    J. Lumbar Puncture

V. Management
    A. Control underlying medical illness.
    B. Place patient in quiet environment with dim light.
    C. Protect patient against injury.
    D. Discontinue possible causative/exacerbating drugs and limit sedation (except in withdrawal states).
    E. Administer intravenous fluid, thiamine, multivitamins, folate, and glucose after thiamine given.
    F. Frequent Vitals

VI. Characteristics of Dementia
    A. Conventionally said to involve impairment in memory and one other cognitive sphere (i.e., language, praxis, calculation, judgment, visuospatial orientation, abstract thinking, concentration, etc.)
    B. May have behavioral abnormalities and personality changes.
    C. Little or no disturbance of consciousness or perception (delirium must be absent)
    D. Definition does not imply a specific cause, progressive course, or irreversibility.
    E. Subcortical Dementia

    1. Characterized by forgetfulness, slowed mentation, apathy, depression, psychomotor retardation, perhaps a disorder of movement, etc.

    2. Relative sparing of "cortical" functions (i.e., memory, language, praxis, naming, calculation, etc.)

    3. Prototype: AIDS dementia complex, Huntington's disease

    4. Predominant pathology is usually in basal ganglia and thalamus, although no form of dementia is strictly cortical or subcortical.

VII. Relative Frequency of Types
  A. Alzheimer's Disease (AD)—60%
  B. AD + Other Disorders—10%
  C. Vascular Disease—5%
  D. Other Degenerative Diseases—5%
  E. Treatable Causes (i.e., tumor, ETOH-alcohol, etc.)—10%
  F. Reversible Dementia (i.e., depression, drugs, metabolic)—5%
  G. Miscellaneous—5%

VIII. Causes of Dementia
  A. Neurodegenerative
    1. Alzheimer's disease
    2. Dementia with Lewy bodies
    3. Pick's disease and other frontotemporal dementias
    4. Huntington's disease
    5. Progressive supranuclear palsy
    6. Parkinson's disease, Shy-Drager syndrome
    7. Olivopontocerebellar atrophy (OPCA)
    8. Familial dementia with spastic paraparesis
    9. Parkinson–ALS dementia complex of Guam
    10. Cerebro/cerebellar or cerebrobasal ganglionic degenerations
    11. Progressive hemiatrophy
  B. Vascular
    1. Multiinfarct (including Binswanger's disease) and bilateral cortical infarcts or unilateral cortical infarcts in eloquent areas
    2. Hypoperfusion following cardiac arrest
  C. Structural/Traumatic
    1. Hydrocephalus—communicating or noncommunicating
    2. Chronic subdural hematoma
    3. Brain tumor
    4. Midbrain hemorrhage
    5. Cerebral contusion
    6. Postradiation
    7. Brain abscess
  D. Metabolic/Nutritional/Endocrine/Toxic
    1. Hypothyroidism
    2. Cushing's syndrome
    3. Wernicke-Korsakoff syndrome (thiamine deficiency)
    4. Subacute combined degeneration (Vitamin B_{12} deficiency)

5. Pellagra—nicotinic acid deficiency
6. Wilson's disease
7. Hepatic encephalopathy
8. Porphyria
9. Uremia
10. Electrolyte disorders (e.g., hypercalcemia)
11. Thiamine deficiency
12. Chronic drug intoxication
13. Chronic heavy metal toxicity (e.g., lead)
14. Carbon monoxide poisoning (chronic)

E. Infections
1. HIV-associated dementia
2. Neurosyphilis
3. Subacute sclerosing panencephalitis (SSPE)
4. Progressive multifocal leukoencephalopathy (PML)
5. Whipple's disease
6. Cryptococcosis
7. Postviral encephalitic states
8. Chronic fungal or tuberculous meningitis

F. Disorders of Myelin
1. Multiple sclerosis (MS)
2. Marchiafava-Bignami disease
3. Leukodystrophies (see section on inherited disorders)

G. Neoplastic
1. Meningeal carcinomatosis
2. Limbic encephalitis

H. Inherited Neurometabolic Disorders
1. Leukodystrophies (Krabbe's disease, metachromatic, adrenoleukodystrophy, etc.)
2. Lipid storage diseases (Tay-Sachs disease, Niemann Pick disease, etc.)
3. Myoclonic epilepsy (neuronal ceroid lipofuscinosis)

I. Epilepsy
J. Depression—pseudodementia
K. Collagen-Vascular/Inflammatory
1. Sjögren's syndrome
2. SLE
3. Neurosarcoidosis, etc.

L. Miscellaneous (Prion diseases)
1. Creutzfeldt-Jakob disease (sporadic, iatrogenic, new variant, and familial types)
2. Gerstmann-Sträussler-Scheinker disease
3. Fatal familial and fatal sporadic insomnia
   Note: Remember the mnemonic for causes of dementia: DEMENTIA
   D—degenerative, depression, drugs
   E—endocrine
   M—metabolic, myelin
   E—epilepsy
   N—neoplasm, nutrition

T—toxic, trauma
I—infection, inflammation, inherited disorders, infarction
A—atherosclerotic/vascular
S—structural, systemic

IX. Dementia and Delirium Quick Reference Table

Feature	Cortical Dementia	Subcortical Dementia	Delirium
Onset	Insidious	Insidious	Sudden
Duration	Months to years	Months to years	Hours to days
Course	Progressive	Progressive	Fluctuating
Attention	Normal	Normal	Fluctuating
Speech	Normal	Hypophonic, dysarthric	Slurred, incoherent
Language	Aphasic	Normal or anomic	Anomia, dysgraphia
Memory	Learning deficit (AD)	Retrieval deficit	Encoding deficit
Cognition	Acalculia, concrete	Slow, delapidated	Impaired
Awareness	Impaired	Preserved	Impaired
Demeanor	Disinhibited	Apathetic	Apathetic, agitated
Psychosis	Possible	Possible	Often florid
Motor signs	None	Tremor, dystonia	Tremor, asterixis
EEG	Diffuse slowing	Normal or mild slowing	Moderate-to-severe slowing

X. Dementia Deficits Table

	AD	PD	HD	PSP
Orientation	I	N	N	N
Memory				
Immediate	I	I	I	N
Delayed	SI	I	I	N
Recognition	SI	N	N	N
% Retained	<50	50–80	50–80	50–80
Executive function	SI	SI	SI	SI
Language				
Naming	SI	N	N	N
Fluency	I	SI	SI	SI
Visuospatial	I	I	SI	I

AD, Alzheimer's disease; HD, Huntington's disease; I, impaired; N, normal; PD, Parkinson's disease; PSP, progressive supranuclear palsy; SI, severely impaired.

XI. Evaluation
  A. Good history and physical, with family and good mental status examination
  B. CT without contrast initially
  C. EEG
  D. EKG
  E. Urinalysis
  F. Serum for the following: CBC, chem 18 (with electrolytes and LFTs), TFTs, B12, RPR, ESR, ANA, RF
  Note: Consider the following in younger patients or if initial work-up is negative: cortisol, Wilson's work-up, porphyria work-up, 24-hour urine for heavy metals, HIV, PPD, ACE level, vitamin E, VLCFA
  G. Lumbar puncture if indicated (with cytology, AFB and fungal stains, ACE level, MS profile, etc.)
  H. Neuropsychologic testing if trouble with diagnosis, etc.
  I. Arteriogram/Brain biopsy as indicated

XII. General Management (Specifics depend on underlying etiology)
   A. Rule out treatable causes early.
   B. Incurable Dementias
      1. Pharmacologic treatment of neuropsychiatric symptoms (see table below)

Psychosis

Drug	Trade name	Starting dose	Max dose
Atypical antipsychotics			
Risperidone	Risperdal	0.5 mg/d	1–3 mg/d
Olanzapine	Zyprexa	2.5 mg/d	5–10 mg/d
Quetiapine	Seroquel	12.5–25 mg/d	50–150 mg/d
Clozapine	Clozaril	6.25–12.5 mg/d	25–100 mg/d
Typical neuroleptic (high potency)			
Haloperidol	Haldol	0.25–0.5 mg/d	2–4 mg/d
(mid potency)			
Loxapine	Loxitane	2.5–5 mg/d	10–20 mg/d
(low potency)			
Thioridazine	Mellaril	10–30 mg/d	100–300 mg/d

Agitation/Aggression

Class	Drug	Trade name	Starting dose	Max dose
Antipsychotics (same as listed in previous table)				
Anticonvulsants	Divalproex	Depakote	125 bid	1,500–2,000 mg/d
	Carbamazepine	Tegretol	50–100 mg/d	500–800 mg/d
Antidepressants	Trazadone	Deseryl	25–50 mg/d	200–300 mg/d
	Paroxetine	Paxil	5–10 mg/d	40 mg/d
	Sertraline	Zoloft	25–50 mg/d	150–200 mg/d
	Citalopram	Celexa	10–20 mg/d	40 mg/d
Anxiolytics	Buspirone	Buspar	5 mg bid	45 mg/d
	Lorazepam	Ativan	0.5 mg/d	4–6 mg/d
Others	Propranolol	Inderal	10 mg bid	50–240 mg/d

Depression

Drug	Trade name	Starting dose	Max dose
Selective Serotonin Reuptake Inhibitors			
Fluoxetine	Prozac	10 mg/d	20–40 mg/d
Paroxetine	Paxil	5–10 mg/d	40 mg/d
Sertraline	Zoloft	25–50 mg/d	150–200 mg/d
Citalopram	Celexa	10–20 mg/d	40 mg/d
Fluvoxamine	Luvox	50 mg/d	300 mg/d
Tricyclics			
Nortriptyline	Pamelor	10 mg/d	50–100 mg/d
Desipramine		50 mg/d	150 mg/d
Others			
Nefazodone	Serzone	150 mg bid	600 mg/d
Venlafaxine	Effexor	75 mg/d	375 mg/d

Anxiety

Drug	Trade name	Starting dose	Max dose
Buspirone	Buspar	5 mg/d	30–45 mg/d
Lorazepam	Ativan	0.5 mg/d	2–6 mg/d
Oxazepam	Serax	10 mg/d	30 mg/d

Sleep Disturbance

Drug	Trade name	Starting dose	Max dose
Trazadone	Deseryl	50 mg/d	300 mg/d
Zolpidem	Ambien	5–10 mg/d	10 mg/d
Temazepam	Restoril	15 mg/d	30 mg/d
Zaleplon	Sonata	5–10 mg/d	10 mg/d

   2. Nonpharmacologic treatment of neuropsychiatric symptoms
     a. Increased daytime activities
     b. Music therapy
     c. Environmental enhancement
     d. Daycare
     e. Specific caregiver-focused interventions
     f. Interaction with knowledgeable professional and nonprofessional caregivers
   3. Cognitive symptoms (see Alzheimer's Disease treatment)

CENTRAL NERVOUS SYSTEM DEGENERATIVE DISEASES

I. Dementias
  A. Alzheimer's Disease (AD)
    1. Epidemiology
      a. The most common degenerative disease of the brain
      b. 10% of people over age 65 years have AD, and approximately two-thirds of new cases of dementia over age 65 are attributable to AD.
      c. Male = Female, onset usually after age 60 years but can begin earlier.
      d. Risk factors: Advanced age, family history, Down's syndrome (all patients over age 35 years have AD), low educational level, chromosomal mutations on chromosomes 1, 14, and 21, apolipoprotein E ε - 4 genotype, history of brain injury, history of depression, female gender
    2. Pathophysiology
      a. Cleavage of the amyloid precursor protein by beta and gamma secretases produces the potentially cytotoxic Aβ fragment (primarily Aβ 40 and Aβ 42).
      b. Extracellular aggregates of Aβ deposit in an insoluble β-pleated sheet configuration, which may damage neuronal structure, inhibit synaptic transmission, and incite a cytotoxic inflammatory cascade: this produces many of the pathologic changes seen in the brains of AD patients.
      c. Most familial cases are associated with one of four genetic defects: amyloid precursor protein, apoE ε 4 (most common mutation, lower age of onset), and presenilin 1 and 2 (associated with aggressive early onset).
      d. Decreased choline-acetyltransferase in the hippocampus and neocortex due to loss of cholinergic projections from the nucleus basalis of Meynert
    3. Clinical features
      a. Gradual decline of intellectual function
      b. Poor short-term memory
      c. Visuospatial disorientation
      d. Language/speech problems—aphasia, anomia, and later echolalia, mutism
      e. Apraxias—dressing, ideomotor

     f. Personality changes and paranoid delusions not uncommon
     g. Eventually bedbound, immobile, and mute
     h. Motor and sensory functions spared until very late in disease
     i. Seizures occur in approximately 10% of patients.

4. Imaging
     a. CT/MRI: Atrophy of temporal, frontal, and parietal lobes (with relative sparing of the primary motor and sensory cortices), symmetric widening of the sylvian fissures and dilatation of the temporal horns
     b. PET: Decreased metabolism in the bilateral parietal and temporal lobes
     c. SPECT: Decreased blood flow in the bilateral parietal and temporal lobes

5. Pathology
     a. Senile plaques—argyrophilic with central amyloid core. Correlate best with severity of dementia. Contain extracellular deposits of amyloid β proteins.
     b. Neurofibrillary tangles— intraneuronal cytoplasmic bundles of paired helical filaments (PHF); subunit of PHF is the microtubule associated protein, tau (tau in tangles is hyperphosphorylated, insoluble, and paired with ubiquitin)
     c. Granulovacuolar degeneration—seen in pyramidal cells of hippocampus
     d. Amyloid—stains with congo red and has apple-green birefringence under polarized light. Found in plaque cores and in blood vessels (amyloid congophilic angiopathy)
     e. Hirano bodies—eosinophilic, cytoplasmic inclusions in hippocampal cells
     f. Decreased synaptic density, widespread loss of neurons in the cortex, nucleus basalis of Meynert (substantia innominata) and locus ceruleus
     g. Tau-staining positive—increased in cells destined to undergo fibrillary degeneration
     h. Formation of plaques and tangles represents one of several cytologic responses by neurons to the gradual accumulation of $A\beta$ and $A\beta$ associated proteins.

6. Other disorders with neurofibrillary tangles
     a. Down's syndrome (increased plaques and tangles)
     b. Parkinson's disease (helps to explain why approximately 30% of patients with PD also develop dementia)
     c. Dementia pugilistica—occurs in boxers, increased neurofibrillary tangles but not plaques
     d. Postencephalitic Parkinsonism
     e. Progressive supranuclear palsy
     f. PD/dementia/ALS complex of Guam
     g. Subacute Sclerosing Panencephalitis (SSPE)
     h. Kufs' disease

7. Diagnosis
     a. DSM IV criteria are reliable to diagnose dementia of the AD type.
     b. No imaging (functional or structural), genetic, or biochemical laboratory test can be routinely recommended for diagnosing AD (2001 AAN Practice Parameter).

8. Treatment (Currently available treatments are based on cholinergic hypothesis, which states that there is a selective loss of cholinergic cell bodies and enzymes necessary for normal cognition.)
     a. Rule out reversible causes of dementia.
     b. Tacrine (tetrahydroaminoacridine, or THA)—a reversible acetylcholinesterase inhibitor.

(1) Dosage schedule
    (a) 10 mg qid for 6 weeks, then
    (b) 20 mg qid for 6 weeks, then
    (c) 30 mg qid for 6 weeks, then
    (d) 40 mg qid
Note: Must closely monitor LFTs which increase in 50% of patients
c. Donepezil (Aricept)
    (1) Not associated with significant hepatotoxicity
    (2) Mild cholinergic side effects (nausea, vomiting, diarrhea, etc.)
    (3) Begin at 5 mg q day and increase to 10 mg q day after 4 weeks.
d. Rivastigmine (Exelon)
    (1) Not associated with significant hepatotoxicity
    (2) Inhibits acetylcholinesterase and butyrylcholinesterase.
    (3) Substantial cholinergic side effects with rapid titration (should be given with food)
    (4) Begin at 1.5 mg bid and titrate to 3 to 6 mg bid
e. Galantamine (Reminyl)
    (1) Not associated with significant hepatotoxicity
    (2) Acetylcholinesterase inhibitor and nicotinic receptor modulator
    (3) Begin at 4 mg bid and increase to 8 to 12 mg bid, with 4 weeks between dose increases (lessens the likelihood of cholinergic side effects)
f. All the cholinesterase inhibitors have a broad range of efficacy, which includes cognition, behavior, and function.
g. These drugs provide temporary stabilization of AD-related deterioration.
h. Vitamin E —1000 I.U. bid significantly delayed functional decline, institutionalization, and death in moderate AD in one study.
i. Selegiline
    (1) Same results as with Vitamin E
    (2) 5-mg bid dose
j. Symptomatic treatment of behavioral problems and agitation
k. Supportive care for the patient and caregivers

9. Prevention
  a. Postmenopausal estrogen replacement may be effective, although studies are not in agreement.
  b. Antiinflammatory drugs—observational studies show an approximate 50% reduction in AD risk for users of NSAIDs for 2 or more years.
  c. Potentially preventative—red wine, HMG-CoA reductase inhibitors, antioxidants

B. Pick's Disease (a frontotemporal dementia)
  1. Epidemiology
    a. Rare
    b. Onset usually in sixth decade of life
    c. Females > males
  2. Clinical features
    a. Personality changes and behavioral problems—apathy, abulia, frontal release signs (frontal lobe involvement). Poor judgment is a hallmark.
    b. Aphasia (temporal lobe involvement)

     c. Klüver-Bucy–type syndrome may occur (hypersexual, hyperoral, docile)

     d. Generalized cognitive decline (usually sparing praxis and visuospatial function)

     e. Disturbed behavior is usually the presenting symptom.

  3. Imaging—CT/MRI: Characteristic atrophy of the frontal and temporal lobes ("Pick's at poles") with relative sparing of the posterior third of the superior temporal gyrus and primary motor and sensory cortices

  4. Pathology

     a. Neuronal loss in layers I through III

     b. Pick's bodies—argyrophilic, intracytoplasmic inclusions

     c. Ballooned neurons (also seen in cortical–basal ganglionic degeneration)

C. Other frontotemporal dementias

  1. All clinically similar to Pick's, but lack its distinctive pathology

  2. Are progressive

  3. Involve loss of judgment, accompanied by disinhibition, social misconduct, and apathy and/or aphasia

  4. Behavioral changes are worse than memory loss

  5. Variants include primary progressive aphasia, dementia plus upper or lower motor neuron dysfunction, progressive subcortical gliosis, familial form localizing to chromosome 17.

  6. Account for 5% to 10% of dementias in most neurology practices

  7. Onset in the sixth decade

D. Dementia with Lewy Bodies

  1. Epidemiology

     a. Thought to be second leading cause of dementia; underrecognized

     b. Age at onset typically 50 to 80 years (average age 72)

     c. Male > Female (2:1)

  2. Clinical features

     a. Triad: (1) Dementia (2) Psychosis (3) Mild extrapyramidal symptoms

     b. Presenting symptoms: Commonly neurobehavioral; disinhibition and psychiatric problems in 30% to 50%, frank psychosis in approximately 30%, mild delusions and visual hallucinations as well as executive dysfunction are early features

     c. Extrapyramidal symptoms: Mostly rigidity and bradykinesia; tremor is rare and occurs late if at all. Dementia is far worse than the movement disorder. May have transient lapses of consciousness

  3. Pathology

     a. Lewy bodies—eosinophilic, cytoplasmic inclusions found throughout the cortex and in pigmented neurons of the brain stem

     b. Stain with ubiquitin (especially in CA 2 and 3 regions of hippocampus)

     c. Tau negative, amyloid negative, Alzheimer's-type pathologic changes are seen in 50% to 75% of cases (mainly plaques)

D. Vascular Dementia—can be due to ischemic stroke of any type, cerebral hemorrhage, anoxic/ischemic injury, or vasculitis

  1. Epidemiology

     a. Usually in those with history of stroke, risk factors for vascular disease

     b. Frequency is approximately 10% of all dementias

     c. Male > female

2. Clinical features
   a. Clinical features can be scored using the Hachinski scale:
      A score of > 7 suggest multiinfarct dementia
      A score of ≤ 4 indicates probable primary degenerative dementia.

Clinical Finding	Score
Abrupt onset	2
Fluctuating course	2
History of stroke	2
Focal neurologic symptoms	2
Focal neurologic signs	2
Stepwise deterioration	1
Nocturnal confusion	1
Preservation of personality	1
Depression	1
Somatic complaints	1
Emotional incontinence	1
Hypertension	1
Evidence of atherosclerosis	1

   b. May be associated with pseudobulbar palsy (dysphagia, dysarthria, emotional and urinary incontinence, increased jaw jerk and facial reflexes) due to multiple bilateral lacunar infarctions. Gait disturbance may also be present.
   c. Prominent frontal/executive function with less language impairment than in AD
3. Imaging and pathology
   a. Usually evidence of bilateral cerebral infarctions
   b. MRI evidence of disease of > 25% of cerebral white matter
4. Treatment—Aimed at stroke prevention (control of HTN, etc.)
E. Other Diseases Associated with Dementia
   1. Prion diseases (Creutzfeldt-Jakob, Gerstmann-Sträussler-Scheinker, etc.)
   2. Thalamic dementia (rare syndrome of pure degeneration of the thalamus, subacute dementia, choreoathetosis)
   3. Mitochondrial disorders (MERRF, MELAS)
   4. Hydrocephalic dementia (NPH: dementia, gait disturbance, urinary incontinence)
   5. Posttraumatic dementia (usually static, nonprogressive)
   6. Postencephalitic dementia (e.g., Herpes encephalitis may result in decreased memory as a sequela due to destructive lesions in the bilateral inferomedial temporal lobes.)

Comparison of the Common Dementias

	Diffuse Lewy Body Disease	Alzheimer's Disease	Pick's Disease
Male:female ratio	M > F	M = F	F > M
Symptoms	Psychiatric	Apraxia, aphasia	Personality changes
	Mild EPS	Visuospatial abnormality	Aphasia
Cortex involvement	Diffuse	Parietal lobes	Frontal pole
	Mesial temporal	Temporal pole	
Inclusion bodies	Lewy bodies	NF tangles	Pick bodies
		Plaques	
		Granulovacuolar degeneration	
		Hirano bodies	
Tau	Negative	Positive	Positive
Ubiquitin	Positive	Negative	Negative
Amyloid	Negative	Positive	Negative

II. Movement Disorders
  A. Parkinson's Disease
    1. Epidemiology
      a. Onset: ages 20 to 80 years; peaks in sixth decade of life
      b. Juvenile and familial cases have been described
      c. Common; affects 1% of the population over age 50 years
      d. Male: female ratio—3:2
    2. Clinical features
      a. Four characteristic features
        (1) Rigidity—"cogwheeling"
        (2) Bradykinesia— slowness of movement, festinating gait
        (3) Resting tremor—3 to 5 Hz "pill rolling" tremor, often asymmetric, usually initial symptom
        (4) Postural instability—the most difficult symptom to treat
      b. Other features: Decreased blink rate, stooped posture, drooling, soft monotonous voice, "masked facies," micrographia, failure to inhibit blinking in response to tapping the bridge of the nose (Myerson's sign), widening of the palpebral fissures (Stellwag sign), decreased arm swing, "freezing"
      c. 30% of patients have dementia.
      d. Unilateral onset and good response to L-dopa support the diagnosis.
      e. Depression incidence 2% per year
      f. Sensory symptoms (dysesthetic pain, tingling) and restless legs are common.
      g. Dysautonomia is often seen.
      h. Seborrhea and seborrheic dermatitis are common.
    3. Pathology
      a. Loss of pigmented neurons in the substantia nigra pars compacta and other pigmented neurons (locus ceruleus, dorsal motor nucleus of vagus)
      b. Lewy bodies—eosinophilic, cytoplasmic inclusions in pigmented neurons
    4. Pathophysiology
      a. Depletion of dopamine containing cells in the substantia nigra leads to decreased dopamine (and relative increased acetylcholine) in the striatum.
      b. MPTP model: MPTP is converted to MPP+ by MAO-b and is toxic to dopaminergic cells. This is the basis for using MAO-b inhibitors in treatment of PD and serves as an animal model for study of the disease.

Genetic Forms of Parkinson's Disease

Name of protein	Gene location	Transmission pattern
α-Synuclein	4q21–q22	Autosomal dominant
Parkin	6q25.2–q27	Autosomal recessive
Ubiquitin carbonyl-terminal hydrolase-L1	4p	Autosomal dominant
Iowa pedigree: PD/ET	4q	Autosomal dominant
Tau; frontotemporal dementia	17q21	Autosomal dominant
Susceptibility gene	2p13	
GTP cyclo-hydrolase I (dopa-responsive dystonia)	14q22	Autosomal dominant
Maternal inheritance	Mitochondrial DNA	Mitochondrial

   c. Genetics
     (1) Onset before age 50–higher likelihood of genetic etiology
     (2) Most common gene defect causing PD is PD2 on chromosome 6q25–q27, coding for protein parkin; autosomal recessive

5. Treatment
   a. Levodopa (L-dopa)
     (1) Clinical form—Sinemet (carbidopa/levodopa)
     (2) Dose: Start at one 25/100-tab bid-tid
     (3) Crosses blood–brain barrier (BBB) and is metabolized via L-aromatic-amino acid decarboxylase to dopamine; mainstay of treatment
     (4) Combined with carbidopa (peripheral decarboxylase inhibitor) to decrease the peripheral conversion of L-dopa to dopamine. This allows more L-dopa to cross the BBB, decreases the dosage of L-Dopa needed, and decreases side effects.
     (5) Side effects: Dose-related, reversible
       (a) Nausea/vomiting, orthostatic hypotension
       (b) Dose-related dyskinesias, restlessness, dystonia, athetosis
       (c) Insomnia, hallucinations, anxiety, nightmares, mania
     (6) Should be taken 30 minutes before or 1 hour after meals because protein decreases absorption and transport of L-dopa.
     (7) Drug interactions
       (a) Vitamin B_6—decreases effective dose of L-dopa because it increases peripheral metabolism
       (b) MAO inhibitors—can exaggerate central dopamine effects by decreasing metabolism of dopamine
       (c) Reserpine—depletes central dopamine
       (d) Antipsychotics (D2 blockers)—decrease efficacy of the drug
     (8) After 5 years of L-dopa therapy, approximately 75% of patients have some complication (see tables)
   b. MAO inhibitors: (Deprenyl, Eldepryl/Selegiline)
     (1) Selective inhibitors of MAO-b
     (2) Decrease degradation of dopamine
     (3) Some studies suggest that early treatment with these drugs may have a neuroprotective effect. Delays need for L-dopa by an average of 9 months.
     (4) Dose: 5 mg bid (in morning and at noon); give second dosage early in the day to avoid insomnia from the drug's stimulant effects
     (5) Side effects: Insomnia, nausea/vomiting, dizziness, psychosis, and dyskinesias
     (6) Do not have to avoid tyramine as with MAO-a inhibitors
   c. Dopamine agonists: Bromocriptine/Parlodel, Pergolide/Permax, Ropinirole/Requip, Pramipexole/Mirapex
     (1) Directly stimulate D2 and D3 receptors
     (2) Can improve "on-off" phenomenon when combined with L-dopa. Can be used with L-dopa to potentiate effect
     (3) Can improve some adverse effects of long-term L-dopa use.

(4) Can allow for reduction in L-dopa dosage.

(5) Can be used as monotherapy in early stages to delay the need for L-dopa (potential neuroprotective effect?)

(6) Side effects: drowsiness, edema, sleep attacks, orthostatic hypotension, hallucinations, dyskinesias, nausea/vomiting. Pleuropulmonary fibrosis and erythromelalgia (tender, red, edematous extremity) are rare side effects of the ergot derivatives pergolide and bromocriptine

(7) Dosing:

    (a) Bromocriptine: start at 1.25 mg q.h.s.; increase by 2.5 mg q 3–7 days to max of 10–30 mg per day in 3 divided doses

    (b) Pergolide: start at 0.05 mg q day; increase by 0.1 to 0.15 mg per day q 3 days to goal of 3 mg per day in 3 divided doses

    (c) Pramipexole: start at 0.125 mg tid; increase by 0.25 mg q week to maximum of 1.5 mg per day in 3 divided doses

    (d) Ropinirole: start at 0.25 mg tid; increase by 0.25 to 0.5 mg tid q week to a maximum of 24 mg per day in 3 divided doses

(8) All less effective than L-dopa, but less likely to produce dyskinesias

d. Anticholinergics (Trihexyphenidyl/Artane, Benztropine/Cogentin)

(1) More effective for tremor than rigidity or bradykinesia

(2) Less expensive than other Rx but the elderly may not tolerate

(3) Side effects: CNS—decreased memory, confusion, psychosis; peripheral—dry mouth, constipation, urinary retention, blurred vision, exacerbation of glaucoma

(4) Dose:

    (a) Benztropine = 0.5 mg bid Max 4 to 6 mg/d

    (b) Trihexyphenidyl = 1 mg bid Max 6 to 10 mg/d

e. Amantadine/Symmetrel

(1) Antiviral agent, blocks reuptake of dopamine

(2) Less efficacious than other treatment

(3) Side effects: Dry mouth, confusion, nausea, and livedo reticularis

(4) Dose: 100 mg bid; maximum 200 mg bid

f. COMT inhibitors (catechol–o-methyl transferase inhibitors)—prolong half-life of L-dopa

(1) Tolcapone—dose: 100–200 mg p.o. tid; risk of liver failure has limited its use

(2) Entacapone—dose: 200 mg p.o. given with each L-dopa dose

g. Surgical treatment—reserved for drug failures

(1) Cerebral implantation of fetal adrenal medullary tissue or fetal nigral cells has provided improvement in some; controversial

(2) Thalamotomy/Thalamic stimulation—best for contralateral intractable tremor; 70% effective; stimulation is safer

(3) Pallidotomy—best for contralateral dopamine induced dystonia and chorea; some benefit for bradykinesia and tremor

(4) Subthalamic nucleus stimulation—best for contralateral bradykinesia and tremor; allows reduction in L-dopa dosage; helps symptoms that are helped by L-dopa

Specific Management of Some Parkinsonian Symptoms

Symptom	Management
Depression	Tricyclics, other antidepressants
	Electroconvulsive therapy
Dysarthria	Clonazepam
Sialorrhea	Anticholinergics, tympanic neurectomy
Action tremor	Beta blockers, primidone, alcohol
Painful dystonia	Baclofen, lithium
Painful rigidity	Muscle relaxants (cyclobenzaprine, orphenadrine)
Myoclonus	Clonazepam, methysergide
Akathisia	Anxiolytics, propranolol, naltrexone
Unilateral tremor/Rigidity	Thalamotomy/pallidotomy
Nausea	Diphenidol, cyclizine, carbidopa, benserazide, domperidone
Orthostatic hypotension	Fludrocortisone, yohimbine
Paroxysmal drenching sweats	Beta blockers
Incontinence	Hyoscyamine, oxybutinin, bethanechol
Constipation	Stool softeners, laxatives

Clinical Fluctuations in Parkinson's Disease

Clinical Condition	Management
End-of-dose deterioration	Decrease interval between levodopa doses
	Use sustained-release levodopa
	Use dopamine agonists
	Increase carbidopa levodopa or lisuride infusions
Delayed onset of response	Give before meals or with high carbohydrate meals
	Give antacids
	Administer levodopa or lisuride infusions
Drug-resistant "off" periods	Increase levodopa dosage and frequency
	Give before meals
	Administer levodopa or lisuride infusions
Random oscillation (on-off)	Levodopa or lisuride infusions
	Encourage levodopa withdrawal ("drug holiday")
Freezing	Increase levodopa
	Administer dopamine agonists
	Administer desipramine
	Encourage pacing
	Encourage gait modification

Dyskinesias in Parkinson's Disease

Dyskinesia	Management
Peak-dose dyskinesia	Decrease each dose of levodopa
	Add dopamine agonist
Diphasic dyskinesia	Decrease between-dose intervals
	Increase each dose
Early morning and off-period	Administer baclofen, dopamine agonists, nighttime levodopa, anticholinergics, tricyclics, and/or lithium
Myoclonus	Administer clonazepam, methysergide
	Decrease levodopa
Peak-dose pharyngeal dystonia	Decrease dose of levodopa
	Use anticholinergics
Dystonic posture	Increase levodopa
	Use anticholinergics
	Perform thalamotomy
Orofacial dyskinesias	Decrease levodopa
	Use anticholinergics
Akathisia	Use anxiolytics, propranolol, and/or naltrexone
	Might not be related to levodopa therapy

B. Multiple system atrophy (MSA)—encompasses 10% of patients with Parkinsonism
  1. MSA is a neuropathologic term that encompasses four overlapping syndromes (known as the Parkinson's plus syndromes):
    a. Shy-Drager syndrome
      (1) Parkinsonism + dysautonomia
      (2) Orthostatic hypotension, impotence, bowel/bladder dysfunction
      (3) Due to degeneration of the preganglionic sympathetic neurons in the intermediolateral cell columns and dorsal motor nucleus of the vagus (as well as the substantia nigra and striatum)
    b. Striatonigral degeneration
      (1) Parkinsonism (tremor usually absent), pyramidal signs, laryngeal stridor
      (2) Due to degeneration primarily in the putamen and caudate with secondary changes in the substantia nigra and pallidum (loss of striatopallidal and striatonigral fibers)
      (3) L-dopa has no effect and may provoke dystonic reactions.
    c. Olivopontocerebellar atrophy
      (1) Mild Parkinsonism, pyramidal signs, cerebellar findings
      (2) Familial (cerebellar findings predominate) or sporadic
      (3) Degeneration of cerebellum, pons, and inferior olives, as well as the substantia nigra and striatum
    d. Parkinsonism-amyotrophy syndrome—Degeneration of the substantia nigra and anterior horn cells
  2. Suspect a Parkinson's plus syndrome when the patient has Parkinsonism plus one or more of the following:
    a. Prominent dysautonomia
    b. Ataxia
    c. Corticospinal tract findings
    d. Bilateral, symmetric onset of symptoms
    e. Lack of resting tremor
    f. Poor response to L-Dopa
  3. Pathology (common to all disorders in the MSA category)
    a. Glial cytoplasmic inclusions
      (1) Composed of altered microtubules
      (2) Found in oligodendrocytes
      (3) Relatively specific for MSA
  4. Imaging—Fluorodeoxyglucose PET scanning often shows striatal and frontal lobe hypometabolism in MSA
  5. Treatment—trial of L-dopa to maximum tolerated dose or up to 2 g per day (± anticholinergics)
C. Progressive Supranuclear Palsy (Richardson-Steele-Olszewski syndrome)
  1. Epidemiology
    a. Onset: After age 40 years (usually in the sixth decade of life)
    b. Not familial
    c. Male > female
  2. Clinical features

   a. Decreased balance with unexplained falling ("toppling phenomenon")
   b. Supranuclear gaze palsy—first lose voluntary downgaze, then upgaze, then horizontal movements
   c. Dysphagia, dysarthria, pseudobulbar palsy
   d. Axial dystonia (erect posture)
   e. Mild dementia (prominent executive dysfunction)
   f. Akinetic rigid Parkinson-like syndrome with paucity of tremor (axial > limb)
   g. Poor L-dopa response
3. Pathology
   a. Pons and midbrain atrophy
   b. The cortex and cerebellum are usually spared.
   c. Neurofibrillary tangles are found in residual midbrain neurons.
4. Imaging
   a. Atrophy of the pons and midbrain
D. Cortical–Basal Ganglionic Degeneration
1. Epidemiology
   a. Male = Female
   b. No family history
   c. Usually occurs in the seventh decade
   d. Average survival 5 to10 years
2. Clinical features
   a. Corticospinal tract and extrapyramidal involvement
   b. Asymmetrical, unilateral onset
   c. Usually begins in the upper extremity (more commonly on the left)
   d. Extrapyramidal rigidity (akinetic-rigid), action and postural tremor, apraxia, and "alien hand syndrome" of the involved upper extremity
   e. Reflex myoclonus and dystonia
   f. Cortical sensory loss, "clumsiness"
   g. Very mild dementia (late and in only some cases)
   h. Supranuclear gaze palsy and apraxia of gaze and eyelid opening (late)
   i. Slowly spreads to involve both sides of the body
   j. Signs of corticospinal tract disease usually present (i.e., increased DTRs in 65% of patients and upgoing toes in 50%)
3. Imaging
   a. MRI: Asymmetrical parietal lobe atrophy (greatest on the side contralateral to the involved limb, usually the right parietal lobe)
   b. PET: Decreased metabolism in the thalamoparietal and medial frontal areas, greatest on the involved side
4. Pathology
   a. Cortical atrophy, neuronal loss, and gliosis greatest in the parietal and frontal (premotor) lobes on the side contralateral to the involved limb
   b. Degeneration of the substantia nigra and striatum
   c. Achromasia of the residual neurons (swollen cells with eccentric nuclei and loss of the Nissl substance)
   d. No Pick bodies, tangles, plaques, GVD, amyloid, or Lewy bodies

        e. EM: Cytoplasm filled with 10 nm intermediate filaments

     5. Other potential causes of the alien hand syndrome

        a. Parietal lobe lesions

        b. Supplementary motor area lesion

        c. Corpus callosum lesion

E. Parkinson–Dementia–ALS Complex of Guam (Lytico-Bodig disease)

     1. Epidemiology

        a. Onset: Middle-to-late adulthood

        b. Male > female

        c. Found in the Chamorro Indian population; incidence decreasing

        d. May be related to exposure to a neurotoxin found in the cycad nut

     2. Clinical features

        a. Combination of symptoms characteristic of Parkinsonism, dementia, and motor neuron disease/ALS (weakness, spasticity)

        b. Supranuclear gaze palsy may occur.

     3. Pathology

        a. Characteristic neurofibrillary tangles in degenerating neurons

        b. Lewy bodies and senile plaques are absent.

F. Dystonia Musculorum Deformans (Torsion Spasm)

     1. Epidemiology

        a. Two patterns of inheritance:

           (1) AR: Restricted to Jewish patients, begins in early childhood, progressive over a few years, usually normal or superior IQ

           (2) AD: Not limited to any ethnic group, begins in late childhood or adolescence, progresses more slowly

     2. Clinical features

        a. Dystonia begins intermittently, usually after activity late in the day.

        b. Usually begins with inversion of the foot

        c. Soon the spine and shoulder/pelvic girdles become involved.

        d. Gradually, the spasms become more frequent and then continuous, and the body may become grotesquely contorted.

        e. Cranial muscles also involved (leads to dysphagia and dysarthria)

        f. Hands are characteristically spared.

        g. No other neurologic deficits present

     3. Pathology

        a. No specific changes

     4. Treatment

        a. High-dose anticholinergics (Artane 30 mg/d or more)

        b. VL thalamotomy

G. Hallervorden-Spatz Disease

     1. Epidemiology

        a. AR inheritance

        b. Onset: Late childhood or early adolescence

        c. Progresses slowly over 10 to 20 years

        d. Linkage to chromosome 20p12.3–p13 reported

2. Clinical features
   a. Spasticity, increased DTRs, upgoing toes (corticospinal tract signs)
   b. Rigidity, dystonia, choreoathetosis (extrapyramidal tract signs)
   c. Spasticity and rigidity are most prominent in the legs; the child walks with stiff gait on toes with arms held stiff and fingers hyperextended.
   d. Facial and bulbar muscles also affected; patients often have frozen, pained expression and speak through clenched teeth.
   e. Eventually anarthric
   f. General cognitive decline
   g. ± Pigmentary degeneration of the retina and optic atrophy
3. Imaging
   a. CT: Lesion in lenticular nuclei
   b. MRI T2: Striking hypointensity of the medial globus pallidus (Eye of the tiger sign)
   c. Increased uptake of radioactive iron in the basal ganglia after IV injection of labeled ferrous citrate
4. Pathology
   a. Hallmark is olive or golden-brown discoloration of the medial globus pallidus. (There is also pigmentary degeneration of the SN and red nucleus.)
   b. Swollen axon fragments resembling those found in neuroaxonal dystrophy

H. Huntington's Disease
   1. Epidemiology
      a. AD, chromosome 4
      b. Trinucleotide repeat disease (normal # of repeats = 11 to 34; > 37 = disease)
      c. 90% of child patient cases inherit the disease from their father (anticipation).
      d. Average age of onset is 35 to 40 years, with death usual within 15 years.
      e. Childhood onset can occur and is more rapidly progressive.
      f. Males > Females
      g. Spontaneous mutations may occur, causing sporadic disease
      h. Mutation results in abnormal expression of the protein huntingtin, which accumulates in cells
   2. Clinical features
      a. Triad: (1) Personality disorder/behavior changes, (2) dementia, (3) chorea
      b. The behavioral/personality changes typically appear before the chorea or dementia. Patients may become depressed, suspicious, irritable, impulsive, eccentric, or emotionally labile.
      c. The movement disorder may first appear as restless or fidgety behavior that later evolves into more severe chorea.
      d. "Westphal variant"—childhood form, akinetic/rigid state with mental retardation and seizures. Rapidly progressive.
   3. Imaging
      a. MRI/CT: Large boxcar-shaped ventricles with caudate atrophy, mild cortical atrophy
      b. PET: Hypometabolism in caudate and putamen
   4. Pathology

    a. Atrophy of the caudate (most prominent), putamen, cortex (especially layer 3)

    b. Pathophysiology: Degeneration of GABA, GAD, and cholinergic neurons in the striatum with relative preservation of dopaminergic connections

    c. Striatum eventually replaced by gliosis

5. Treatment

    a. Haloperidol (2 to 10 mg/d) most effective in suppressing the movement disorder, but the disease is relentlessly progressive despite this. (Atypical antipsychotics can also be used.)

    b. Genetic counseling is essential.

    c. Symptomatic treatment of depression

I. Wilson's Disease (hepatolenticular degeneration)

1. Epidemiology

    a. AR, chromosome 13

    b. Prevalence: 1/35,000 of general population; 1/100 are heterozygous for the gene

    c. Onset of neurologic symptoms: Ages 11 to 25 years, rarely beyond third decade

2. Clinical features

    a. The liver is affected first in all cases with hepatitis and eventually cirrhosis.

    b. Neurologic symptoms are classically described as dysphagia, dysarthria, drooling, and various movement disorders.

    c. Rigidity and slowness of movement, mouth hangs open, slow saccadic eye movements

    d. The motor disorders tend to begin in the bulbar muscles then spread caudally.

    e. Coarse "wing-beating" tremor seen in outstretched limbs

    f. Kayser-Fleischer rings—(deposition of copper in Descemet's membrane of the cornea); seen in 100% of patients with CNS disease and 75% of those with only liver disease. Slit lamp examination may be necessary.

    g. Lab: Decreased serum ceruloplasmin, increased serum free copper, increased urinary copper excretion, abnormal LFTs, increased ammonia

3. Imaging

    a. CT: Diffuse cerebral, cerebellar, and brain stem atrophy. Hypodensity of the thalamus and basal ganglia

    b. MRI: increased T1 signal in basal ganglia

4. Pathology

    a. Brick-red discoloration and atrophy of the basal ganglia

    b. Spongy degeneration and cavitation in the putamen

    c. Alzheimer type II cells (large protoplasmic astrocytes)

    d. Opalski cells (large phagocytic cells)

    e. Pathophysiology: Defect in copper-binding P-type ATPase leading to decreased biliary excretion of copper. This leads to storage of copper in the liver, CNS, and cornea. (Note — Menkes' Disease is also caused by a mutated copper-transporting ATPase)

5. Treatment

    a. Ideally should begin treatment before onset of neurologic symptoms

    b. Copper-poor diet, K sulfide with meals (to decrease copper absorption)

    c. D-Penicillamine (copper chelating agent) 1 to 2 g/d + pyridoxine 25 mg/d

    d. If intolerant of D-Penicillamine, use zinc acetate or ammonium tetrathiomolybdate or triethylene tetramine. (Use zinc acetate 50 mg tid for maintenance therapy and presymptomatic treatment.)

    e. Treatment should continue for life.

    f. 10% to 50% of patients may actually worsen with D-penicillamine treatment.

    g. Consider liver transplant.

    h. Improvement begins after 5 to 6 months and is usually complete by 2 years.

III. Inherited Ataxias—Early onset

  A. *Friedreich's Ataxia*

    1. Epidemiology

      a. Autosomal recessive (the only autosomal recessive trinucleotide repeat disease identified thus far)

      b. Trinucleotide repeat disease

      c. Chromosome 9

      d. Mutation in gene encoding a mitochondrial protein, frataxin

      e. Onset of symptoms before 25 years of age in most cases

      f. 50% of cases have onset before age 10

    2. Clinical Features

      a. Usually begins with gait ataxia; difficulty in standing steadily and running is early symptoms. Upper extremity ataxia and dysarthria appear later.

      b. Peripheral neuropathy with pes cavus, hammer toes

      c. Kyphoscoliosis

      d. Cardiomyopathy in 50% of cases, diabetes mellitus in 10%

      e. Physical examination: Ataxia, dysarthria, decreased or absent DTRs, loss of vibratory and position sense, positive Rhomberg, up going toes. Sensorineural hearing loss and optic atrophy occur in a minority of patients.

    3. Prognosis

      a. Progressive limb and gait ataxia. Most patients are unable to walk by age 25 to 30.

      b. Dysarthria progressive, intellect remains intact

      c. Cardiomyopathy and arrhythmias major threat to life

      d. Most patients live into their 30s, usually dying from cardiac disease or infection.

      e. Some patients with minimal scoliosis or cardiac disease may live into their 50s and beyond.

    4. Diagnostic Studies

      a. NCVs—sensory NCVs absent in lower extremities, slowed in upper extremities

      b. Genetic testing—the larger the gene expansion (larger number of repeats), the more severe the disease

      c. CT/MRI not helpful

    5. Pathology

      a. Spinal cord degeneration in 3 key areas

        (1) Posterior columns, dorsal root ganglia (leads to loss of vibratory and position sense, loss of reflexes, positive Rhomberg)

           (2) Corticospinal tracts—weakness, upgoing toes

           (3) Spinocerebellar tracts—ataxia, dysarthria

      b. Clarke's column, lower cranial nerve nuclei, dentate nuclei, and superior cerebellar peduncles may also show degeneration

      c. Myocardial muscle fiber degeneration

B. *Non-Friedreich's Ataxia, diseases with similar phenotypes to FA*

  1. Ataxia with Vitamin E Deficiency (AVED)

      a. Abnormalities in Vitamin E absorption or metabolism can cause syndromes clinically indistinguishable from FA.

      b. AVED is autosomal recessive.

      c. Low or undetectable levels of Vitamin E, without fat malabsorption

      d. Due to mutation in gene encoding for alpha-tocopherol transfer protein (alpha-TTP)

  2. Abetalipoproteinemia (Bassen-Kornzweig Syndrome)

      a. Rare autosomal recessive disorder of lipoprotein metabolism

      b. Malabsorption of Vitamin E

      c. Absence of apolipoprotein B containing proteins (chylomicrons, LDL, VLDL)

      d. Presence of retinopathy distinguishes from FA

      e. Diagnostic studies that also help in distinguishing from FA: low serum cholesterol levels, acanthocytosis on peripheral blood smear, abnormal serum protein electrophoresis

  3. Acquired Vitamin E deficiency

      a. Associated with severe malabsorption in diseases such as cystic fibrosis, cholestatic liver disease, celiac disease, short bowel syndrome

  4. Early Onset Cerebellar Ataxia with retained reflexes (EOCA)

      a. Heterogeneous group of disorders, most autosomal recessive

      b. Childhood onset resembling FA but with retained reflexes

      c. Limbs may even be spastic

      d. Negative FA triplet repeat test

      e. Diabetes, cardiac disease, and skeletal deformities absent

      f. Better prognosis than FA

      g. Diagnosis of exclusion (exclude other biochemical defects such as those listed below and FA)

  5. Progressive Ataxia associated with biochemical abnormalities

      a. Multiple inherited diseases cause progressive ataxia including ceroid lipofuscinosis, cholestanolosis, ataxia-telangiectasia, xeroderma pigmentosum, Cockayne's syndrome, GM-2 gangliosidosis, adrenoleukodystrophy, metachromatic leukodystrophy, mitochondrial diseases (MERRF, KSS, NARP), sialidosis, Niemann-Pick and sphingomyelin storage disorders, and some others

C. *Ataxia Telangiectasia (Louis-Bar Syndrome)*

  1. Epidemiology

      a. Autosomal recessive

      b. Mutation in the ATM gene (leads to defect in DNA repair)

      c. Chromosome 11

      d. ATM protein serves as a regulator of cell cycle check-point in response to DNA damage

2. Clinical Features
   a. Begins earlier than FA, usually in infancy
   b. Progressive truncal ataxia, usually wheelchair bound by age 12
   c. Hallmark oculocutaneous telangiectasias appear at age 3 to 5, well after the onset of ataxia. Rarely the first sign of the disease.
   d. Dysarthria, nystagmus, oculomotor dyspraxia, dystonia, athetosis, myoclonic jerks
   e. Polyneuropathy
   f. Cognitive dysfunction or arrested intellectual development
   g. Delayed growth and development, but signs of premature aging (gray hair) can occur
3. Prognosis
   a. Immunodeficiency leads to recurrent respiratory infections
   b. Associated with cancer—leukemias and lymphomas most common, but can affect any organ
   c. Mean age of death is 20, usually from infection or neoplasm
4. Diagnostic studies
   a. Elevated AFP and CEA levels (alpha-fetoprotein and carcinoembryonic antigen)
   b. Decreased or absent IgA levels
   c. Fibroblasts can be screened for increased x-ray sensitivity and radioresistant DNA synthesis
5. Pathology
   a. Cerebellar degeneration
   b. Loss of myelinated fibers in:
      (1) Posterior columns
      (2) Peripheral nerves
      (3) Spinocerebellar tracts
   c. Degeneration of:
      (1) Dorsal roots and sympathetic ganglia
      (2) Anterior horn cells
   d. Loss of pigmented cells in:
      (1) Substantia nigra
      (2) Locus ceruleus
      (3) Lewy bodies in some pigmented cells
D. Progressive Myoclonic Ataxias
   1. Heterogenous group of childhood disorders
   2. Progressive cerebellar ataxia and action myoclonus
   3. Most due to mitochondrial disorders (MERRF, KSS, NARP). (See section on mitochondrial disorders.)
   4. Rare cases of polyQ disease and DRPLA have juvenile onset (see following information and the section on triple repeat diseases).
IV. Inherited Ataxias—Late Onset
   A. *Spinocerebellar ataxias (Types 1–14)* (see table)—General information:
      1. Most are caused by a CAG repeat (CAG/polygutamine diseases or "polyQ" diseases) and are Autosomal Dominant.

2. Progressive cerebellar ataxia, with varying degrees of bulbar dysfunction, ophthal-moparesis, pyramidal and extrapyramidal signs, optic atrophy, dementia.
3. SCA types 2,3,6 appear to be the most common (accounting for approximately half of all cases worldwide)
4. SCA3 is also known as *Machado-Joseph disease.*
   a. The most common dominantly inherited ataxia in the world.
   b. Clinical Features
      (1) Begins in 30s or 40s with gait ataxia
      (2) Can begin before age 20 or after age 60 rarely
      (3) Within 3 years of onset, have progressive supranuclear ophthalmoparesis
      (4) Bulging eyes due to lid retraction and decreased blink
      (5) Parkinsonian features common, especially with younger onset disease (rigidity and dystonia)
      (6) Dysarthria, dysphagia seen later
      (7) Facial fasciculations can be seen
      (8) Death within 15 to 25 years typically

The Dominant Spinocerebellar Ataxias

Disease and Chromosome	Locus	Genetic Mutation	Frequently Associated Clinical Features (Besides Ataxia, Dysarthria, Dysphagia also common.)
SCA1	6	CAG/polyQ	Dysarthria, dysphagia, ophthalmoparesis, pyramidal findings, neuropathy, choreoathetosis. Parkinson's features uncommon. Intellect spared until late. Frontal lobelike syndrome may occur late in disease.
SCA2	12	CAG/polyQ	Dysarthria, slow saccades, neuropathy, areflexia, facial myokymia, dementia
SCA3	14	CAG/polyQ	Machado-Joseph disease. Bulging eyes, ophthalmoparesis, facial fasciculations. Parkinsonism common. Dysarthria, dysphagia seen later.
SCA4	16	Unknown	Prominent sensory axonal neuropathy, early areflexia, pyramidal tract signs, eye movements preserved.
SCA5	11	Unknown	Pure cerebellar ataxia and dysarthria. Milder disease than SCA types 1–4.
SCA6	19	CAG/polyQ	Late onset (range age 30–70), slow progression, often pure cerebellar syndrome, prominent gaze-evoked and vertical nystagmus, mild neuropathy
SCA7	3	CAG/polyQ	Retinal degeneration, blindness
SCA8	13	CTG repeat	Variable. Bulbar findings, sensory neuronopathy.
SCA9	?	?	?
SCA10	22	ATTCT repeat	Seizures. So far found only in Mexican families. Large pentanucleotide repeat.
SCA11	15	Unknown	Mild disease. Hyperreflexia without extrapyramidal features or sensory loss. Normal life expectancy.
SCA12	5	CAG nonencoding	Arm and head tremor. Paucity of movements, abnormal eye movements. Dementia in elderly patients.
SCA13	19	Unknown	Early childhood onset. Motor dysfunction, mental retardation.
SCA14	19	Unknown	Axial myoclonus, tremor. Single Japanese family.

B. *Dentatorubral-pallidoluysian atrophy* (DRPLA)
   1. Epidemiology
      a. Very rare
      b. Also a polyQ disease—Autosomal dominant, triple repeat

2. Clinical Features
   a. Usually begins in adulthood, resembles Huntington's disease
   b. Cerebellar ataxia, choreoathetosis, dystonia (pseudo-HD form)
   c. Early onset disease may have myoclonus and ataxia (myoclonic-epilepsy form)
3. Pathology
   a. Degeneration of the dentatorubral and pallidoluysian systems

C. *Olivopontocerebellar Atrophy* (OPCA)
   1. Epidemiology
      a. Can be familial (usually AD, can be AR or sporadic)
   2. Clinical Features
      a. Familial form: Onset in fifth decade. Ataxia first in legs, then arms, then bulbar musculature. 50% develop parkinsonian features. May have associated nystagmus, optic atrophy, retinal degeneration, ophthalmoplegia, and urinary incontinence.
      b. Sporadic form: Older age at onset, pure cerebellar syndrome, without the above associated symptoms

V. Degenerative Diseases of the Spinal Cord—Predominantly Upper Motor Neuron
   A. Primary Lateral Sclerosis
      1. Epidemiology
         a. Rare, accounts for < 5% of all cases of motor neuron disease.
      2. Clinical Features
         a. Onset usually after age 40
         b. Slowly progressive spasticity and weakness of the limbs
         c. May stabilize with time, or may progress rapidly in some cases
         d. Rarely lose the ability to walk with cane or other assistance
         e. Most have no sphincter symptoms (rare spastic bladder)
         f. Dysarthria and dysphagia may occur
      3. Pathology
         a. Degeneration of corticospinal tracts
         b. Corticobulbar tracts may be affected
      4. Diagnostic Studies
         a. MRI usually normal, but helps to rule out other causes of spastic paraparesis
         b. No denervation seen on electromyography or muscle biopsy
      5. Differential diagnosis of adult onset spastic paraparesis
         a. Multiple Sclerosis
         b. Cervical stenosis/cervical myelopathy
         c. Amyotrophic lateral sclerosis
         d. Adrenoleukodystrophy
         e. Tropical Spastic Paraparesis
         f. HIV-associated myelopathy
         g. Paraneoplastic myelopathy
         h. Combined Systems Degeneration (Vitamin B_{12} deficiency)
         i. Familial spastic paraparesis

VI. Degenerative Diseases of the Spinal Cord—Predominantly Lower Motor Neuron
   A. Spinal Muscular Atrophy—Type I. Werdnig-Hoffmann Syndrome.
      1. General characteristics of Types I, II, and III

      a. All Autosomal Dominant
      b. Chromosome 5
      c. All show denervation on EMG and muscle biopsy
      d. Nerve conduction velocities normal
      e. CPK usually elevated (usually 1 to 2 times normal)
      f. No sensory loss or cerebral dysfunction (no mental retardation)
  2. Clinical Features of Type I—Werdnig-Hoffmann Syndrome
      a. Symptoms evident at birth or soon after, before age 6 months
      b. One of the most common causes of "floppy infant syndrome"
      c. Muscle weakness, hypotonia progresses to flaccid quadriplegia
      d. Tongue fasciculations (usually not seen in limb muscles)
      e. Areflexia
      f. Ocular muscles spared
      g. Normal reaction to sensory stimuli, alert appearance
      h. 85% die by age 2 years
B. Spinal Muscular Atrophy—Type II.
  1. Clinical Features
      a. Similar to Werdnig-Hoffmann, except that onset is later
      b. Onset from age 6 months to 1 year
      c. Can develop the ability to sit, but very delayed
      d. Finger trembling, flaccidity, alert, cognitively normal
      e. 70% lack deep tendon reflexes
      f. May survive past age 2 years
C. Spinal Muscular Atrophy—Type III
  1. Clinical Features
      a. Onset in late childhood or adolescence
      b. Falling, trouble walking up and down stairs at age 2 to 3 years
      c. Proximal limb weakness, legs more severely affected than arms
      d. Absent deep tendon reflexes in most cases
      e. Fasciculations of tongue and limb muscles
      f. More benign course, may have near normal life span
      g. Sensation, bulbar muscles, and intellect spared
D. Childhood Bulbar Muscular Atrophy—Fazio-Londe Syndrome
  1. Clinical Features
      a. Onset late childhood, adolescence
      b. Dysfunction limited to lower cranial nerves
      c. Selective dysarthria, dysphagia, facial diplegia
      d. Tongue wasting with fasciculations
      e. Symptoms may remain restricted for years, but weakness of arms and legs can occur later.
      f. Progresses to death in 1 to 5 years
E. Adult Bulbar Muscular Atrophy—Kennedy Disease
  1. Genetics
      a. X-linked recessive
      b. Trinucleotide (CAG) repeat disease

    2. Clinical Features

        a. Symptoms begin after age 40 years

        b. Dysarthria, dysphagia appear first, followed by limb weakness

        c. Tongue fasciculations

        d. Absent deep tendon reflexes

        e. Gynecomastia, reduced fertility (androgen insensitivity)

        f. Sensory neuropathy

        g. May have congenital fractures, joint contractures

VI. Degenerative Diseases of the Spinal Cord—Mixed Upper and Lower Motor Neuron

    A. Amyotrophic Lateral Sclerosis—Lou Gehrig's Disease

        1. Epidemiology

            a. Male to Female ratio is 2:1

            b. Onset usually after age 50

            c. About 5% to 10% of cases are familial (autosomal dominant).

            d. 20% of familial cases are due to a defect in the SOD1 (superoxide dismutase) gene on chromosome 21.

        2. Clinical Features

            a. Weakness, atrophy, fasciculations (lower motor neuron signs)

            b. Hyperreflexia, spasticity, up going toes (upper motor neuron signs)

            c. May have asymmetric onset involving hands, extremities (e.g., foot drop). Then generalizes to involve legs, arms, and bulbar muscles (dysphagia, dysarthria).

            d. Muscle cramps

            e. Weight loss

            f. Sensation, extraocular muscles, and sphincter function are spared

            g. Death usually occurs within 3 to 5 years (90% die within 6 years)

            h. Hemiplegic (Mills) variant—begins with weakness on one side

        3. Diagnostic Studies

            a. EMG—widespread denervation in at least three limbs. Giant motor unit potentials, polyphasic MUPs, fasciculations

            b. NCS—usually normal

            c. Neuroimaging—usually normal

        4. Pathologic Findings

            a. Degeneration of anterior horn cells and corticospinal tracts

            b. Bunina bodies—intracytoplasmic, eosinophilic inclusions in anterior horn cells

            c. Muscle biopsy—fascicular atrophy, neurogenic atrophy

        5. Treatment

            a. Riluzole (must monitor LFTs)

               (1) Slows course of disease (minimally)

               (2) Diminishes glutamate release from neuronal terminals

            b. Supportive care

TREMOR

I. Definition, Phenomenology, and Classification

    A. Definition and general information

1. Tremor is the most common of all movement disorders.
2. The two most prevalent diseases associated with tremor are Essential Tremor and Parkinson's Disease.
3. Defined as an involuntary, rhythmic oscillation of a functional body region produced by activation of reciprocally innervated agonistic and antagonistic muscles.
4. Patterned and rhythmic (unlike chorea, dystonia, myoclonus, or tics)
5. Amplitude is variable and increases with emotional activation (fear, anxiety, excitement).
6. Frequency usually remains stable.

B. Classification
   1. Rest Tremor
      a. Seen when the affected body part is completely supported against gravity, such as when hands are resting in the lap, or hanging freely during ambulation.
      b. Frequency usually from 3 to 6 Hz
      c. Most commonly associated with:
         (1) Idiopathic Parkinson's Disease
         (2) Parkinsonism
   2. Action Tremor
      a. Occurs during voluntary contraction of skeletal muscle
      b. Categorized as postural, kinetic, or isometric
      c. Postural—seen when body part is voluntarily maintained against gravity, such as holding arm out in front of body
      d. Kinetic—oscillation during guided voluntary movement. Demonstrated on finger-to-nose test, eating, drinking, etc.
         (1) Simple Kinetic tremor—during directed voluntary movements
         (2) Intention tremor—increasing amplitude during pursuit of a target
         (3) Isometric tremor—evoked by voluntary muscle contractions without movement (push against wall, make fist, hold up weight)
         (4) Task specific tremor—only with specific task such as writing, speaking.

Tremor type	Frequency	Rest	Posture	Movement
Physiologic	8–12 Hz	+	++++	++
Parkinsonian	4–6 Hz	++++	++	++
Essential	4–11 Hz	+	+++	++
Cerebellar	3–5 Hz	+	+++	++++

II. Specific Tremor Syndromes
   A. Physiologic Tremor
      1. Usually nonvisible, asymptomatic for most activities
      2. Can be seen with amplification, such as holding a piece of paper on the outstretched hand, or when using a laser pointer on a distant screen.
   B. Enhanced Physiologic Tremor (EPT)
      1. Visible, postural, high frequency tremor. No other neurologic disease.
      2. May be enhanced by drugs, emotional states, stress, exercise, fatigue, hypothermia, hypoglycemia, hyperthyroidism, drug or alcohol withdrawal.

      3. Resolves with withdrawal of enhancing factor.

      4. Beta-blockers can help decrease EPT.

C. Essential Tremor (ET)

  1. Epidemiology

     a. The most common involuntary movement disorder

     b. About 5 million people in the U.S. affected

     c. Prevalence increases with age, as many as 10% of those over age 65 may have ET.

  2. Genetics

     a. Autosomal dominant

     b. Positive family history in at least 60% to 70% of patients

  3. Diagnostic criteria

     a. Bilateral action tremor of the hands and forearms OR

     b. Isolated head tremor without dystonia or abnormal posturing

     c. No additional neurologic signs, other than "cogwheeling"

     d. Secondary criteria include:

        (1) Long duration (greater than 3 years)

        (2) Positive family history

        (3) Beneficial response to alcohol

        (4) No underlying disease or drugs present known to cause tremor.

  4. Clinical Features

     a. Affects hands in 90%, head in 50%, voice in 30%, legs and chin in 15%.

     b. Isolated head tremor in 34%.

     c. Kinetic component common. Rarely, rest component seen (5%).

     d. May begin unilaterally, but becomes bilateral over time. It is generally symmetric, although minor asymmetry is common.

     e. Slowly progressive

     f. Worsens with stress, anxiety, fatigue, CNS stimulants

     g. Produces functional disability with writing, drinking, eating, etc

  5. Treatment

     a. Primidone

        (1) 70% of patients will get reduction in tremor

        (2) Typical dose is 50 to 350 mg/d, usually at bedtime

        (3) Tolerance occurs in about 13%

        (4) Head tremor responds less well than arm tremor

        (5) Acute side effects: vertigo, nausea, and unsteadiness.

        (6) Chronic side effects: drowsiness, depression

     b. Beta-Adrenergic Antagonists

        (1) Reduce tremor in 40% to 50% of patients

        (2) Propanolol dose usually 80 to 320 mg/d

        (3) Again more effective for arm tremor than head tremor

        (4) Side effects: fatigue, impotence, bradycardia, and depression

        (5) Contraindicated with CHF, DM, asthma, heart block

     c. Ethanol

        (1) Temporarily reduces ET in 50% to 90% of patients

        (2) May be a rebound effect when it wears off

      d. Benzodiazepines
         (1) Alprazolam and clonazepam have shown limited benefit.
      e. Clozapine
         (1) Some benefit in several case reports
         (2) Dose usually 18 to 36 mg/d
         (3) 1% to 2% risk of fatal agranulocytosis. Must monitor CBC weekly for first 6 months then biweekly thereafter.
      f. Other agents with variable results
         (1) Topiramate, mirtazapine, gabapentin, glutethimide, methazolamide
      g. Surgical treatment
         (1) Thalamotomy (VIM nucleus)—69% to 83% of patients responded with total resolution or significant improvement in contralateral tremor in recent studies.
         (2) Deep Brain Stimulation (DBS)—Unilateral or Bilateral. Recent study suggests that Thalamotomy and DBS are about equally effective in relieving tremor, but DBS has fewer adverse events.

D. Parkinson's Tremor
  1. Clinical Features
      a. 50% of Parkinson's patients report tremor as initial symptom
      b. Rest tremor with frequency of 4 to 6 Hz
      c. Classic "pill-rolling" movement of fingers, pronation-supination of the forearm, flexion-extension at the elbow
      d. Approximately 10% of PD patients do not have tremor
      e. Commonly has both postural and kinetic components, in addition to the classic resting component.
  2. Treatment
      a. Anticholinergics
         (1) Trihexyphenidyl, Benztropine
         (2) Decreases tremor by more than 50%
         (3) Side effects: dry mouth, blurred vision, hallucinations, memory problems/confusion, prostatism.
      b. Dopaminergic agents
         (1) Levodopa, dopamine agonists
         (2) Better for rigidity and bradykinesia than for tremor
         (3) May improve tremor by about 50%
      c. Beta-Adrenergic antagonists
         (1) Propanolol, nadolol
         (2) May reduce postural component
      d. Clozapine
         (1) May be useful when other measures have failed.
         (2) Dosages and precautions about agranulocytosis same as for ET.
      e. Surgical treatment
         (1) Thalamotomy
         (2) Deep Brain Stimulation
E. Cerebellar Tremor
  1. Clinical Features

          a. Usually affects proximal muscles, worsens as the extremity approaches the target.
          b. Demonstrated on finger-to-nose and heel-to-shin testing
          c. Titubation is a cerebellar postural tremor of the trunk and head, caused by lesions of the cerebellar vermis.
          d. Multiple sclerosis is most common cause, but can occur with a variety of tumors, strokes, degenerative diseases, paraneoplastic disorders, etc.
     2. Treatment
          a. No well-established pharmacotherapy
             (1) Thalamic VIM DBS may be of benefit
  F. Holmes' Tremor
     1. Clinical Features
          a. "Rubral" or midbrain tremor
          b. Combination of rest, postural, and kinetic tremors
          c. Frequency is slower that most other tremors (2 to 4 Hz)
          d. Caused by interruptions in the midbrain tegmentum
          e. Other brain stem and cranial nerve findings usually present
          f. May be a delay in the occurrence of the lesion and onset of tremor.
     2. Treatment
          a. Limited benefit, limited data, questionable efficacy
             (1) Benzodiazepines, valproic acid, beta-blockers, anticholinergics, dopamine agonists, levodopa
             (2) VIM Thalamotomy, VIM DBS
  G. Dystonic Tremor
     1. Clinical Features
          a. Tremor superimposed on dystonia
          b. Commonly associated with torticollis
          c. Tremor is exacerbated by moving in the direction opposite the force of contraction caused by the dystonia
     2. Treatment
          a. Botulinum Toxin into involved muscles
  H. Voice Tremor
     1. Clinical Features
          a. Most notable with attempt to produce long words or sounds
          b. Occurs in 15% to 25% of patients with Essential Tremor (ET)
          c. Other disorders associated with voice tremor:
             (1) Parkinson's Disease
             (2) Amyotrophic Lateral Sclerosis
             (3) Cerebellar Disorders
          d. Must be differentiated from spasmodic dysphonia
     2. Treatment
          a. Usually difficult, with variable effectiveness
          b. Medications: primidone, propanolol, benzodiazepines
          c. Surgical: VIM DBS
          d. Botulinum Toxin injections may be effective for voice tremor associated with adductor spasmodic dysphonia and severe voice tremor associated with ET

I. Primary Writing Tremor
   1. Clinical Features
      a. Tremor only appears while writing or adopting hand position for writing
      b. Asymmetric
      c. No other neurological signs
      d. Frequency ranges from 5 to 7 Hz
   2. Treatment
      a. Medications: primidone, propanolol, anticholinergics
      b. Surgical: VIM DBS
      c. Botulinum Toxin injections
J. Palatal Tremor (Palatal Myoclonus)
   1. Clinical Features
      a. Rare movement disorder comprised of rhythmic involuntary movements of the soft palate.
      b. Two types:
         (1) Symptomatic palatal tremor (SPT)
             (a) Persists through coma and sleep
             (b) Due to brain stem or cerebellar lesion
             (c) Hypertrophic degeneration of the inferior olives
             (d) Abnormalities of the dentato-rubro-olivary pathways
             (e) Lifelong condition
         (2) Essential palatal tremor (EPT)
             (a) Monosymptomatic disorder
             (b) Neurological exam is normal other than for palatal tremor
             (c) Inferior olives and brain stem are normal
             (d) Usually a chronic condition
   2. Treatment
      a. No currently effective treatment for SPT
      b. EPT may respond to phenytoin, barbiturates, benzodiazepines, anticholinergics, 5-hydroxytryptophan
K. Orthostatic Tremor
   1. Clinical Features
      a. Rare tremor disorder of the legs and trunk that occurs on standing and stops with walking or sitting
      b. On standing, the tremor increases in a crescendo fashion over seconds to minutes to the point that the patient cannot continue to stand and must either sit or walk.
      c. Usually occurs in middle aged or elderly
      d. EMG shows 16 Hz burst pattern in weight bearing muscles
   2. Treatment
      a. Clonazepam is drug of choice. Dose 0.5 to 2.0 mg per day
      b. Other: primidone, phenobarbital, valproic acid
L. Tardive Tremor
   1. Clinical Features
      a. Part of the spectrum of tardive dyskinesia

        b. Caused by treatment with neuroleptics or other dopamine blocking agents
        c. May affect the head, lips, arms, or legs
        d. Worsens after withdrawal of the neuroleptic
    2. Treatment
        a. Tetrabenazine (dopamine-depleting agent)
        b. Atypical neuroleptics (e.g., clozapine)
M. Drugs and other agents that can cause tremor
    1. Drugs:
        a. Alcohol (tremor can occur with ETOH use, or withdrawal)
        b. Amphetamines
        c. CNS stimulants (theophylline, albuterol, caffeine)
        d. Anticonvulsants (valproic acid)
        e. Lithium
        f. Amiodarone
        g. Corticosteroids
    2. Chemical and other agents
        a. Heavy metals
        b. Metal chelators
        c. Carbon tetrachloride

NEUROCUTANEOUS SYNDROMES

I. Tuberous Sclerosis
  A. Epidemiology: 1:10,000
  B. Inheritance: AD, chromosome 9 (occasionally chromosome 16)
  C. Clinical Features
    1. Voigt's classical triad—present in only one-third of patients
        a. Epilepsy
        b. Adenoma sebaceum
        c. Mental deficiency
    2. Primary criteria
        a. Adenoma sebaceum (90% over age 4 years)
        b. Ungual fibroma (appear at puberty)
        c. Cerebral cortical tubers
        d. Subependymal nodules (candle gutterings)
        e. Fibrous forehead plaques
    3. Secondary criteria
        a. Infantile spasms—start at 4 to 7 months (75%) and EEG may show hypsarrhythmia
        b. Ashleaf spots (90%)
          (1) Hypomelanotic lesions
          (2) May be the earliest skin manifestation of tuberous sclerosis
          (3) Requires Wood's lamp for diagnosis
        c. Shagreen patches (subepidermal fibrous patches)
          (1) Usually found in the lumbosacral region

(2) Orange peel appearance
    d. Retinal hamartomas, phakomas
    e. Bilateral renal cysts
    f. Angiolipomas of the kidney
    g. Rhabdomyosarcomas of the heart
    h. First degree relative with tuberous sclerosis
  4. Renal failure is the most common cause of death.
D. Imaging
  1. Cortical tubers
    a. Measure 5 mm to 3 cm
    b. Hypodense on CT
  2. Candle gutterings
    a. Appear on walls of lateral ventricles
    b. Frequently calcified
  3. Subependymal giant-cell astrocytoma
    a. Occur most frequently at the foramen of Monro
    4. Hydrocephalus secondary to obstruction of the foramen of Monro
E. Pathology
  1. Cortical tubers
    a. Giant cells
    b. Gliosis
    c. Disorganized myelin
    d. Hamartomas
  2. Heterotopic islands
  3. Subependymal giant-cell astrocytomas
F. Treatment
  1. Lesion resection
  2. Adrenocorticotropic hormone
  3. Antiepileptic drugs
II. Neurofibromatosis Type I (Peripheral)
  A. Inheritance: AD, chromosome 17
  B. Clinical Features
    1. Café au lait spots—six or more
    2. Axillary freckles
    3. Lisch nodules (white hamartomas in iris)
    4. Multiple cutaneous (molluscum fibrosum) tumors
    5. Multiple subcutaneous tumors
      a. Firm nodules
      b. Plexiform neuromas (bag of worms)
    6. Acoustic neuromas
    7. Trigeminal neuromas
    8. Optic gliomas
    9. Spinal root tumors
   10. Bone cysts, pathologic bone fractures (pseudoarthrosis)
   11. Pheochromocytoma

        12. Scoliosis

        13. Precocious puberty

        14. Syringomyelia

        15. Obstructive hydrocephalus from glial overgrowth

        16. Seizures: 20 times rate for general population

        17. Hyperactivity

        18. Intellectual impairment in 40%

   C. Pathology

        1. Cutaneous tumors—loosely arranged elongated connective tissue cells

        2. Café au lait spots

           a. Normal number of melanocytes

           b. Increased number of melanosomes

        3. Neurofibromas—malignant degeneration in 2% to 5%

III. Neurofibromatosis Type II (Central)

   A. Inheritance: AD, chromosome 22

   B. Clinical Features

        1. Paucity of cutaneous lesions

        2. Bilateral acoustic neuromas

           a. Neuroma grows on vestibular portion of CN VIII.

           b. First symptom is hearing loss secondary to compression on cochlear component of CN VIII.

        3. Meningiomas

IV. Stürge-Weber Syndrome (Encephalotrigeminal Angiomatosis)

   A. Inheritance: Sporadic

   B. Clinical Features

        1. Port wine nevus of the face (rarely bilateral)

           a. Extent of nevus usually mirrors intracranial involvement.

           b. Nearly all that involve the upper eyelid have associated cerebral lesions.

        2. Contralateral hemiparesis

        3. Contralateral hemiatrophy

        4. Glaucoma

        5. Seizures (often intractable)

        6. Mental retardation

   C. Imaging

        1. Tram-line calcifications on radiographs by age 2 years

           a. Secondary to calcification of cortex

        2. Cerebral atrophy

        3. Thickened calvarial diplöe

        4. MRI with gyriform enhancement

   D. EEG: Decreased potentials over affected area

   E. Pathology

        1. Occipital lobe most frequently affected

        2. Leptomeningeal angiomas

        3. Calcification of cortex

        4. Calcification of blood vessel walls

V. Familial Telangiectasia (Osler-Rendu-Weber Syndrome)
   A. Inheritance: AD
   B. Clinical Features
      1. Angiomas in skin, CNS, GI tract, GU tract, mucous membranes
      2. Bleeding
   C. Pathology
      1. Defect in blood vessel walls results in mechanical fragility.
VI. Incontinentia Pigmenti
   A. Inheritance: X-linked dominant
   B. Clinical Features
      1. Lesions begin as linear vesiculobullous lesions and progress to hyperkeratosis and hyperpigmentation with linear streaks and whorls.
      2. Slate-gray pigmentation
      3. Alopecia
      4. Delayed motor development
      5. Spastic hemiparesis
      6. Mental retardation
      7. Seizures
   C. Pathology
      1. Atrophy
      2. Microgyria
      3. Focal necrosis in white matter
   D. Lab
      1. Eosinophilia (65%)
VII. von Hippel-Lindau Disease (Hemangioblastoma of the Cerebellum)
   A. Inheritance: AD
   B. Clinical Features
      1. Ataxia
      2. Obstructive hydrocephalus
   C. Pathology
      1. Cerebellar hemangioblastomas—multicystic tumor
      2. Retinal hemangioblastomas
      3. Hepatic cysts
      4. Pancreatic cysts
      5. Renal tumors
      6. Polycythemia because of increased erythropoietin
      7. Pheochromocytoma
VIII. Ataxia-Telangiectasia (Louis-Bar Syndrome)
   A. Inheritance: AR
   B. Defect: Defect in DNA repair
   C. Clinical Features
      1. Normal development for first few years
      2. Ataxia—limb, gait, speech by age 4 to 5 years
      3. Choreoathetosis
      4. Absent optokinetic nystagmus

      5. Apraxia of voluntary gaze
      6. Mild intellectual decline
      7. Polyneuropathy (absent DTRs by age 9 years)
      8. Subpapillary venous plexus telangiectasias after age 3 to 5 years
      9. Neoplasia especially lymphomas and gliomas
    10. Absent of decreased immunoglobulins
    11. Death by second decade from neoplasia or infection

D. Pathology
    1. Cerebellar degeneration
    2. Loss of myelinated fibers in:
      a. Posterior columns
      b. Peripheral nerves
      c. Spinocerebellar tracts
    3. Degeneration of:
      a. Dorsal roots
      b. Sympathetic ganglia
      c. Anterior horn cells
    4. Loss of pigmented cells in:
      a. Substantia nigra
      b. Locus ceruleus
    5. Lewy bodies in pigmented cells

E. Lab
    1. Decreased immunoglobulins

TRINUCLEOTIDE REPEAT DISEASES

I. Basic Principles
  A. May be inherited as Autosomal Dominant, Recessive, or X-Linked traits
  B. Variable phenotype, even within the same family
  C. *Amplification*—The larger the number of repeats, the more severe the disease.
  D. *Anticipation*—The tendency for disease to worsen in successive generations.
  E. Paternal transmission is more likely to result in a significant increase in repeat length. Therefore, juvenile-onset disease is more likely to be paternally inherited.

II. Trinucleotide repeat diseases
  A. *CAGpolyglutamine (polyQ) Diseases*
    1. SCA 1
    2. SCA 2
    3. SCA 3 / MJD
    4. SCA 6
    5. SCA 7
    6. Huntington's Disease
    7. Dentatorubral-pallidoluysian atrophy (DRPLA)
    8. Spinal and Bulbar Muscular Atrophies
  B. *Disorders with repeats outside of protein coding region*
    1. Friedreich's Ataxia

2. Myotonic Dystrophy
3. Fragile X Syndromes (FraXA and FraXE)
4. SCA 8
5. SCA 12

Disease	Trinucleotide	Normal Range	Disease Range	Protein
Huntington's	CAG	<37	37–121	Huntintin
Fragile X (A, E, F, 16A)	CGG	6–54	50–1,500	FMR-1
Myotonic dystrophy	CTG	5–37	44–3,000	Myotonin
Spinocerebellar atrophy type 1	CAG	25–36	43–81	Ataxin-1
Spinobulbar muscular atrophy	CAG	13–30	30–62	Androgen receptor
Dentatorubral–Pallidoluysian atrophy	CAG	30 or less	>31	CTG-B37
Machado-Joseph	CAG	30 or less	>31	Unknown
Friedreich's ataxia	GAA	<200	200–900	Frataxin

MITOCHONDRIAL DISORDERS

I. Genetics

Disorder	Inheritance	Mutation Type	Ragged Red Fibers
MELAS	Maternal	Point mutation at tRNA(leu)	+
MERRF	Maternal	Point mutation at tRNA(lys)	+
MIMyCa	Maternal	Point mutation at tRNA(leu)	+
LHON	Maternal	Point mutation at ND1, ND4, or cytochrome b genes (possibly others)	–
CPEO	Sporadic/AD	Single deletion/multiple deletions	+
KSS	Sporadic	Single deletion or insertion	+

Abbreviations of disorders are listed on page 280–281.

II. Clinical Presentation
   A. Mitochondrial Encephalomyopathy, Lactic Acidosis, and Stroke-like Syndrome (MELAS)
      1. Epidemiology
         a. Childhood onset—diffuse disease
         b. Adult onset—focal disease
      2. Clinical features
         a. Mitochondrial myopathy
         b. Encephalopathy
         c. Stroke-like episodes—usually occipital cortex
         d. Episodic vomiting
         e. Cerebral blindness
         f. Hemiparesis
         g. Hemianopia
      3. Pathology: Ragged red fibers on muscle biopsy
      4. Lab: Lactic acidosis
   B. Myoclonic Epilepsy with Ragged Red Fibers (MERRF)
      1. Epidemiology: Childhood onset
      2. Clinical features
         a. Myoclonic epilepsy
         b. Myoclonus/Ataxia
      3. Pathology
         a. Neuronal loss in dentate, inferior olive, substantia nigra

      b. Gliosis in cerebellar cortex
      c. Degeneration of posterior columns
      d. Ragged red fibers on muscle biopsy
C. Maternally Inherited Myopathy and Cardiomyopathy (MIMyCa)
    1. Epidemiology: Maternally inherited; adult onset
    2. Clinical features
      a. Myopathy
      b. Cardiomyopathy
    3. Pathology: Ragged red fibers on muscle biopsy
D. Leber's Hereditary Optic Neuropathy (LHON)
    1. Epidemiology
      a. Male: female = 2:1
      b. Affects males in second or third decade of life
      c. Females pass the gene to their sons and the carrier states to their daughters.
      d. Males do not transmit the disease.
    2. Clinical features: Painless unilateral central vision loss
    3. Pathology: No ragged red fibers on muscle biopsy
E. Chronic Progressive External Ophthalmoplegia (CPEO)
    1. Epidemiology: Onset before age 20 years
    2. Clinical features
      a. Insidiously progressive immobility of the eyes with ptosis
      b. Pupils are spared.
      c. Can be an isolated disease or occur as part of:
          (1) Oculopharyngeal dystrophy—CPEO + dysphagia
          (2) Kearns-Sayre syndrome
          (3) Ophthalmoplegia plus—CPEO
             (a) Mental retardation
             (b) Hearing loss
             (c) Slow EEG
             (d) Spongiform degeneration of cerebrum and brainstem
    3. Pathology: Ragged red fibers on muscle biopsy
    4. Laboratory: + increased CSF protein
F. Kearns-Sayre Syndrome (KSS)
    1. Epidemiology: Onset before age 20 years
    2. Clinical features
      a. CPEO
      b. Retinal degeneration (pigmentary retinopathy)
      c. Cardiac conduction defects (heart block)
      d. Cerebellar syndrome
    3. Pathology: Ragged red fibers on muscle biopsy
    4. Laboratory: CSF protein > 100 mg/dL
G. Leigh's Disease—subacute necrotizing encephalomyelopathy
    1. Epidemiology
    2. Clinical features
      a. Respiratory disorders (episodic hyperventilation, apnea)
      b. External ophthalmoplegia

        c. Paralysis of deglutition

        d. Abnormal movements (ataxia, chorea, jerks)

    3. Pathology

        a. Demyelination

        b. Gliosis

        c. Necrosis

        d. Neuronal sparing

        e. Location: Basal ganglia → brainstem → cerebellum → cortex

        f. Due to many defects in mitochondrial function, such as:

           (1) Decreased cytochrome C oxidase

           (2) Decreased pyruvate dehydrogenase

    4. Lab: Increased lactate and pyruvate

III. Treatment

  A. Carnitine, 2 to 3 g/d

  B. Coenzyme Q 60 to 300 mg/d

  C. Vitamin K_3, 40 to 80 mg/d

  D. Vitamin C, 500 mg/d

NORMAL AGE-RELATED NEUROLOGIC CHANGES

  A. Vibration for 10 to 12 seconds in the great toe

  B. Benign forgetfulness of aging (dates, names)

  C. Limited upgaze after age 60 years

  D. Decreased smooth pursuit

  E. Smaller pupils

  F. Decreased olfaction and taste

  G. Decreased high-frequency hearing (consonants)

  H. Mild iliopsoas weakness

  I. Slightly decreased tandem gait

  J. Mild increase in physiologic tremor

  K. Decreased ankle reflexes

  L. Increased reaction time

  M. Neuronal number decreases

  N. Synapse number decreases

  O. Dendritic spines decrease

  P. Brain weight decreases 10%

BEHAVIORAL NEUROLOGY

I. Aphasia

  A. Broca's Aphasia

    1. Description: Disordered grammar, nonfluent, linguistic dysprosody, poor naming, poor repetition, and paraphasias

    2. Lesion: Frontal operculum lower motor cortex, anterior division of left middle cerebral artery

  B. Chronic Broca's Aphasia

    1. Description: Mutism or hyperkinetic, spastic

       2. Lesion: Dorsolateral frontal, opercular subcortical extension

C. Wernicke's Aphasia
       1. Description: Paraphasic or empty content, neologisms, circumlocutions, paragrammatism, poor naming, apraxia, poor repetition
       2. Lesion: Superior temporal gyrus

D. Conduction Aphasia
       1. Description: Poor repetition, hesitation, variable naming, and decreased auditory short-term memory
       2. Lesion: Supramarginal gyrus (arcuate fibers)

E. Transcortical Motor Aphasia
       1. Description: Imitation block, echolalia, normal repetition, poor syntax, improves with direct dopamine agonists
       2. Lesion: Large dorsolateral frontal lesions that spare the perisylvian cortex

F. Transcortical Sensory Aphasia
       1. Description: Fluent semantic paraphasias circumlocutions, jargon, normal repetition, poor comprehension, poor naming, and poor reading
       2. Lesion: Middle or inferior temporal gyrus that spares the perisylvian cortex

G. Aphemia
       1. Description: Mutism or very effortful speech, but writing is preserved
       2. Lesion: Anterior or medial frontal or white matter undercutting Broca's area, but sparing the perisylvian cortex

II. Dyslexia

A. Alexia without Agraphia
       1. Description: Inability to read with preserved ability to write
       2. Lesion: Left occipital lobe with splenium of corpus callosum

B. Neglect Dyslexia
       1. Description: Failure to identify initial letters in a letter string; neglect syndrome component
       2. Lesion: Right neglect dyslexia sometimes seen with left brain damage

C. Attentional Dyslexia
       1. Description: Preserved single words, disrupted composition, sometimes preserved single letter reading with compromised letter string reading
       2. Lesion: Alzheimer's disease (AD), attention disorder

D. Deep Dyslexia
       1. Description: Semantic errors, concrete words easier, difficulty with functors (articles and pronouns), unable to read nonwords such as "PRAT"
       2. Lesion: Large perisylvian lesions, usually associated with aphasias

E. Phonologic Dyslexia
       1. Description: Reading without print to sound conversion, impaired reading of nonword letter strings
       2. Lesion: Dominant perisylvian cortex, superior temporal lobe, angular gyrus

F. Surface Dyslexia
       1. Description: Inability to pronounce words of nonphonologic pronunciation (i.e., irregular words such as cough, rough, bough)
       2. Lesion: AD, poorly localized

III. Agraphia

A. Apraxic Agraphia
   1. Description: Difficulty writing letters (motor control)
   2. Lesion: Superior parietal lobe dominant
B. Spatial Agraphia
   1. Description: Spatial orientation abnormal, sometimes associated with neglect
   2. Lesion: Nondominant parietal lobe
C. Parkinsonian Agraphia
   1. Description: Micrographia, slow, may have motor perseveration
   2. Lesion: Poorly localized
D. Callosal Agraphia
   1. Genu: Apraxic agraphia with inability to type
   2. Body: Apraxic agraphia with ability to type
   3. Splenium: unilateral aphasic agraphia (incorrect spellings)
E. Dementia Agraphia
   1. Description: Semantic errors, homophone errors (night for knight), spatial agraphia
   2. Lesion: AD
F. Isolated Agraphia
   1. Description: Spelling errors
   2. Lesion: Possibly second frontal gyrus (Exner's area)
G. Acalculia
   1. Description: Abnormalities of number processing
   2. Lesion: Left posterior hemisphere

IV. Apraxia
A. Limb Kinetic Apraxia
   1. Description: Loss of finely graded finger movements (subtle form of weakness)
   2. Lesion: Contralateral parietal lobe
B. Ideomotor Apraxia
   1. Description: Movement production errors (positional or spatial errors)
   2. Lesion: Dominant inferior parietal lobe, ± corpus callosum, ± SMA
C. Disassociation Apraxia
   1. Description: No recognizable action or command, but use objects well
   2. Lesion: Callosal disconnections
D. Conduction Apraxia
   1. Description: More impaired with imitating than when positioning
   2. Lesion: Unknown
E. Ideational Apraxia
   1. Description: Movement sequence errors, required to complete a task
   2. Lesion: Dementia
F. Conceptual Apraxia (sometimes referred to as Ideational apraxia)
   1. Description: Decreased tool—object action knowledge
   2. Lesion: Dementia, left parietal

V. Visual Agnosia
A. Apperceptive Agnosia
   1. Description: Unable to see objects properly (perception), unable to copy
   2. Lesion: Diffuse brain damage (carbon monoxide), left occipitotemporal lesion
B. Associative Agnosia

      1. Description: Impaired object visual recognition (memory of names and function), able to copy drawings

      2. Lesion: Occipitotemporal

  C. Prosopagnosia

      1. Description: Inability to recognize faces

      2. Lesion: Right (emotional faces) or bilateral PCA infarction

  D. Central Achromatopsia

      1. Description: Disorder of color perception (faded)

      2. Lesion: Occipitotemporal junction (lingual and fusiform gyri); may accompany other lesions with hemianopsia, alexia, etc.

  E. Color Agnosia

      1. Description: Disorder of color recognition

      2. Lesion: Occipitotemporal lesion

  F. Color Anomia

      1. Description: Disorder of color naming

      2. Lesion: Left occipitotemporal

VI. Auditory Agnosia

  A. Cortical Deafness

      1. Description: Disorder of audiometric sensitivity, speech comprehension, speech repetition, recognition of familiar sounds, musical perception, vocal prosody

      2. Lesion: Bilateral Heschl's gyrus

  B. Pure Word Deafness

      1. Description: Disorder of speech comprehension, speech repetition, musical perception

      2. Lesion: Bilateral anterior superior temporal gyrus

  C. Auditory Sound Agnosia

      1. Description: Disorder of recognition of familiar sounds, musical perception

      2. Lesion: Temporoparietal junction

  D. Sensory Amusia

      1. Description: ± Musical perception, recognition of prosody

      2. Lesion: Nondominant hemisphere

  E. Expressive Aprosodia

      1. Description: Inability to produce emotional intonations (anger, fear)

      2. Lesion: Right frontal

  F. Receptive Aprosodia

      1. Description: Inability to comprehend emotional intonations (anger, fear)

      2. Lesion: Right posterior

VII. Sensory Agnosia

  A. Astereognosis

      1. Description: Impaired tactile perception

      2. Lesion: Disruption of somatosensory pathways, right hemisphere

  B. Tactile Agnosia

      1. Description: Impaired tactile object recognition unilateral

      2. Lesion: Inferior parietal cortex contralateral, posterior insula, lateral somatosensory association cortex

  C. Optic Ataxia

      1. Description: Inability to accurately reach for visually perceived objects

      2. Lesion: Intraparietal sulcus and superior parietal lobule, usually bilateral

D. Phantom Body Parts

      1. Description: Sensation that missing body part remains

      2. Lesion: No CNS lesion; probable cortical reorganization of the representation of the missing limb

E. Autotopagnosia

      1. Description: Inability to localize one's own body parts

      2. Lesion: Left posterior parietal lobe

F. Finger Agnosia

      1. Description: Inability to recognize fingers

      2. Lesion: Contralateral hemisphere lesions, usually left

G. Constructional Apraxia

      1. Description: Inability to copy drawings, disorder of analysis and reproduction of spatial arrangement

      2. Lesion: AD, poorly localized

H. Topographical Disorientation

      1. Description: Inability to find one's way in a familiar environment or learn new paths

      2. Lesion: Right parietal, dementia

I. Reduplicative Amnesia

      1. Description: Recognize immediate surroundings but believe they are in a different location

      2. Lesion: Right frontal and parietal, AD

J. Neglect

      1. Description: Spatial neglect

      2. Lesion: Inferior parietal lobe, medial frontal, dorsofrontal contralateral, also thalami, basal ganglia and midbrain

K. Balint's Syndrome

      1. Description: Simultagnosia, optic ataxia, optic apraxia, spatial disorientation, impaired depth perception

      2. Lesion: Bilateral parietal occipital junction

L. Anton's Syndrome

      1. Description: Denial of blindness, confabulatory responses

      2. Lesion: Bilateral occipital lobe lesions

M. Anosognosia (Hemiplegia)

      1. Description: Unawareness of a neurologic deficit

      2. Lesion: Nondominant parietal lobe, frontal, basal ganglia

N. Gerstmann's Syndrome

      1. Description: Agraphia, acalculia, right/left confusion, finger agnosia

      2. Lesion: Left angular gyrus

O. Callosal Syndrome

      1. Description: Unable to name objects in left hand; mimic position of one hand with the other in absence of visual feedback, apraxic left upper extremity, mirror movements, alien hand

      2. Lesion: Corpus callosum

13

Transplant Neurology

TRANSPLANT NEUROLOGY—COMPLICATIONS

I. Glucocorticoids
   A. Opportunistic Infections
   B. Steroid Myopathy
   C. Psychosis
   D. Delirium
II. Methotrexate
   A. Intrathecal
      1. Aseptic meningitis
      2. Acute transverse myelopathy
   B. IV high dose
      1. Stroke
      2. Encephalopathy
III. Anti-CD3
   A. Cytokine release
   B. Aseptic meningitis
IV. Cytarabine
   A. Myelopathy
   B. Neuropathy
   C. Cerebellar toxicity (often reversible)
V. Cyclosporine
   A. Skin—hypertrichosis
   B. GI Tract—anorexia, nausea, vomiting
   C. Liver—cholestasis
   D. Hematologic—thrombosis, thrombotic thrombocytopenia purpura, hemolytic uremic syndrome
   E. Endocrine System—hyperglycemia
   F. Neoplasia—primary central nervous system (CNS) lymphoma
   G. Central Nervous System
      1. Confusion
      2. Psychosis
      3. Coma
      4. Tremor in 20% to 40% of cases
      5. Seizures in 2% to 5% of cases

      6. Encephalopathy
      7. Focal
         a. Aphasia
         b. Cortical blindness
         c. Movement disorders
         d. Ataxia
         e. Paresis
   H. Peripheral Nervous System
      1. Dysesthesias and neuropathy
   I. Side effects usually reverse rapidly with decreasing dose.
   J. MRI changes are reversible
VI. FK-506—similar to cyclosporin
VII. Graft Versus Host Disease (GVHD)—usually in bone marrow transplant patients
   A. Neuro-autoimmune
      1. Myasthenia gravis
      2. Inflammatory myositis
   B. Acute Transverse Myelitis

14
Neuro-Ophthalmology

OPHTHALMOLOGY

I. Nystagmus
  A. Congenital
    1. Decreased with convergence
    2. Increased with fixation
    3. Optokinetic nystagmus (OKN) inversion
    4. Uniplanar in all directions
  B. Latent
    1. Seen only when one eye covered
    2. Fast component away from covered eye
    3. Decreased visual acuity
  C. Downbeat—cervicomedullary junction
    1. Arnold-Chiari syndrome
    2. Spinocerebellar degeneration
    3. Brain stem stroke
    4. Multiple sclerosis (MS)
  D. Upbeat
    1. Localizes weakly to medulla
  E. Rotary
    1. Localizes to thalamus
  F. See-saw
    1. Localizes to suprasellar region
  G. Convergence—retraction
    1. Dorsal midbrain (Parinaud's syndrome)
    2. Poor OKNs downward
    3. Differential diagnosis by age
      a. 10 years: Pinealoma
      b. 20 years: Head trauma
      c. 30 years: Vascular malformation
      d. 40 years: MS
      e. 50 years: Basilar stroke
  H. Gaze-evoked
    1. Drugs: Antiepileptic drugs or sedatives
    2. Bilateral brain stem lesions

3. Cerebellar lesions
I. Ocular Myoclonus
   1. Localizes to Mollaret's triangle
J. Ocular Bobbing
   1. Rapid downward jerk with slow drift to primary gaze
   2. Localizes to pons
   3. Differential diagnosis
      a. Hydrocephalus
      b. Metabolic encephalopathy
K. Opsoclonus (dancing eyes)
   1. Localizes to dentate nucleus
   2. Differential diagnosis
      a. Neuroblastoma
      b. Postinfectious
      c. Visceral carcinoma
II. Cerebellar Lesions
   A. Ipsilateral smooth pursuit defect (becomes saccadic)
   B. Transient eye deviation contralateral to lesion
III. Frontal Lesions
   A. Ipsilateral eye deviation
   B. Intact slow pursuit
   C. Eyes can doll past palsy
   D. OKNs abnormal toward lesion
   E. Frontal abnormalities are typically transient (days to weeks)
   F. PPRF lesions result in permanent abnormalities
IV. Parietal Lesions
   A. Contralateral Homonymous Hemianopia
   B. Normal Saccades
   C. Pursuit abnormal toward side of lesion
   D. OKNs abnormal toward side of lesion
V. Parinaud's Syndrome
   A. Supranuclear Upgaze Palsy
   B. Lid Retraction
   C. Convergence—retraction Nystagmus
   D. Light—near Dissociation
VI. Tolosa-Hunt Syndrome
   A. Painful Ophthalmoplegia
   B. Elevated Erythrocyte Sedimentation Rate (ESR)
   C. Positive Lupus Erythematosus (LE) Prep
   D. V1 Sensory Changes
   E. Treat with high-dose prednisone (100 mg/d)
VII. Miller-Fisher Variant of Guillain-Barré Syndrome/Guillain-Barré Syndromes
   A. Oculomotor Palsy
   B. Areflexia

      C. Ataxia

      D. GQ-1b Antibody Positive

VIII. Pituitary Apoplexy

      A. Multiple Extraocular Muscle Palsies

      B. Severe Headache

      C. Bilateral Blindness

  IX. Argyll-Robertson Syndrome

      A. Small, Irregular Pupils

      B. Light—near Dissociation

      C. Intact Visual Acuity

      D. Poor Dilation

   X. Balint's Syndrome

      A. Paralysis of Visual Fixation

      B. Optic Ataxia

      C. Simultagnosia

  XI. Optic Disc Edema

      A. Swelling of the disc often associated with hemorrhages

        1. Papilledema—optic disc edema associated with increased intracranial pressure

        2. Papillitis—optic disc edema associated with inflammatory or demyelinating diseases

        3. Bilateral optic disc edema differential diagnosis

          a. Papillitis

          b. Optic neuritis

          c. Ischemic optic neuropathy

          d. Neuroretinitis (disc edema with a macular star, inflammatory)

          e. Papilledema (until proven otherwise—90% of cases)

          f. Inflammatory disease

          g. Infiltrative disease

        4. Unilateral optic disc edema differential diagnosis

          a. Optic neuritis

          b. Asymmetric papilledema

          c. Anterior ischemic optic neuropathy

          d. Inflammatory disease

          e. Infiltrative disease

          f. Foster Kennedy syndrome (ipsilateral disc edema and contralateral disc atrophy caused by frontal masses)

          g. Pseudo-Foster Kennedy syndrome

          h. Neuroretinitis

      B. Optic Neuritis

        1. Associated with afferent pupillary defect, decreased visual acuity, and pain on motion of that eye

        2. Treatment

          a. The Optic Neuritis Treatment Trial showed equal visual outcome for placebo, PO steroids, and IV steroids.

          (1) PO steroids increase the risk of subsequent MS.

          (2) IV steroids decrease the risk of subsequent MS.

  C. Ischemic Optic Neuropathy

     1. Usually caused by giant-cell arteritis, polymyalgia rheumatica, etc.

     2. Painless vision loss, more common in older adults

XII. Functional Ophthalmology

  A. Malingerer hits all obstacles.

  B. Hysteric misses all obstacles.

  C. Hysteric/malingering blindness eyes move with rocking mirror.

  D. Decreased visual acuity—check VEP (visual evoked potential).

     1. Electroretinogram (ERG) checks rods and cones.

  E. Constricted fields—hysterical

     1. Tubular field—field same as distance increases

     2. Spiral fields

  F. Ocular Motility

     1. Polyopia

     2. Voluntary nystagmus—rapid oscillation with blepharospasm

     3. Conjugate eye abnormalities (move independently)

  G. Accommodative/Convergence Disorder

     1. Accommodative spasm

  H. Chromotopia—all things one color

  I. Micropia—everything small

  J. Asthenopia—eyes tired

Pupil Characteristics

	General	Light-Near	Anisocoria Greater	Mydriatics	Miotics
Essential anisocoria	Round, regular	Both brisk	No change	Dilates	Constricts
Horner's syndrome	Small, round, unilateral	Both brisk	Darkness	Dilates	Constricts
Tonic pupil (Holmes-Adie syndrome)	Larger in bright light 90% unilateral	Absent to light Tonic to near	Light	Dilates	Constricts
Argyll-Robertson syndrome	Small, irregular, bilateral	Poor to light Better to near	No change	Poor dilation	Constricts
Midbrain	Mid-dilated, bilateral	Poor to light Better to near	No change	Dilates	Constricts
Atropine	Very large, round, unilateral	Fixed	Light		No
Oculomotor palsy (non-diabetic)	Mid-dilated, unilateral	Fixed	Light	Dilates	Constricts

15
Pain

HEADACHE

I. Headache Classification
  A. Migraine
    1. Migraine without aura
    2. Migraine with aura
      a. Migraine with typical aura
      b. Migraine with prolonged aura
      c. Familial hemiplegic migraine
      d. Basilar migraine
      e. Migraine aura without headache
      f. Migraine with acute-onset aura
    3. Ophthalmoplegic migraine
    4. Childhood periodic syndromes associated with migraine
      a. Benign paroxysmal vertigo of childhood
      b. Possibly alternating hemiplegia
    5. Complicated migraine
      a. Status migranosis
      b. Migrainous infarction
  B. Tension-type Headache
    1. Episodic tension-type headache
    2. Chronic tension-type headache
  C. Cluster Headache
    1. Episodic cluster headache
    2. Chronic cluster headache
      a. Unremitting from onset
      b. Evolved from episodic
    3. Chronic paroxysmal hemicrania
  D. Miscellaneous
    1. Idiopathic stabbing headache
    2. External compression headache
    3. Cold stimulus headache
    4. Benign cough headache
    5. Benign exertional headache
    6. Headache associated with sexual activity

     7. Rebound headache
     8. Trigeminal neuralgia
     9. Postdural puncture headache
    10. Meningeal headache
    11. Subarachnoid hemorrhage
    12. Brain masses
    13. Temporal arteritis
    14. Pseudotumor cerebri

II. Headache Description
  A. Migraine without Aura
    1. At least five attacks
    2. Duration 4 to 72 hours
    3. Characteristics (at least two of the following)
      a. Unilateral location
      b. Pulsating or throbbing quality
      c. Moderate to severe intensity
      d. Aggravated by activity
    4. Associated with at least one of the following:
      a. Photophobia
      b. Nausea/vomiting
      c. Phonophobia
    5. Frequently beginning in sleep
    6. Epidemiology
      a. Females:Males = 3:1
      b. 60% familial
      c. Migraine without aura, 85% of total migraines
  B. Migraine with Aura
    1. At least two attacks
    2. Duration 4 to 72 hours
    3. Characteristics (at least three of the following)
      a. One or more aura symptoms are fully reversible.
      b. At least one aura develops slowly over 4 minutes.
      c. No one aura symptom lasts more than 1 hour.
      d. Headache follows aura within 1 hour.
      e. Visual auras include leading edge of scintillating light followed by central scotoma, central achromatopsia, ophthalmoplegia.
    4. Headache characteristics
      a. Unilateral location
      b. Pulsating or throbbing quality
      c. Moderate-to-severe intensity
      d. Aggravated by activity
    5. Associated symptoms
      a. Photophobia
      b. Nausea/vomiting

      c. Phonophobia
    6. Epidemiology
      a. Migraine with aura comprises 15% of total migraines.
C. Cluster Headache
   1. At least five attacks
   2. Duration 15 to 180 minutes
   3. Characteristics
     a. Unilateral orbital or temporal location
     b. Severe pounding quality
   4. Associated ipsilateral symptoms (at least one of the following)
     a. Lacrimation
     b. Conjunctival injection
     c. Nasal congestion
     d. Rhinorrhea
     e. Facial sweating
     f. Miosis
     g. Ptosis
     h. Eyelid edema
   5. Usually occurs at night
   6. Frequency: Clusters separated by weeks or months
   7. Occurs in clusters with from one to eight attacks qd
   8. Epidemiology
     a. Male:Female = 4:1
     b. Onset: During one's 30s
D. Rebound Headache
   1. Occurs with chronic use of analgesics or narcotics
   2. Severe global headache
   3. Abortive agents ineffective
E. Trigeminal Neuralgia (Tic Douloureux)
   1. Episodic sharp stabbing pain in V2 and V3 > V1
   2. Usually unilateral
   3. Triggered by stimulation of face or mouth
   4. Pain may result in facial spasm.
   5. Possible association with demyelinating diseases, such as multiple sclerosis
F. Postdural Puncture Headache
   1. Epidemiology
     a. Follows 20% of lumbar punctures.
     b. Rarely occurs spontaneously.
   2. Dull, throbbing, diffuse headache
   3. Worse with sitting or standing
G. Meningeal Headache
   1. Global steady and severe
   2. Meningismus, fever, leukocytosis, altered consciousness
   3. Kernig and Brudzinski's signs

H. Subarachnoid Hemorrhage
   1. Sudden, explosive headache
   2. Meningismus, altered consciousness
   3. CT positive in 80% of cases
   4. Lumbar puncture positive in more than 90% of cases
I. Brain Mass
   1. Dull, constant, progressive over weeks
   2. Worse with cough
   3. Early AM nausea and headache
   4. Associated focal neurologic deficits
J. Temporal Arteritis
   1. Dull unilateral headache
   2. Thick, tortuous, temporal artery with decreased pulse
   3. Jaw claudication, low-grade fever, anemia, increased erythrocyte sedimentation rate (ESR)
   4. Results in acute monocular blindness and ophthalmoplegia
   5. Diagnosed by temporal artery biopsy
   6. Epidemiology: Usually more than 60 years of age
K. Pseudotumor Cerebri
   1. Dull, constant headache
   2. Blurred vision, diplopia, papilledema
   3. Visual field constriction, initially inferior nasal
   4. Most common in young obese females
   5. Related to multiple medications
      a. Oral contraceptive pills, lithium, tetracycline, Vitamin A

III. Treatment
   A. Migraine
      1. Prophylactic
         a. Beta blockers, calcium channel blockers, tricyclic antidepressants, methysergide, clonidine, valproate, serotonin reuptake inhibitors, levetiracetam, topiramate, gabapentin, antipsychotic agents, mirtazapine, venlafaxine, botulinim toxin injections, etc.
         b. Adjust order for treatment of concomitant diseases.
         c. Verapamil works well in complicated migraine.
      2. Abortive
         a. DHE (dihydroergotamine) 45 protocol
            (1) Prochlorperazine (Compazine) 10 mg IV prior to DHE
            (2) Metoclopramide (Reglan) 10 mg IV prior to DHE
            (3) DHE 0.5 mg IV over 2 to 3 minutes q8h
            (4) If ineffective, increase to DHE 1 mg q8h for 3 days
            (5) Monitor blood pressure and pulse q4h.
            (6) Contraindicated for patients with cardiac disease and age over 60 years
         b. DHE 45 injection or nasal spray
         c. Compazine, Phenergan, Thorazine, Droperidol

      d. Sumatriptan (Imitrex) injection, nasal spray or tablet
        (1) 6 mg SC autoinjector
        (2) 25- to 100-mg tablets
        (3) 5- to 20-mg nasal spray
      e. Zolmitriptan (Zomig) tablet and orally disintegrating wafer
        (1) Tablets of 2.5 to 5 mg
      f. Naratriptan
        (1) Tablets of 1 to 2.5 mg
      g. Rizatriptan (Maxalt) tablet and orally disintegrating wafer
        (1) Tablets of 5 to 10 mg
        (2) 5 milligrams if taking propranolol
      h. Almotriptan (Axert)
        (1) Tablets of 6.25 to 12.5 mg
      i. Common triptan side effects include tingling, warmth, flushing, chest discomfort
      j. Triptan contraindications include ischemic heart disease, stroke, basilar migraine, uncontrolled hypertension, use of MAO-I antidepressants, pregnancy category C
      k. Fiorinal or fioricet (barbiturate and analgesic combinations)
      l. Prednisone/Methylprednisolone
      m. Nonsteroidal antiinflammatories (NSAIDs)
      n. Narcotics in special cases (pregnancy, CAD, stroke)
   3. Dietary
      a. Avoid caffeine, chocolate, cheese, nuts, processed meats, alcohol, MSG, citrus fruits, lima beans, yeast
B. Cluster
   1. Oxygen 10 L/NC
   2. Lithium 300 mg qd and titrate
   3. Prednisone 80 mg qd and taper
   4. Indomethacin 25 mg qd
   5. Methylsergide (Sansert) 2 mg qd
   6. Viscous lidocaine nasal spray
   7. Verapamil titrate
   8. Sphenopalatine nerve block
   9. Gasserian ganglion rhizotomy
C. Rebound
   1. Discontinue offending drugs
D. Trigeminal Neuralgia
   1. Carbamazepine (Tegretol)
   2. Phenytoin (Dilantin)
   3. Baclofen
   4. Amitriptyline
   5. Ganglion rhizotomy
E. Postdural Puncture Headache

1. IV fluids
2. Trendelenburg position
3. Bedrest
4. Blood patch

F. Pseudotumor Cerebri
   1. Beta blocker
   2. Calcium channel blocker
   3. Tricyclic antidepressants
   4. Digoxin
   5. Steroids
   6. Serial lumbar punctures
   7. Acetazolamide
   8. Furosemide

IV. Indications for Imaging headache Patients
   A. First or worst headache
   B. Change in headache
   C. Abnormal neurologic examination
   D. Progressive headache
   E. Headache always occurring on the same side
   F. No response to therapy

16
Neuroimaging

NEUROIMAGING

I. CT Density

Moiety	Hounsfeld Units
Bone	1,000
Calcium	100
Acute blood	85
Tumor	Possibly 30–60
Gray matter	35–40
White matter	25–30
CSF	0
Adipose	−100
Air	−1,000

II. Computed Tomography (CT) in Stroke

Duration	Without Contrast	With Contrast
Hyperacute	Normal or blurring of gray-white junction	No enhancement
Acute	Poorly defined hypodensity, maximal edema	No enhancement or mild gyral enhancement
Subacute	Hypodensity, less edema	Gyral enhancement
Remote	Sharply defined hypodensity	Enhancement in 6 weeks

III. CT in Hemorrhage

Duration	Without Contrast
Acute	Hyperdensity, mass effect
Subacute	Hypodense periphery with hyperdense center, mass effect
Remote	Hypodense

IV. Magnetic Resonance Imaging (MRI)
   A. Repetition Time (TR)—time between successive radio frequency (RF) pulses
   B. Echo Time (TE)—time between giving the RF pulse and measuring the tissue's RF signal
   C. Relaxation Time—time required to return to equilibrium after an RF pulse
   D. MRI—based primarily on the relaxation times of various tissues

    E. Diffusion weighted images are positive in more than 90% of ischemic strokes within minutes of the event

    F. Diffusion perfusion images can be obtained to show the mismatch between the images (ischemic and hypoperfused regions).

V. T1-Weighted Imaging

Dark (long T1)	Bright (short T1)
Cerebrospinal fluid (CSF)	Fat
Intracellular deoxyhemoglobin	Contrast
Calcium	Methemoglobin
Air	Proteinaceous material
Water (edema)	Hypoxic changes
Most tumors	Melanoma
	Hepatic failure

VI. T2-Weighted Imaging

Dark (short T2)	Bright (long T2)
Cortical bone	CSF
Calcium	Water (edema)
Hemosiderin	Most tumors
Intracellular deoxyhemoglobin	
Methemoglobin	
Ferritin	
Mucinous material	
Air	

VII. MRI in Hemorrhage

MRI Modality	T1	T2
Acute (3 hours to 3 days)	Isodense/Hypointense	Isodense/Hypointense
Subacute (3 to 7 days)	Hyperintense	Hypointense
Subacute (> 7 days)	Hyperintense	Hyperintense
Chronic		
Hemosiderin	Hypointense	Hypointense
Resorbed	Hypointense	Hyperintense

VIII. Ultrasonography

    A. Brightness Modulation (B mode)

        1. Based on reflection of sound waves off of tissue interfaces

        2. Best used to view anatomy

        3. Used to measure vessel diameter and evaluate plaque

    B. Doppler Ultrasonography

        1. Based on reflection of sound waves off of moving targets such as RBCs

        2. Best used to evaluate blood velocity and flow dynamics

        3. Blood velocity increases in the segment of stenosis.

    C. Power Doppler

        1. Uses the power of the signal to identify possible flow.

IX. Positron Emission Tomography (PET)
   A. Uses nucleides containing positrons such as oxygen-15, fluorine-18, carbon-11, nitrogen-13.
   B. These nucleides are incorporated into tracers.
      1. FDG (containing glucose) to measure brain metabolism
      2. Oxygen-15 measures cerebral blood flow and cerebral metabolic rates.
X. Single Proton Emission Computed Tomography (SPECT)
   A. Uses radioactive tracers to measure cerebral blood flow.
   B. Ictal SPECT usually shows increased blood flow in the region of the seizure focus.
   C. Interictal SPECT usually shows decreased blood flow in the seizure focus.
   D. SPECT usually shows decreased temporoparietal blood flow in Alzheimer's disease patients.

17

Autoimmune Antibodies

I. Paraneoplastic Autoantibodies
   A. Yo (anti-Purkinje cell antibody)
      1. Indication: Cerebellar degeneration
      2. Tumor: Breast, ovarian, endometrial, cervical
      3. Clinical Features: Cerebellar symptoms evolve over weeks to months and then stabilize.
         a. Only one-third of patients can walk unassisted.
         b. Neurologic symptoms precede tumor diagnosis in 50%.
         c. Cerebellar degeneration occurs in less than 1% of the patients at risk.
      4. Pathology: Destruction of cerebellar Purkinje cells
      5. Cerebrospinal fluid (CSF): Lymphocytic pleocytosis, increased protein and IgG.
      6. Levels: Positive at 1:2,000
      7. Treatment: Fewer than 10% responsive to plasmapheresis, IV IgG, steroids, cyclophosphamide
   B. Hu
      1. Indication: Sensory neuropathy, limbic encephalitis
      2. Tumor: Small-cell lung cancer, prostate
      3. Clinical Features: Sensory neuropathy, limbic encephalitis, ataxia, autonomic dysfunction, and mononeuritis multiplex are the most common presentations.
         a. Neurologic symptoms precede tumor diagnosis in 75%.
         b. Anti-Hu antibodies have been found in fewer than 1% of cancer patients.
      4. Pathology: Sensory neuronopathy. Limbic encephalitis
      5. CSF: Pleocytosis, increased protein and IgG, Hu antibodies
      6. Levels: Positive at 1:2,000. Most are more than 1:100,000.
      7. Treatment: None found effective
   C. Ri
      1. Indication: Opsoclonus, truncal ataxia
      2. Tumor: Breast, small-cell lung cancer
      3. Clinical features: Abrupt onset of opsoclonus and truncal ataxia
         a. Neurologic symptoms precede tumor diagnosis in 50%.
         b. 20% of patients with opsoclonus have a tumor.
         c. Half of children with opsoclonus/myoclonus have a neuroblastoma.
      4. CSF: Pleocytosis, increased protein and IgG
      5. Treatment: Opsoclonus in children with neuroblastoma has a good prognosis with treatment of the neuroblastoma.

    D. CAR (VPS)
       1. Indication: Rapid visual loss
       2. Tumor: Small-cell lung cancer, prostate, cervical, colon, and melanoma
       3. Clinical features: Rapid visual loss and retinal degeneration
II. Peripheral Neuropathy Antibodies
    A. GM-1 (anti-ganglioside antibody)
       1. Indication: Motor neuropathy, including amyotrophic lateral sclerosis, Guillain-Barré syndrome, multifocal motor neuropathy, and lower motor neuron disease
       2. Clinical features: Monoclonal gammopathy is present in one-third of patients.
       3. Treatment: IV IgG acutely followed by cyclophosphamide
          a. Steroids and plasmapheresis have not shown benefit.
    B. Myelin-associated Glycoprotein (MAG)
       1. Indication: Pure demyelinating neuropathy or gammopathy-associated sensory neuropathy
       2. Clinical features: Half of patients with IgM monoclonal gammopathy and neuropathy have IgM MAG.
       3. Pathology: Antibodies bind to myelin.
       4. Treatment: Plasmapheresis, IV IgG, cyclophosphamide
    C. Sulfatide
       1. Indication: Axonal predominantly sensory neuropathy

18

Autonomic Nervous System Testing

I. Anatomy and Physiology
  A. Preganglionic sympathetic neurons are located in the intermediolateral cell column in the spinal cord from T2 to L1.
  B. Preganglionic parasympathetics are present in the nuclei of cranial nerves III, VII, IX, X and in the spinal cord from S2 to S4.
  C. Primary postganglionic neurotransmitter for sympathetic neurons is norepinephrine.
  D. Primary postganglionic neurotransmitter for parasympathetic neurons is muscarinic acetylcholine.
  E. Primary postganglionic neurotransmitter for sweat glands is acetylcholine.
  F. Denervation hypersensitivity is a sign of a postganglionic lesion.
II. Valsalva Maneuver
  A. Pressure of approximately 40 mm Hg for 15 seconds produces the ideal stimulus.
  B. The Valsalva maneuver has four phases
    1. Phase I—increased blood pressure secondary to increased intrathoracic pressure
    2. Phase II early—reduced blood pressure and cardiac output secondary to decreased venous return
    3. Phase II late—4 to 5 seconds later, increased blood pressure because of increased sympathetic tone
    4. Phase III—onset with a sudden release of intrathoracic pressure, causing a decrease in blood pressure for 1 to 2 seconds
    5. Phase IV—overshoot of blood pressure lasting less than 10 seconds caused by increased venous return during persistent vasoconstriction
  C. The Valsalva maneuver should not be performed in patients with proliferative retinopathy.
  D. Valsalva may induce syncope, angina, or arrhythmia.
  E. Longest R-R interval during phase IV, compared with the shortest R-R interval during phase II, should be less than 1.51. This may be decreased in normal elderly patients.
  F. Exaggerated decrease in phase II suggests sympathetic vasomotor dysfunction.
  G. Absent overshoot during phase IV indicates the inability to increase the cardiac output and cardiac adrenergic dysfunction.
III. Heart Rate Response to Deep Breathing
  A. Precise reflex mechanism is unclear.
  B. Heart rate increases during inspiration.
  C. Heart rate decreases during expiration.
  D. Test is maximized with patient lying flat with deep respirations.

     E. Monitor heart rate or R-R interval.

     F. Normal is more than a 14-beat-per-minute difference.

     G. Borderline is a difference of 11 to 14 beats per minute.

     H. Abnormal is a differences of fewer than 11 beats per minute.

     I. This is a very sensitive test for early cardiovagal dysfunction.

IV. Heart Rate Response to Standing

     A. Initial tachycardia followed by a subsequent bradycardia

     B. Compare R-R interval at fifteenth beat to R-R interval at thirtieth beat

     C. Normal ratio, >1.03

     D. Borderline ratio, 1.01 to 1.03

     E. Abnormal ratio, <1.01

V. Tilt Table Testing

     A. Measurement of blood pressure following standing or tilting

     B. Tilting to 80° should occur within 4 seconds.

     C. Patient should remain supine for at least 20 minutes prior to tilt.

     D. Patients with significant sympathetic dysfunction have a progressive decline in blood pressure during the tilt.

     E. Normal if <11 mm Hg change

     F. Borderline if 11 to 29 mm Hg change

     G. Abnormal if >29 mm Hg change

VI. Blood Pressure Response to Hand Grip

     A. Blood pressure is obtained at rest.

     B. Blood pressure is obtained after 5 minutes of sustained grip at 30% of maximal grip.

     C. The increase in diastolic grip from rest to conclusion of hand grip is measured.

     D. Normal if >15 mm Hg increase

     E. Borderline if 11 to 15 mm Hg increase

     F. Abnormal if <11 mm Hg increase

VII. Thermoregulatory Sweat Test

     A. This is a qualitative test of sudomotor function.

     B. Dust patient with Alizarin-Red.

     C. Subject the patient to whole-body heating.

     D. The pattern of sweating is then recorded.

     E. This test cannot differentiate between preganglionic and postganglionic lesions.

VIII. Silastic Imprint Test

     A. Sweat glands are stimulated with iontophoresis of pilocarpine.

     B. Silastic is spread over the stimulated region.

     C. The imprint of the sweat droplets is then analyzed for size and number.

     D. This is a sensitive, quantitative test for sudomotor neuropathy in diabetes.

IX. Quantitative Sudomotor Axon Reflex Test (QSART)

     A. Test of postganglionic sympathetic sudomotor function

     B. Iontophoresis of acetylcholine onto the skin stimulates sympathetic C-fibers and causes an axon reflex.

     C. A sudomoter then measures the humidity from the sweat response (a quantitative measure).

     D. Anhidrosis on the Thermoregulatory test and the QSART indicates a preganglionic lesion.

19

Head Injury

I. Glasgow Coma Scale

Eye opening
    Spontaneous   4
    To voice   3
    To pain   2
    None   1
Best motor response
    Obeys commands   6
    Localizes pain   5
    Withdraws to pain   4
    Flexor posturing   3
    Extensor posturing   2
    None   1
Best verbal response
    Conversant and oriented   5
    Conversant and disoriented   4
    Inappropriate words   3
    Incomprehensible sounds   2
    None   1

II. Diffuse Axonal Injury

	Mild	Moderate	Severe
Loss of consciousness	Immediate	Immediate	Immediate
Length of unconsciousness	6–24 hr	>24 hr	Days to weeks
Decerebrate posturing	Rare	Occasionally	Present
Amnesia	Hours	Days	Weeks
Memory deficit	Mild	Moderate	Severe
Outcome at 3 months			
Good recovery	63%	38%	15%
Severe deficit	6%	12%	14%
Death	15%	24%	51%

III. Elevated intracranial pressure management
    A. Monitor with CT
    B. Sedation
    C. Pressor management if CPP < 70 mm Hg
    D. Blood pressure reduction if CPP >120 mm Hg
    E. Mannitol 0.25 to 1 g/kg q2 to 6h
    F. Albumin and lasix
    G. Hyperventilate to keep PCO_2 levels at 28 to 32 mm Hg
    H. Pentobarbital for burst suppression with continuous EEG
    I. Systemic hypothermia

20

Sleep

I. Parasomnias

	Sleep Terror	Nightmare
Prevalence	Uncommon	Common
Sleep stage	SWS	REM
Onset	First 90 minutes of sleep	Second half of night
Features	Intense; vocalization, fear, motor activity	Less intense; vocalization, fear, motor activity
Mental content	Sparse	Elaborate
Violent behavior	Common	None
Injury	More likely	Unlikely
Amnesia	Often	Rare
Ability to arouse	Difficult	Easy
On awakening	Confused	Oriented

	Confusional Arousals	Sleep Walking	REM Sleep Behavior Disorder
Prevalence	Uncommon	Common	0.5%. More common in Parkinson's
Sleep stage	SWS	SWS	REM
Onset	First one-third of the night	First one-third of the night	Last one-third of the night
Features	Complex behavior; slow confused speech	Complex behaviors not limited to walking	Acting out dreams; may be violent. Increased EMG tone.
Violent behavior	Occasional	Rare	Frequent
Injury	Rare	Rare	Occasional
Treatment	Benzodiazepines	Benzodiazepines; TCAs	Clonazepam, Carbamazepine

II. Narcolepsy
  A. Prevalence is one in 2,000 (0.02%) with narcolepsy–cataplexy syndrome.
  B. Peaks in the second decade.
  C. Monozygotic twins are discordant for narcolepsy.
  D. More common in Japan
  E. Male:female = 1:1
  F. Symptoms
    1. Excessive daytime somnolence but typically awaken feeling refreshed
    2. Sleep attacks
    3. Cataplexy (67% to 80% of narcoleptics)
      a. Elicited by emotion
      b. Severity varies
      c. Extraocular muscles typically not involved but blurred vision may occur

      e. Duration seconds to 30+ minutes

      f. Monosynaptic H-reflex inhibited

      g. Weakness caused by emotion or excitement (when you tell or hear a joke)

      h. Weakness most frequently occurs at the knee.

      i. Adrenergic uptake inhibition mediates the anticataplectic effect of antidepressants and strongly inhibits REM.

      j. TCA—Vivactil the best (blocks reuptake of norepinephrine)

      k. Anafranil, Tofranil, Imipramine, Fluoxetine, Zoloft have been used.

      l. MAO inhibitors (phenylzine) reduce cataplexy.

    4. Sleep paralysis (64% of narcoleptics)

      a. Inability to move while awakening, able to move with stimulation

      b. Seconds to 10-minute duration

    5. Hypnogogic hallucinations (67% of narcoleptics)

      a. Vivid dreams during wakefulness

      b. Usually visual

      c. Auditory hallucinations possible

      d. Cenesthopathic—sensation of picking or rubbing or a sense of levitation

    6. Only about 15% have the whole tetrad (EDS with sleep attacks, cataplexy, sleep paralysis, hallucinations).

    7. Nocturnal sleep disruption is common with repeated awakenings and frightening dreams.

    8. Increased PLMs on nocturnal sleep studies

    9. REM behavior disorder is more common in narcoleptics.

    10. Automatic behavior with amnestic episodes

  G. Genetics

    1. 86% of narcoleptics with definite cataplexy have HLA DQB1-0602 on chromosome 6.

    2. Orexin or hypocretin is also frequent.

III. Idiopathic Hypersomnia

  A. Excessive daytime sleepiness

  B. Undisturbed nocturnal sleep possible

  C. Difficult awakenings

  D. Short 1- to 4-sec microsleeps

  E. Automatic behavior

  F. Onset usually age

  G. Multiple Sleep Latency—usually longer in idiopathic hypersomnia than narcolepsy

Appendix

GENERALIZED CONVULSIVE STATUS EPILEPTICUS

I. Treatment Protocol
  A. Make Diagnosis
    1. Two or more convulsions without full recovery of consciousness or a single seizure lasting greater than 10 minutes.
  B. Treatment Based on Convulsion/Seizure Status
    At **0 to 10 minutes** :
    1. Ensure airway. Nasal O_2. Oximeter.
    2. Vital signs, EKG monitor
    3. Start IV with normal saline.
    4. Draw blood for dextrostick, FBP, CBC, AED levels, toxin screen
    5. Thiamine 100 mg IV
    6. Glucose 50 mL of 50% solution
    At **10 to 30 minutes** :
    1. Lorazepam 0.1 mg/kg IV at 2 mg/min
    2. Monitor BP, HR, RR q 5 min during this and all drug infusions.
    3. If seizures continue:
        a. Adults: Fosphenytoin 20 mg/kg IV in NS at 150 mg/min
        b. Children: 1 mg/kg/min
        c. Elderly: 15 mg/kg
    4. If the seizures continue, IV valproate (Depacon 20 mg/kg)
    5. If seizures still continue: Intubate. Phenobarbital 20 mg/kg IV at 100 mg/min
    At **30 to 60 minutes:**
    1. Intensive care unit admission. Arterial line. Continuous EEG monitoring.
    2. Pentobarbital 10 mg/kg over 1 hour or 250 mg microboluses
    3. Pentobarbital 1 to 2 mg/kg/h titrated to burst suppression on EEG
    4. Stop pentobarbital and monitor at 12, 24, and 72 hours.
  C. Complications
    1. Hypotension
        a. Stop infusion.
        b. Pressors as needed
        c. Trendelenburg position
    2. Respiratory depression
        a. Intubate.
        b. Slow or stop infusion if needed.
    3. Cardiac dysrhythmias

        a. Phenytoin sometimes causes heart block or increased QT interval.
        b. Slow infusion as needed
  D. Maintenance
    1. Begin maintenance drug within first 12 hours.
    2. Assess etiology of status as indicated with CT, LP, EEG, etc.

BRAIN DEATH CRITERIA

  I. Prerequisites
    A. Cause is known and irreversible.
    B. No severe overlying medical condition
      1. Electrolytes, acid/base disturbances, endocrine abnormalities
    C. No Drug Intoxication or Poisoning
    D. Core temperature at least 32°C (90°F)
  II. Cardinal Features
    A. Unresponsive (i.e., no motor response to pain)
    B. No Brain Stem Reflexes
      1. No pupil response to light
      2. No oculocephalic reflex (doll's eyes maneuver)
      3. No caloric vestibular reflex (response to cold calorics)
        a. Fifty milliliters of H_2O; allow 1 minute each ear; allow 5 minutes between ears.
      4. No corneal reflex; no grimacing to pain
      5. No gag; no cough or bradychardia with suction
    C. Apnea Test
      1. Temperature at least 36.5°C (97°F); SBP at least 90; no diabetes insipidus or positive fluid balance in past 6 hours
      2. Preoxygenate the patient to get PO_2 at least 200 and PCO_2 to 40 or lower.
      3. Shut off vent for 8 minutes. Stop test if you see respiratory movements, SPB <90, PO_2 significant desaturation, or cardiac arrythmia.
      4. Draw ABG: Test is positive if PCO_2 is at least 60 or 20 mm Hg increase over baseline value.
  III. Optional Confirmatory Tests
    A. Angiography—no filling at level of carotid bifurcation or circle of Willis
    B. EEG—electrocerebral silence
    C. Transcranial Doppler U/S—no signal
    D. Tech 99 HMPAO Brain Scan—no uptake
    E. SSEPs—no response of N20 to P22
    F. Repeat examination in 6 hours.
  IV. Medical Record Documentation
    A. Etiology and irreversibility of condition
    B. Absence of brain stem reflexes
    C. Absence of motor response to pain
    D. Absence of respirations with PCO_2 at least 60
    E. Justification for confirmatory test and result
    F. Result of repeat examination in 6 hours (optional)

Subject Index